The Foundations of
Unani Medicine

The Foundations of
Unani Medicine

Principles, Diagnosis, and
Treatments in Unani Medicine

SHAHID H. BUKHARI

Copyright © 2024, Shahid H Bukhari

Paperback ISBN: 978-1-7385214-0-1
Hardback ISBN: 978-1-7385214-2-5

All rights reserved. No part of this book may be reproduced or utilized in any form or by any means, electronic or mechanical, including photocopying, recording, or by any information storage and retrieval system, without permission in writing from the publisher.

Note to the reader: This book is intended as an informational guide. The remedies, approaches, and techniques described herein are meant to supplement, and not to be a substitute for, professional medical care or treatment. They should not be used to treat a serious ailment without prior consultation with a qualified healthcare professional.

First Printing Edition 2024

Published by CUTAM Press, Manchester, UK.

www.cutam.org.uk

بسم الله الرحمن الرحيم

CONTENTS

Forewords 21

Preface 24

SECTION 1

GENERAL FACTORS OF THE EXISTENCE 29

A Brief History of Unani Medicine 30

Medicine during the Islamic empires 30

THE SCIENCE OF MEDICINE 31

Definition of medicine 31

Theoretical aspect of medicine (Tibb Nazari) 31

Practical aspect of medicine (Tibb 'Amali) 32

Subject matter of medicine 32

Material Causes 32

Efficient Causes (Asbab Fa'iliyya) 33

The six essential factors (Asbab Sitta Daruriyya): 33

Non-essential Causes (Asbab Ghair Daruriyya): 33

Formal Causes 33

Final Causes (Asbab Tamamiyya) 34

The subject of Unani medical science 34

Factors of Existence (Umar Tabiyya) 34

Medicatrix Naturae 34

- Elements (Arkan) 37
- Temperament (Mizaj) 40
- Temperament types 41
- Humours (Akhlat) 48
  - Blood Humour (Khilt Dam) 51
  - Phlegm Humour (Khilt Balgham) 52
  - Yellow Bile Humour (Khilt Safra) 55
  - Black Bile Humour (Khilt Sawda) 57
- Organs (Udw) 61
- Compound organs 61
- Pneumas (Arwah) 68
- Faculties/power (Quwwa) 70
  - Mental faculty (Quwwat Nafsaniyah) 71
  - Vital faculty (Quwwat Haywanniya) 76
- Natural/Physical faculty (Quwwat Tabi'iyya) 76
  - Nutritive faculty (Quwwat Ghadhiya) 77
  - Transformative faculty (Quwwat Mughayyira) 78
  - Absorptive faculty (Quwwat Jhadiba) 79
  - Digestive faculty (Quwwat Hadima) 80
  - Expulsive faculty (Quwwat Dafi'a) 82
- Functions (Af'al) 85
  - Mental or psychic functions (Af'al Nafsaniyya) 85
  - Vital functions (Af'al Haywaniyya) 86
  - Physical/Natural functions (Af'al Tabi'iyya) 86

SECTION 2

DISEASES, CAUSES AND SIGNS 90

States Of The Human Body 91

Health (Sihhat) 91

Disease (Marad) 91

Intermediate state 93

Diseases 94

Types of diseases 95

Compound diseases 97

Types of Simple Diseases 97

Impaired temperament (Su-e-Mizaj) 98

Structural Diseases (Amrad Su-e-Tarkib) 101

Loss of continuity (Tafarruq Ittisal) 103

Compound Diseases (Amrad Murakkab) 105

Swellings (Awram) 105

Complex and Simple Disease Classifications 113

Study of Causations (Ilm al-asbab) 115

Definition and classification of causes 115

Definition of causes 115

Cause (Sabab) 116

The Six Essential Factors (Asbab Sitta Dharruriyya) 119

Air 119

Seasons 121

Four seasons and their qualities (Fusul Arba'a Kayfiyat) 121

Characters of the four seasons 122

- Celestial factors 124
- Earthly factors 124
- Wind Direction and its effects 127
- Effects of different types of air: 128
- Food and Drinks 129
  - Water 129
  - Effects food and drinks 131
  - Types of diet 134
- Bodily Movement and Repose (Haraka wa Sukun Badani) 135
- Mental Activity and Repose (Haraka wa Sukun Nafsaniyya) 136
- Sukun nafsaniyya (Mental repose) 137
- Sleep And Wakefulness (Nawm wa Yaqza) 137
- Retention And Evacuation (Ihtibas Wa Istifragh) 137
- Non-essential Factors (Asbab Ghayr Daruriyya) 139
  - Hammam (Therapeutic bath /Turkish bath) 139
  - Sunbathing 140
  - Splashing water 141
  - Oiling (Tadhin) 141
  - Therapeutic massage (dalk) 141
  - Exercise (Riyadat) 143
- Fatigue (I'ya') 145
- Causes Related To The Four Qualities 146
- Causes of obstruction and constriction of ducts 148
- Causes of duct dilatation (asbab ittisa majari) 148
- Causes of roughness (asbab khushunat) 148

Causes of smoothness in skin or mucous membranes (asbab malasat) 149

Causes of dislocation and separation of structures 149

Causes of abnormal connections between organs (asbab su mujawirat) 149

Causes of abnormal movements (asbab ghayr tab'i) 149

Causes of increased size and number of organs 150

Causes of discontinuity/separation (asbab tafarruq ittisal) Internal causes .. 150

External causes 151

Causes of ulcers (asbab qarha) 151

Causes of swelling (asbab waram) 151

Pain 152

Causes of pain (asbab waja') 153

Factors Leading to Cessation of Pain 154

Fundamental approach to pain management 155

Causes of congestion 156

Causes of infection 156

Causes of retention and evacuation (Asbab ihtibas wa istifragh) 156

Causes of weakness of organs (Asbab du'f a'da) 157

SIGNS AND SYMPTOMS ('ILM AL-DALA'IL WA'L 'ALAMAT) 159

Clinical Manifestation Of Diseases (A'rad Amrad) 159

Signs of health 159

Signs of disease 159

Signs of external diseases 160

Signs of internal diseases 161

Signs indicating temperament 163

Signs indicating a temporarily acquired temperament 165

Signs of a balanced temperament 165

Signs and symptoms of plethora/fullness ('alamat-i-imtila) 166

Signs that indicate a dominant humour 167

Signs of obstruction ('alamat-i-sudad) 167

Signs of swelling/inflammation ('alamat -i-awram) 168

Signs of reeh 169

Signs of loss of continuity (alamat-i-tafarruqi-ittisa) 169

SECTION 3
PULSE, URINE & STOOL 172

The Pulse (AL-NABD) 173

Movement of pulse 175

Conditions for examination of pulse 176

Methods of examining the pulse 178

Reason for examining the pulse at the wrist 178

Parameters which describe the pulse (adilla nabd): 179

    Amount of Expansion of Pulse 180

    Strength of Pulse (Kayfiy'e Qar') 184

    Duration of the movement of Pulse (Zamana-i-Harakat): 185

    Period of Pause (Zamana-i- Sukun) 185

    Texture of the Arterial Wall (Qiwam-i-Ala) 186

    Emptiness and Fullness (Khala wa Imtila) 187

    The Feel of Touch/ Temperature Sensation (Malmas) 187

    Uniformity and Variability (Istiwa wa Ikhtilaf) 188

    Regularity and Irregularity (Nizam wa' Adm-i-Nizam) 190

    Measurement 190

Compound pulses 192

Normal pulse (Nabd tibbi) 196

Equal pulse - pulsus aequalis (Nabd mustawi) 196

Causes of pulse (Asbab nabd) 197

Causes of pulse types 198

Causes of compound pulse 202

Effects of age on the pulse 203

Differences in the pulse of men and women 204

Effects of temperament on the pulse 204

Effects of seasons on the pulse 205

Effects of a country's climate on the pulse 206

Effects of food and drink on the pulse 206

Effects of alcohol on the pulse 206

Effects of water on the pulse 206

Effects of exercise on the pulse 207

Effects of bathing on the pulse 207

Effects of pregnancy on the pulse 207

Effects of pain on the pulse 207

Effects of swelling on the pulse 207

Effects of emotions on the pulse 209

Condition and diseases of body and their pulses types 210

Disease conditions as seen through the pulse 212

Urine 217

Conditions for examination of urine (mu'ayana qarura) 217

Indications from urine (dala'il bawl) 218

    Indications from colours of urine (dala'il alwan al-bawl) 219

    Complex urine colours 222

    Urine density (qiwam al-bawl) 223

    Urine froth (zubada al-bawl) 224

    Urine sediments 225

    Haematuria (bawl al-dam) 226

    Urine of pregnant women.. 227

    Urine during pregnancy 227

    Colours of urine and related condition and diseases.................................... 228

    Urine smell and Mizaj (Temperament) 229

    Urine sediments and diseases... 229

    Urine types and diseases... 230

    Urine and fevers.. 231

    Diseases with their pulse and urine signs 232

Stool **239**

SECTION 4

COMPENDIUM OF DRUGS 242

Drug, Diet And Zulkhassa **243**

Temperament of Drugs **245**

    Composition of drugs 248

    Potency variations in drug temperaments.. 249

    Effects of drugs 253

    Physical properties of drugs.. 255

    Additional properties for drug identification 255

    Hypothesis and experiments... 257

Other means of discovering drug properties 258

Experiments vs hypothesis 259

Principles for experiments on drugs 259

Consistency and weight of a drug 262

Other physical and chemical properties 263

Effects of drugs on organs 264

Effect of drugs on metabasis and metabolism of the body 283

Causes that increase or decrease metabolism 284

Understanding factors that affect metabolism 284

Classification of drugs based on metabolic impact 285

Metabolism Stimulants: Accelerating Metabolic Processes 285

Mechanism of tonics 286

Heat producing and refrigerant drugs (Musakhkhin wa Mubarrid) 291

Shapes of drugs 292

Overview of Drug Forms in Unani Medicine 296

METHODS OF DRUG ADMINISTRATION 305

Collection Of Drugs 308

Storage Of Drugs 309

Utilisation period of drugs 310

Expiry period of drugs 310

Expiry period of drugs in terms of their sources 311

    Mineral drugs 311

    Metals drugs 311

    Non-Metal drugs 311

    Stone and Clay drugs 311

Plant drugs 311

Drug substitutes (Abdal Advia) 313

Beneficial and adverse effects of drugs 319

Correctives drugs 320

Treatment with single and compound drugs 320

Antagonistic drugs and antagonism 323

    Antagonistic drugs 323

The mixing and synthesis of drugs 324

Drug Types: Their function and characteristics 326

SECTION 5
PRINCIPLES OF TREATMENT 344

Regimental therapy (Ilaj-bil Tadbeer) and Diet-o-Therapy (Ilaj-bil Ghiza) 345

Pharmacotherapy 348

Law on quality of drugs 349

Heteropathy (Ilaj bil Didd) 349

Like for like treatment (Ilaj bil-Misl) 350

The law of quantity of drug 350

Law on drug timings 356

Principles of treatment and other considerations 358

Apparent conflicts in treatment 360

Treatment in cases where the diagnoses is difficult 361

General acting drugs 361

The principle of treatment for abnormal temperaments (su-e-mizaj) 363

Evacuation (Istifragh) 366

Concoction (Nudj) 369

Types of mushhilat (purgatives) 372

Purgation (Ishal) 373

Softening (Talyeen) 374

Purgative prescriptions 378

Enema (Huqna) 380

Suppository (shiyaf) 383

Emesis (Qay) 384

Fasd (Venesection) 387

Important veins for fasd 389

Hijama (Cupping therapy) 390

Leech therapy (Irsaal-e-alaq) 393

Diaphoresis/sweating (Ta'riq) 393

Increasing The Flow (Idrar) 397

    Diuresis (Idrar-i-Bawl) 397

Emmenagogic (Idrar-e-haiz) 399

Emmenagogue 399

Galactagogic (Idrar-e-laban) 400

Expectoration 400

Redirection of matter 402

Cauterization (Kaiyy) 405

Pain management 406

    Pain induction 406

    Pain relief 406

    Pain management and conflict of drug action and treatment: 407

    Sedatives 407

Discontinuity	414
Ulcers	415
Fistula	416
Decayed organ	417
Advice on which treatment to start first	417

FURTHER RESOURCES **424**

SELECTED BIBLIOGRAPHY **423**

INDEX **425**

To my beloved parents, whose hard work and love have been my guiding stars;

To my teachers in the traditions of Unani, Western herbalism, Eastern Herbalism, Homeopathy, Naturopathy, Iridology, and TCM, whose wisdom has been the foundation upon which I stand;

To my fellow practitioners and all who have supported me through this journey;

This book is a tribute to your collective light, which has illuminated the path to healing and knowledge.

Forewords

It is interesting to note that despite the widespread availability and funding of Western Scientific Medicine, older traditions such as Islamic, Ayurvedic, and Chinese medicine, which rely on different paradigms to understand and treat diseases, have continued to thrive. This is particularly true in English-speaking countries.

To my knowledge, leading practitioners of the Islamic tradition of medicine, known as 'Unani Tibb' in the Indian Sub-continent, in the UK and USA have all received traditional training under masters in the Islamic heartlands. However, in the UK, there are now training schools in Unani Tibb, and a growing number of students and practitioners are unable to access key foundational texts due to linguistic reasons. While some traditional works, such as Ibn Sina's 'Canon' and As-Suyuti's 'Medicine of the Prophet', have been translated into English, and there have been some short modern works, such as Hakim Chishti's 'The Book of Sufi Healing' and Salim Khan's 'Islamic Medicine', there has developed a great need for a comprehensive English textbook that summarises all the major sources on Unani Tibb. Hakim Shahid Bukhari has brilliantly fulfilled this need in 'Foundations of Unani Medicine', drawing from major Arabic and Urdu/Persian sources, as well as his experience as a clinician. Bukhari provides a clear and comprehensive description of Unani medical theory and practice and is able to apply it to contemporary diseases, including psychogenic ones.

'Foundations of Unani Tibb', I believe, will become the indispensable textbook for students and practitioners of Tibb in the English-speaking world, as well as being a valuable source for all with an interest in the subject.

Professor Rasjid Skinner,
Consultant Clinical Psychologist,
Clinical Director: Ihsaan Therapeutic Services.

Unani medicine and Ayurveda are two ancient medical systems originating in Asia and sharing various similarities. Both systems utilise the principles of bodily humours and elemental theory and rely heavily on medicinal plants for healing. Further, they both employ diagnostic techniques like pulse and tongue analysis and emphasise the importance of maintaining daily routines and personal hygiene. Additionally, they employ purification methods such as sweating, vomiting, diuretics, and blood-letting and have developed sophisticated alchemical medicines to combat chronic ailments.

Despite Ayurveda being more widely recognised and its texts increasingly prevalent, Unani medicine remains largely unexplored in Western contexts. As an Ayurvedic practitioner and author of 'Rasa Shastra: The Hidden Art of Medical Alchemy', I find it enriching to contribute a foreword to Shahid's 'The Foundations of Unani Medicine'. This book is a treasure trove of insights into Unani medicine, written by someone who not only deeply understands but also actively practices this healing art.

'The Foundations of Unani Medicine' is an indispensable guide to exploring the intricacies of Unani medicine. It meticulously covers key topics such as the aetiology, manifestation, and symptoms of various diseases, highlighting the critical role of pulse, urine, and stool analysis in diagnostics.

This book is a valuable resource for practitioners and students of alternative medicine and those intrigued by holistic health approaches and healing. Adding this book to your library offers a unique opportunity to explore Unani medicine, a system with a rich heritage that has significantly influenced modern medical practices. Despite its pivotal role in the development of contemporary medicine and its widespread use in various cultures, English language literature has represented Unani medicine to a lesser extent. Shahid's 'The Foundations of Unani Medicine' is, therefore, a crucial contribution, bridging this gap and bringing to light the depth and relevance of this enduring medical tradition.

Andrew Mason,
Ayurvedic Practitioner and author of *Rasa Shastra –*
The Hidden Art of Medical Alchemy, 2024, UK.

I first met Shahid over 10 years ago and was struck by his passion and love of Unani medicine, which at that point I was not familiar with. Over the years I have had the privilege of working with him both as a colleague and as a student and, I hope, have the honour of being considered a friend.

His knowledge of Unani Tibb is unparalleled. His deep passion for the subject and dedication to keep this amazing system of medicine not just alive but accepted alongside mainstream medicine and in full public view, is inexhaustible. This involves furthering research in Unani Tibb to gain greater acceptance of this amazing branch of medicine alongside other medical disciplines. One could say that Shahid was 'born to this'; starting with his interest in traditional medicine as a child and later rekindled upon discovery of 'The Book of Sufi Healing'.

His book is most welcome and long overdue for all students and practitioners of Unani Tibb. It is the culmination of many years of diligent study of both English and Arabic Unani medical texts. Until now there are precious few books available on Unani Tibb, and certainly not those written at a student and practitioner level of understanding. His enthusiasm, both as a practitioner and teacher, is palpable. He is an excellent tutor and literally brings the subject of Unani alive and can explain complex aspects of it with ease and simplicity.

This book comes at a perfect time when we need different answers to current beliefs about health and disease. After the Covid-19 pandemic we need to truly understand disease, but also to understand what constitutes health and why. Western medicine does not offer us this information. Indeed, with the rise of allopathic medicine in the 17th and 18th Centuries the 'four humours medicine' which had been the predominant medicine of Europe for centuries, became ridiculed and side lined in favour of the new 'superior' western reductionist medicine. This has no philosophy and works purely on suppressing symptoms and not understanding what those symptoms represent. Clearly it is failing those who put their trust in it. In direct opposition, Unani Tibb is based on a philosophy which has been 'tried and tested', developed and researched by eminent Arabic scholars for centuries. It provides an understanding of health and disease which we all need to become aware of in order to manage our personal health better.

Shahid works tirelessly promoting the wisdom of Unani Tibb lecturing to doctors, healthcare professionals, students, and the public, furthering awareness and the importance of taking responsibility for our health and providing an understanding of disease when it occurs. I have no doubt that his Choleric enthusiasm will place Unani Tibb firmly at the forefront of our journey forward with understanding health and disease.

Mary Sharma, ND
Ayurveda and Naturopathic practitioner

Preface

In the name of Allah, the Compassionate, the Merciful

Over 25 years ago, I was working as an IT consultant in New York, USA, when I came across 'The Book of Sufi Healing'. The profound insights in the book sparked my interest in Unani medicine, which led me to transition to the practice of Unani medicine. I established a clinical practice in London and later opened a clinic and, eventually, a college in Manchester dedicated to Unani medicine. The college is where individuals from different professions, including doctors, nurses, teachers, and those who want a career change, come together to learn and practice this time-honoured approach to health.

While teaching, I realised that there was a significant gap in the availability of comprehensive English-language resources on Unani medicine. Although Ibn Sina's works were invaluable, being primary source material, these didn't fully meet the needs of my students.

This textbook was born out of a clear need and a deep belief in the vitality and relevance of Unani medicine, which is as effective today as it was in ancient times. As you read this book, you will understand the foundation of my conviction and maybe even come to share it.

The text is designed for diploma-level students and anyone interested in exploring this rich medical tradition. It synthesises extensive Unani literature, texts like 'Asssol-e-tibb', the 'Qanoon', 'Firdous Al-hikma', and my own clinical practice into a cohesive and accessible format. Like the classical texts of Unani medicine, this book is divided into sections covering the essentials of existence, disease, diagnostics, pharmacology, and treatment. Original Unani terms are retained and transliterated, ensuring that students are well-prepared for advanced study.

This preface serves as both an introduction to Unani medicine and an invitation to engage with its profound wisdom.

I am presenting this book to all those who are interested in the study of Unani medicine. I would like to express my gratitude to Dr. S. Maryam for her help in translating, to my students for their curious minds, to my colleagues for their unwavering support, and to all my teachers for their patience and wisdom. I also want to extend my thanks to my wife (a woman of great patience and loyalty) and children for enduring the long hours of writing this book. Lastly, I would like to thank the following students and colleagues for reviewing the draft of my book: Muhammad Hussain, Hana Yousaf, Abid Hussain, Frank Pierow, and Elaine Stavert.

May it be your guide to a deeper understanding and a tribute to Unani medicine's enduring legacy. Together, we continue a conversation on healing that transcends the constraints of time and place.

Shahid Bukhari, ND
Principal, CUTAM college, UK, 2023

Disclaimer to the Reader:

This book is a resource for learning about Unani medicine, a traditional medical system widely recognized and practised in certain parts of the world. It is taught at universities on the Indian subcontinent and has a rich history of application.

It is important to note that the approaches, remedies, and techniques described in this book are meant for informational purposes only and should not replace professional medical advice and treatment. These practices are intended to supplement, not replace, the advice of qualified healthcare professionals and should be considered within the context of complementary medicine.

It is important to understand that the field of Unani medicine is continuously evolving, and interpretations and applications may vary depending on the region and practitioner. Therefore, the content in this book only represents the author's understanding and may not necessarily reflect a universal approach.

Readers, particularly those from regions where Unani medicine is not commonly practised, are strongly advised to consult healthcare professionals before adopting any practices or remedies discussed in this book. This is particularly important for individuals with existing health conditions, those taking prescription medications, or anyone requiring specialised medical care.

'There is no disease that Allah has created, except that He also has created its treatment.'[1]

'In the name of Allah, the most gracious and merciful, we offer our praise and thanks to Him, the Lord of all the worlds. We also send our prayers and blessings to the best of his creations, Prophet Muhammad and his family.

As intelligent beings, it is our duty to seek a close relationship with Allah and to pray for His guidance and blessings. We should obey His commands and refrain from anything that is forbidden, as this will bring good to all people and protect us from harm.

Furthermore, we should study the science of medicine, care for the sick, and work towards their healing. By doing so, we can demonstrate our faith in Allah and earn His rewards. We should also explore the wonders of nature and the human soul, seeking knowledge and understanding of His power, generosity, and grace.

May Allah guide us all on the path of righteousness and bless us with His mercy and forgiveness.'

Al-Samarqandi[2]

---

[1] A famous saying (hadith) from Prophet Muhammad as narrated by Abu Hurayrah.
[2] Najib al-Din al-Samarqandi, Abu Hamid Muhammad ibn 'Ali ibn 'Umar (d.1222 AD), from the Medical Formulary of Al-Samarqandi.

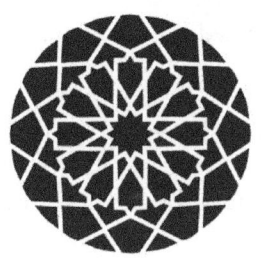

SECTION I

GENERAL FACTORS OF THE EXISTENCE

A Brief History of Unani Medicine

In ancient times, medicine flourished in Egypt, India, China and Greece. In Greece, Hippocrates (460 BC to 377 BC) compiled the rules and principles of medicine and recorded them in a formal way. On this basis, Hippocrates is considered the father of medicine. After Hippocrates, Aristotle (born 384 BC) established the general principles of medicine and Dioscorides compiled the science of drugs and Galen (129-199) clarified the benefits and explanation of the organs.

Medicine during the Islamic empires

Hanain Ibn Ishaq, Masirjuyah, Musa ibn Khalid, Abu Yusuf, Al-Batriq, etc. translated the medical books of Greece physicians into Arabic. This continued till the end of the second Islamic century.

Islamic scholars laid the foundations of a new medicine with the combination of different medicines consisting of Greek, Arabic, Iranian and Indian medicine. At the same time, many diseases underwent new research, new principles were developed and drugs were composed with new methods. Pharmacy was compiled and the science of hygiene was invented. During this period many valuable works were compiled including Abul Hassan Ali bin Rabban Ibtari's Firdous Al-Hikmat, Muhammad bin Zakaria Razi's Hawi Kabir, Ali bin Abbas's Kamil Al-Sana'at, Ibn Sina's Canon of Medicine, Abul Qasim Zahrawi's book Al-Tasrif and Abdul Malik's book Al-Tayseer gained immense popularity.

Ibn Sina (born in 980 AH and died in 1033 AH) was a highly qualified physician and high-class philosopher. His book 'The Canon of Medicine' is a comprehensive and authentic book that covers all fields of medicine and gained international acclaim due to its merits. This book was included in the medical curriculum not only in the Eastern countries but also in the Western countries till the sixteenth century. It has been translated into many languages and many summaries have been written and its translations and interpretations continue to this day. The general part of the Canon is so comprehensive that the teaching of general medicine depends on it in all medical colleges.

Unani medicine also came to India and the study of this medicine was initially started in Arabic and Persian languages and later into Urdu.

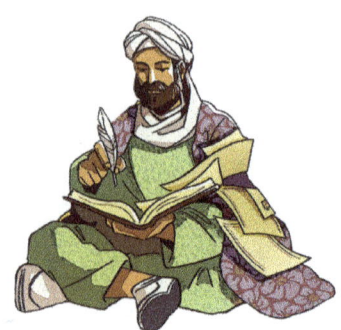

Artist's impression of Ibn Sina.

Foolish the doctor who despises the knowledge acquired by the ancients.

Hippocrates

THE SCIENCE OF MEDICINE[3]

Definition of medicine

Ibn Sina says that medicine is a 'Science by which one learns various states of the human body, in health and when not in health, and means by which health is likely to be lost, and when lost, is likely to be restored'.

From the above definition we can say that the science of medicine is therefore divided into two parts:

    A. Preservation of health (Hafz-e-Sihat[4])
    B. The science of treatment ('Ilaj al-Amraz[5])

There are two aspects of medicine; the theory and the practice.

Theoretical aspect of medicine (Tibb Nazari[6])

In the theory of medicine, the knowledge of medicine is stated but does not relate to its practical application. For example, an explanation of fever is that it increases body temperature and thirst and causes a headache, etc. This is the theoretical information about fever but does not relate to what would be the practical aspects and actions that may need to be taken in case of fever.

---

[3] i.e., Ilm-e-Tibb علم طب Literally (the) knowledge of Tibb. Tibb means medicine.

[4] حفظ صحت Branch of medical science which deals with maintenance, preservation and promotion of health as well as prevention of diseases through various regimens and practices.

[5] علاج الامراض i.e., literally treatment of diseases.

[6] The aspect of medicine concerned with theoretical topics such as temperaments, humours, faculties, various diseases, symptoms and causes.

Practical aspect of medicine (Tibb 'Amali[7])

This field of science informs us about measures and actions. For example, it explains that in a febrile patient, cold water or some antipyretic drugs should be given or that their hands and feet should be massaged – this information is of a practical nature.

Subject matter of medicine

The science of medicine discusses health and disease, and in order to understand the true nature of something, it is important to know its causes. Therefore, for any student of medicine, it is necessary to know the causes of health and disease in order to understand the reality of health and disease.

The causes of health and disease may sometimes be apparent, but at other times, they may not be so easily recognised from the use of our five senses. However, they can be known through the signs and symptoms of a disease. We, therefore, need to understand what signs and symptoms are in order to help diagnose health or disease.

There are four types of causes of health and disease. These are:

1. Material Causes (Asbab Maddiyya)
2. Efficient Causes (Asbab Fa'iliyya)
3. Formal Causes (Asbab Suriyya)
4. Final Causes (Asbab Tamamiyya)

Material Causes (Asbab Maddiyya[8])

In the context of disease, material causes are those factors that directly affect the organs and their vital spirit (pneuma). According to Ibn Sina[9], health and disease are closely related to the organs and pneuma. In contrast, humours and elements can cause health and disease only when they have transformed into organs and pneuma. Thus, the conditions of the organs and pneuma directly affect health and disease and indirectly affect the humours and elements. We will discuss elements, humours, organs, and pneuma in later chapters.

---

[7] The aspect of medicine concerned with knowledge of medical management and practice, e.g., knowledge of methods of preserving health under various conditions and treating every kind of disease.

[8] اسباب مادّیه or physical causes.

[9] Ibn Sina, also known as Avicenna in the West, was a renowned Persian scholar who flourished from 980 to 1037 CE. He was a polymath and is widely recognized as one of the Islamic Golden Age's most significant physicians, astronomers, philosophers, and writers. He is also acknowledged as the father of early modern medicine. His most notable work, The Canon of Medicine, was a comprehensive medical encyclopedia that became a standard text in many medieval universities and remained in use until as late as 1650.

Efficient Causes (Asbab Fa'iliyya[10])

Efficient causes affect and maintain the health of the body. They cause functions to be maintained in the state of health, or they can cause diseases, making bodily functions abnormal.

These causes can be divided into two parts:

The six essential factors (Asbab Sitta Daruriyya[11]):

Six essential factors for maintaining physical, mental, social and spiritual health. These are essential for every person, and an imbalance in any or all of these factors may lead to various disease conditions. The ones that affect all human beings continuously are called essential factors (the others are non-essential). These are as follows:

    a. Air (Hawa)
    b. Foods and drinks (Makulat-o-Mashrubat)
    c. Physical movement and rest (Harakat-o-Sukun Badani)
    d. Mental activity and peace (Harakat-o-Sukun Nafsani)
    e. Sleep and wakefulness (Nawam-o-Yaqza)
    f. Retention and evacuation (Istifragh-o-Ihtibas)

Non-essential Causes (Asbab Ghair Daruriyya[12]):

These causes don't have a continuous effect on the body, but they can cause changes in health or disease. For example:
1. Country
2. Habitat
3. Occupation
4. Habits
5. Age
6. Accidents that come upon the human body
7. Objects entering the human body internally or externally

Formal Causes (Asbab Suriyya[13])

They are of three types:

    a. Temperaments
    b. Faculties, which are formed after temperaments

---

[10] اسباب فاعلیہ or acting causes
[11] اسباب ستہ ضروریہ
[12] اسباب غیر ضروریہ
[13] اسباب ضروریہ or causes related to form.

c. Composition (structure) which are dependent on temperament and faculties.

When all three aspects of health - temperament, faculty, and composition - are normal and natural, a state of health is achieved. In contrast, disease occurs when any one or all three of these aspects are abnormal or unnatural.

Final Causes (Asbab Tamamiyya[14])

Final causes are related to the functions of the body, which can cause dysfunction when affected, such as a blocked artery.

The subject of Unani medical science

The subject of Unani medical science deals with the elements, temperament, humours, organs, pneumas, faculties, functions, and body conditions as they relate to health and disease and their causes. These factors of existence are described under generalities, while diseases, their causes, and presentation, as well as pulse, urine, and faeces, are described under the generalities of their causes.

Factors of Existence (Umar Tabiyya[15])

According to Unani scholars, the factors of existence are related to the Tabi'at (medicatrix naturae). These seven factors are considered to be essential for the composition of the human body, which are responsible for its existence. These seven factors are:

A. Elements/Primary components (Arkan/Anasir)
B. Temperament (Mizaj)
C. Humours (Ikhlat)
D. Organs (A'da)
E. Pneuma (Arwah[16])
F. Faculties (Quwwat)
G. Functions (Af'al)

Medicatrix Naturae (Tabi'a al-Insaniyya[17]/Tabi'at)

Tabi'at (medicatrix naturae) faculty causes movement and relaxation, and it is attributed to the seven factors of existence. For this reason, the Tabi'at is considered as the master of the body. Some of these seven factors are material components, i.e., elements, humours, organs, and pneumas, and some are formal components of the body, such as

---

[14] اسباب تماميه

[15] امور طبيعيه

[16] Light gaseous substances are generated through the interaction of inspired air with the subtle humours present in the organs and fluids of the body. These substances are crucial in supporting the faculties and their respective functions.

[17] الطبيعة الانسانية - Natural power for self-preservation; the power endowed by nature to every individual for self-preservation; it regulates normal functions and is the administrator, protector and healer of the body

temperament, and then some link to both of them, such as faculties and functions. These factors all relate to the body and are known as Mudabbira li'l Badan (factors of the body, i.e., its Tabi'at).

Tabi'at (medicatrix naturae) is the force that performs all the functions for the betterment and growth of the human body. In the case of disease, the Tabi'at is the real physician. It is the Tabi'at that fights disease, and the physician's role is to support the Tabi'at. As a student of Unani medicine and Natural medicine, you need to understand this well.

We know that many diseases are cured without the help of drugs - through the actions of Tabi'at (medicatrix naturae), such as minor wounds, coughs, colds, stomach ailments, weakness, etc. Tabi'at is the force that fights the causes which result in diseases. When this force is weakened, it then becomes difficult to cure a disease.

The faculty that works to protect the body from diseases is referred to in Western medicine as immunity. As long as this faculty remains strong, the bacteria and infections do not affect the body, but when it becomes weak, the environmental bacteria or the bacteria that exists on the external surface of the body, the eyes, nose, ears, mouth, throat, respiratory organs and digestive organs then affects the humours and organs of the body.

Experiments have shown that after bacteria enter the body, some bodies are formed that kill those bacteria and stop their toxic effect on the body. These types of bodies are called antibodies in Western medicine. These bodies are produced in the serum, and the faculty that produces them is the Tabi'at (medicatrix naturae). Therefore, according to this principle, a Western treatment principle, 'treatment with serum', has been invented in which the antibodies of disease are introduced into the body, and the Tabi'at affected by it produces antibodies against the bacteria and their toxins. Tabi'at itself expels substances that are waste and rotten from the body in the form of sweat, eye discharge, ear wax, etc.

Certain substances in the body are useful for repelling diseases. Modern research has shown that body fluids such as the saliva of the mouth, phlegm in the nose, fluid in the eyes and earwax have the effect of killing certain bacteria. The production of these fluids also proves the existence of a medicatrix naturae.

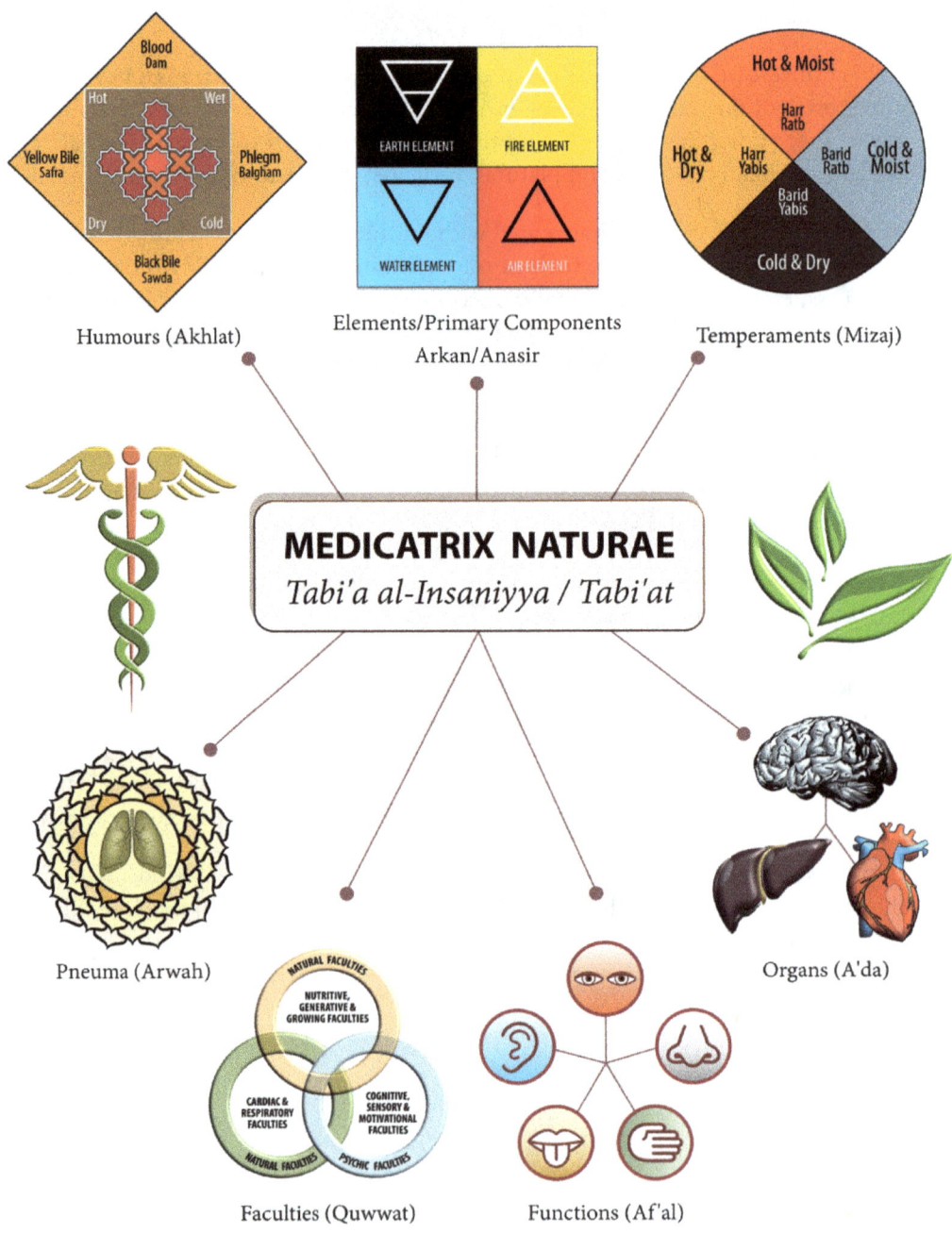

Elements (Arkan)

Definition

Arkan[18] are also known as Anasir[19],[20] and subdivisions. These are simple and unique substances that are the basic components of the human body, etc., that cannot be divided into substances that have different forms and qualities (functions and qualities). The combination and composition of elements produce different species, i.e., the three kingdoms of nature (Animals, minerals, plants). It is important to say here, however, that in the context of Unani medicine, this is not to be understood as the periodic table's elements but as primary components, which we will discuss later.

Conflict among scholars regarding the Anasir (elements)

Throughout history, scholars have held differing views on the number of elements that make up the universe. Some believed in only one element, such as earth or water, and thought that everything in existence was a result of the transformation of those elements. Others believed in a two-element theory, such as fire and earth being the essential components. Still others thought in a three-element theory: fire, air, and earth were the primary elements, and water was considered a combination of air and earth. Then, some believed in a four-element theory consisting of fire, water, air, and earth, which was proposed by Hippocrates in 460 BCE. Finally, a fifth element theory added 'ether' to the mix. However, some scholars believed that the number of elements was too vast to limit them to a specific number and that everything in the universe was a mixture or compound rather than pure elements.

Four physical qualities[21] (Kayfiyat Arba'a)

Unani philosophers believe there are four physical kayfiyat (qualities) in the world, i.e., Heat, Cold, Moisture/wetness and Dryness. Out of these qualities, two physical qualities, namely, heat and cold, are active qualities (Kayfiyat Fa'ila), and the other two qualities, i.e., moisture and dryness, are passive qualities (Kayfiyat Munfa'ila), which are associated with active qualities. So, heat does not exist alone, i.e., any of the passive qualities are associated with it; heat is either associated with dryness or moisture. Similarly, coldness is also associated with some passive qualities, either dryness or moisture. So, there are four compound physical qualities in the world:

1. Kayfiyat Harr Yabis (Hot and Dry) qualities
2. Kayfiyat Yabis Ratb (Hot and Moist) qualities
3. Kayfiyat Barid Yabis (Cold and Dry) qualities

---

[18] اركان
[19] اصر - singular Unsur (عنصر)
[20] Strictly speaking, particles (Anasir) create elements (Arkan), but the terms are often used interchangeably.
[21] Or physical properties /physical states

4. Kayfiyat Barid Ratb (Cold and Moist) qualities

All four of these qualities are associated with a substance. So, the hot and dry qualities are associated with the fire element (Anasir Nar), the hot and moist qualities are associated with the air element (Anasir Hawa), the cold and moist qualities are associated with the water element (Anasir Ma) and the cold and dry qualities are associated with earth element (Anasir Ard). The foundation of Unani medicine is based on these four elements.

(It should be noted that although the ancient philosophers have called fire, water, air and earth simple elements, these, in fact, are all compounds.)

Ibn al-Nafis[22] has presented the following explanation for the four elements:

> *'Only four types of substances are required for the existence of the compounds.*
>
> *Solid matter and then*
>
> *a liquid substance needed to transform into different forms,*
>
> *a need for an aerial substance to create a vacuum in it,*
>
> *and then the use of a hot substance to prepare it.*
>
> *So, these four substances serve this purpose and all compounds are thus formed. Therefore, it must be acknowledged that there are only four basic components of the compounds. These basic components are Earth element, Water element, Air element and fire element.'*

---

[22] Ibn al-Nafis, whose full name was Ala-al-Din Abu al-Hasan Ali ibn Abi-Hazm (1218-1288), was a brilliant polymath who excelled in various fields, including medicine, surgery, physiology, anatomy, and biology. He is famously known as the father of circulatory for his ground breaking work in describing the pulmonary circulation of blood, which he did before William Harvey's De motu cordis in 1628. It is estimated that Ibn al-Nafis wrote over 110 medical textbooks, which is a testament to his vast knowledge and expertise.

GENERAL FACTORS OF THE EXISTENCE | 39

A DIAGRAM REPRESENTING HOW THE CONCEPTS OF ELEMENTS, TEMPERAMENTS, HUMOURS, LIFE STAGES, AND SEASONS INTERCONNECT, OVERLAP, AND INFLUENCE ONE ANOTHER.

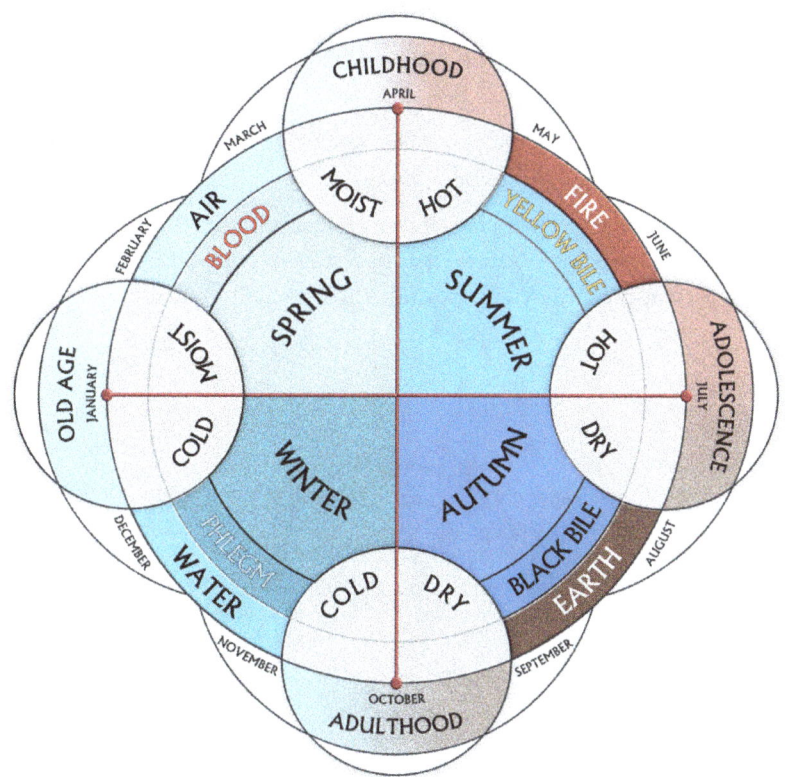

Anasir (Elements) - their states and their existence

1. Earth element:

The Earth Element is defined by its cold and dry nature, making it solid and heavy. It occupies a central position among the elements, serving as a foundation. In the universe, its purpose is to provide stability and structure, forming solid compounds that maintain their shape and weight, ensuring durability and preservation.

2. Water Element:

The water element is characterised by its cold and wet properties. It is believed to surround the earth element but is itself surrounded by the air element. Water is fluid and weighs less than the earth's elements, and it enables the earth element to take on various forms.

3. Air Element:

The air element is hot and moist in temperature, making it airy and less in weight than that of the water element. Its existence in the universe is to cause porosity in compounds and make the compounds lighter and softer.

4. Fire Element:

The Fire Element is hot and dry, positioned above all the other elements. It is associated with the celestial sphere's concave surface, symbolising the limit where material existence transitions and transformations occur. Its function is to concoct or transform substances, facilitating the formation of new compounds through its light and energetic nature.

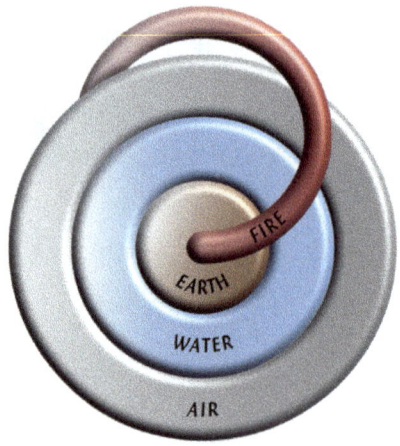

(Figure is a visual representation of the positions of the various elements.)

Temperament (Mizaj)

Definition

The literal meaning of Mizaj[23] (Temperament) is to meet, dissolve and penetrate. The word mizaj originated from the Arabic word imtizaj, meaning intermixture. Although we normally translate Mizaj as temperament, in Unani, Mizaj has a wider meaning.

Mizaj (Temperament) is a quality produced by the action and reaction of opposite qualities of elements, which are broken up into small particles to facilitate their mixing. When these components interact among themselves, a condition is produced, which is

---

[23] مزاج

found in equal proportion in all the particles of the compound. This new formation is known as Mizaj (Temperament).

According to the theory of ancient scholars, there is an attraction in certain elements, which is called Ulfat Kimiyawiyya[24] (chemical affinity), and in some elements, this condition is the opposite, and they do not combine with others; this is called Nafrat Kimiyawiyya[25] (chemical repulsion).

Admixture/Intermixture (Imtizaj)

The force of attraction of the elements is variable. The mutual intermixture of elements and affinity creates a temperament.

There are two types of Intermixtures:

1. Simple intermixture (Imtizaj sadhij)
2. Complex intermixture (Imtizaj haqiqi)

Simple intermixture

A simple intermixture is when two or more elements or components are mixed together in a way that does not change their previous qualities. For instance, if sugar is added to a glass of water, the resulting solution will be sweet and have the properties of both water and sugar. However, if the same solution is heated, the water will evaporate, leaving the sugar behind. This shows that neither the sugar nor the water has been altered, making it a simple admixture.

Complex intermixture

When a few elements mix together in a way that changes their original properties and creates new properties, it is called a compound. For instance, if you heat a glass full of sugar, it will melt and turn red, producing a gas that eventually transforms into black tar. This process is known as compound formation.

Temperament types

There are two types of temperaments in terms of moderation (I'tidal):

1. Normal/Equable temperament (Mizaj Mu'tadil)
2. Abnormal temperament (Mizaj Ghayr Mu'tadil)[26]

---

[24] Property of having chemical attraction present in some primary components/elements or compounds, which enables them to combine with certain other primary components/elements or compounds.
[25] Property of having chemical repulsion present in some primary components or components/elements or compounds, which enables them to repel from combining with other primary components or compounds.
[26] Also known as Inequable temperament, Intemperament or Immoderate temperament.

Normal temperament

It has two types:

1. Real equable temperament (Mizaj Mu'tadil haqiqi)
2. Equable temperament (Mizaj Mu'tadil tibbi)

Real equable temperament

Real Equable Temperament refers to a simple temperament in which the four elements - heat, cold, moisture, and dryness - are equally present in a compound. This results in a moderate temperament. However, such a temperament is not found in any living thing because the number of elements in all compounds found on Earth is not equal. Some elements are present in greater or lesser quantities than others.

Near to Real Equable

According to Ibn Sina, the temperament of the people living on the equator is closer to the Real Equable temperament.

Equable temperament

This is a compound temperament. There are eight types of moderate temperament:

1. The equable temperament of one species as compared to other species (Mizaj Mu'tadil Naw'i bi'l Qiyas ila'l Kharij): Particular temperament provided to a particular species which is normal and most suitable for that species but abnormal for other species.
2. The equable temperament of a member of one species as compared to other members of the same species (Mizaj Mu'tadil Naw'i bi'l Qiyas ila'l Dakhil): This is the temperament of an individual of a specie who is the most moderate among the individuals of that specie.
3. The equable temperament of one race as compared to the others races (Mizaj Mu'tadil Sinfi bi'l Qiyas ila'l Kharij): Equable temperament provided to each race of human, which helps to perform the required functions of each race with maximum completeness.
4. The equable temperament of a person of one race as compared to another person of the same race (Mizaj Mu'tadil Sinfi bi'l Qiyas ila'l Dakhil): This is the temperament of an individual of a race who is the most moderate among the individuals of that race.
5. The equable temperament of a person as compared to other persons (Mizaj Mu'tadil Shakhsi bi'l Qiyas ila'l Kharij): Equable temperament provided to a person which is most suitable for himself to perform his normal functions but is not suitable for any other person.
6. The equable temperament of a person as compared to his own temperament in different states (Mizaj Mu'tadil Shakhsi bi'l Qiyas ila'l Dakhil): Equable

temperament provided to a person which is most suitable for a particular period or state in his life. This is the temperament that a person acquires when he is in good health.

7. Equable temperament of an organ as compared to other organs of the body (Mizaj Muʻtadil Udwi biʼl Qiyas ilaʼl Kharij): Equable temperament furnished to each and every organ of the body.
8. Equable temperament of an organ as compared to its own temperament in different states (Mizaj Muʻtadil Udwi biʼl Qiyas ilaʼl Dakhil): Equable particular temperament provided to an organ in most suitable states which is most ideal as compared to all other states of that organ and the temperament that an organ acquires when it is in good condition.

Abnormal Temperament/ Morbid temperament (Mizaj Ghayr Muʻtadil /Suʼ-i-Mizaj[27])

This is the temperament in which a condition exceeds moderation. This is an imbalance of temperament in terms of its properties (Kayfiyat).[28]

There are two types of abnormal temperament:

1. Simple morbid temperament (Suʼ-i-Mizaj Sada[29])
2. Morbid temperament associated with substance (Suʼ-i-Mizaj Maddi[30])

There are two types of morbid non-substance related temperament:

1. Simple morbid/abnormal non-substance related temperament (Suʼ-i-Mizaj Mufrad Sada), in which a single quality dominates i.e., either hot, cold, dry or wet/moistness.
2. Compound morbid/abnormal non-substance related temperament (Suʼ-i-Mizaj Murakkab Sada), when any two (one active and one passive) of the four physical properties, i.e., hotness, coldness, dryness and moistness dominate abnormally over the others without involving substance in which two qualities dominate

There are also two types of abnormal or morbid substance related temperament:

1. Simple morbid substance related temperament (Suʼ-i-Mizaj Maddi Mufrad), associated with predominance of hot/cold/dry/wet substance.
2. Compound morbid substance related temperament (Suʼ-i-Mizaj Murakkab Maddi), which occurs when any two (one active and one passive) of the four

---

[27] Or impaired temperament.
[28] This can also be a change in terms of qualitative or quantitative predominance of humours (discussed later).
[29] Morbid temperament only changes in four physical properties/qualities, i.e., hotness, coldness, dryness, and wetness/moistness, takes place.
[30] Morbid temperament is a change in any one of four physical properties, i.e., hotness, coldness, dryness and wetness/moistness that takes place with the involvement of a substance.

physical properties, i.e., hot, cold, dry and moist, dominate abnormally over the others due to the predominance of substance.

So, there are four types of Simple abnormal non-substance related temperament:

    a. Abnormal hot temperament: when heat abnormally dominates the body.
    b. Abnormal Cold temperament: when cold abnormally dominates in the body.
    c. Abnormal dry temperament: when dryness abnormally dominates in the body.
    d. Abnormal moist temperament: when moisture abnormally dominates in the body.

And there are also four types of compound abnormal non-substance related temperament:

    a. Abnormal hot and dry temperament caused by only predominance of hot and dry temperament without involving substance.
    b. Abnormal hot and wet temperament caused by only predominance of hot and wet temperament without involving substance.
    c. Abnormal cold and dry temperament caused by only predominance of cold and dry temperament without involving substance.
    d. Abnormal cold and wet temperament caused by only predominance of cold and wet temperament without involving substance.

Similarly, there are eight types of abnormal madda (substance – i.e., containing a corrupted matter) temperament. But the difference between the abnormal non-substance related temperament and abnormal substance related temperament is that the substance is not included in the abnormal non- substance related temperament; only the property increases. But in abnormal substance-related temperament, the substance also increases along with properties, and the substance

These conditions are due to the excess of properties. These conditions will also be present due to a decrease in the properties (hot/cold/dry/moist).

Temperament of Organs (Mizaj A'da)

By Mizaj A'da (temperament of organs) we mean the mizaj obtained by the organs after the intermixture of the Anasir (elements) because different Anasir are involved in the synthesis of organs in different amounts. Therefore, human organs are divided into five groups according their mizaj.

   a. Organs that are equable (A'da' Mu'tadil)
   b. Organs that are hot (A'da Harr)
   c. Organs that are cold (A'da' Barid)
   d. Organs that are moist (A'da' Ratb)
   e. Organs that are dry (A'da' Yabis)

Organs that are equable:

If you look at the organs in terms of equable or moderate temperament, it will be clear that the skin is the most moderate or equable. This is why the skin is considered one of the sensory organs, as it can sense heat, cold, moisture, and dryness. Among the skin, the hand skin is the most moderate, followed by the skin of the palm, fingers, and the skin of the index finger. However, the skin of the distal phalange of the index finger is the most equable, which is why it is used to check the pulse.

Organs that are hot:

Certain organs in our body generate more heat than other organs. This heat generation is more pronounced in organs where blood circulation is higher. Out of all the organs in our body, the heart is the hottest because it pumps the most blood and is the most active organ. Following the heart, the liver is the next hottest organ since it is responsible for preparing nutrients for all the other organs in the body.

The third hottest organ is the flesh, which refers to the muscular or glandular tissues. Numerous blood vessels in the flesh generate a considerable amount of heat, making it the third hottest organ after the heart and liver.

Organs that are cold:

The coldest organs in the body are bones, followed by ligaments, nerves, and the brain. The term 'cold organs' refers to those organs which produce the least amount of heat. Compared to 'hot organs', cold organs have a slower rate of metabolism and transformation, and less blood flows through them. Consequently, less heat is produced in these organs, resulting in their classification as 'cold organs'.

Organs that are moist:

The brain and spinal cord are highly moist, followed by the breasts and testicles, which are also rich in moisture, aiding their reproductive roles. Though the lungs appear moist, they mostly derive their wetness from external sources such as the vapours that ascend from the digestive system and the secretions that descend from the head.

It is necessary to have a certain amount of bodily heat to metabolise fat. If the body does not have enough heat, fat will not be burned for energy but will accumulate in the body. People with a higher amount of body fat are believed to have a cold temperament.

Organs that are dry:

Hair is the driest among all organs, followed by bones, cartilage and ligaments. Dry organs are those that have low moisture, such as hair and bones. Physicians have generally said that hardness equates to dryness. That is, those organs that are hard and solid are also dry.

Temperament according to age

Age is divided into four stages of age:

STAGE OF AGE	MIZAJ	AGE RANGE
Growing Age (Sinn-i-Numu)	Hot and moist	Up to 25 years
Adulthood (Sinn-i-Shabab)	Hot and dry	From 25-45 years
Age of decline (Sinn-i-Kuhulat)	Cold and dry	From 45-65 years
Age of elderly /geriatric age (Sinn-i-Shaykhukhat)	Cold and moist	From 65 onwards

1. **Growing age:**
   The age at which the body continues to grow has a hot and moist temperament needed for growth, extending from birth and lasting for 25 years.
2. **Adulthood:**
   The age at which the body becomes fully mature. This age is from 25 years to 45 years. The temperament of this age tends to be hot and dry.
3. **Age of decline:**
   At the age when innate heat starts to decline, the body inclines to adopt a cold and dry temperament, loses its stability and starts to deteriorate, but it is not significant. This age ranges from 45 to 65 years, and the temperament tends to be cold and dry.
4. **Advanced age:**
   The age when innate heat has declined extends from sixty-five years onward. The body adopts a cold and dry temperament, and there is an excess of abnormal moisture in the body, hence why some say that this age is cold and moist.

TYPES OF TEMPERAMENT IN UNANI MEDICINE

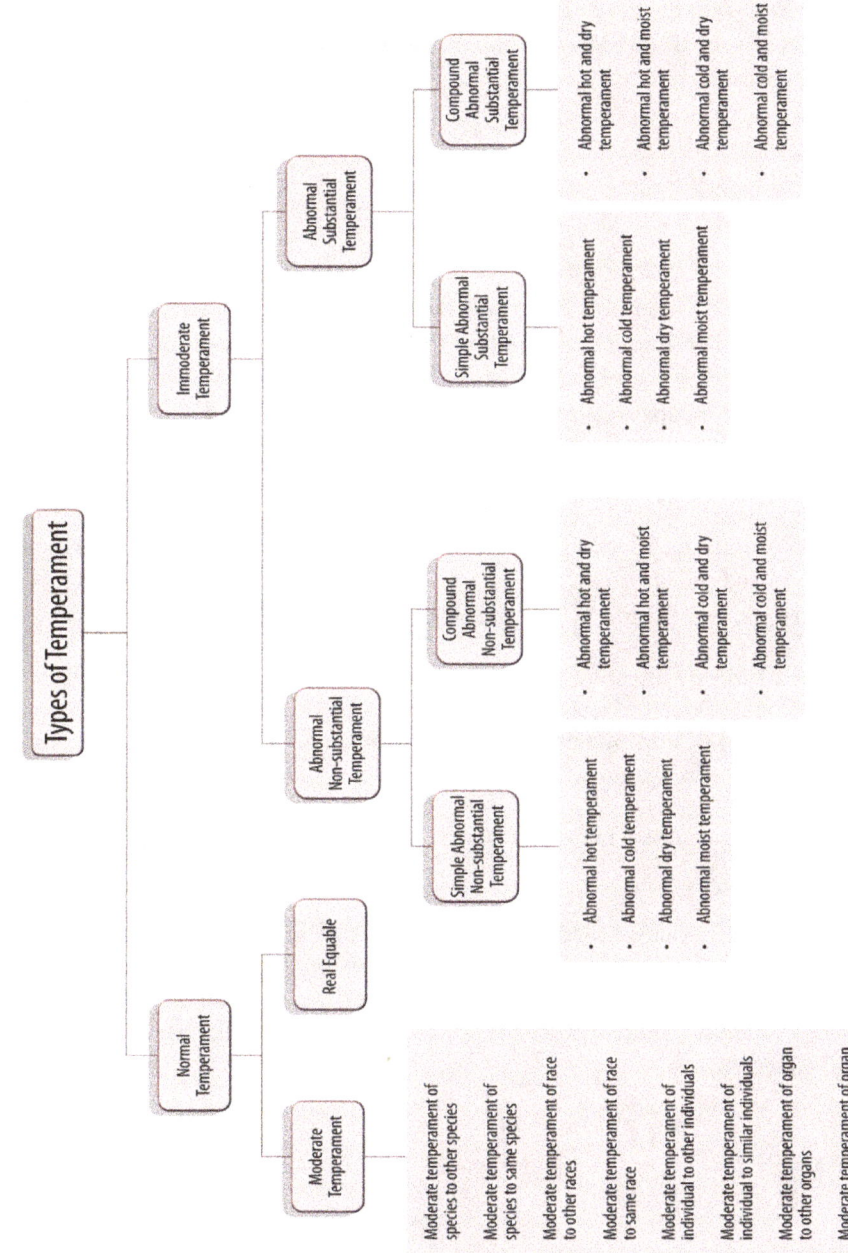

Humours (Akhlat)

The word khilt[31] means a mixed substance. As blood is mixed with different types of fluids, these components are called khilt (humour/mixture). The plural of khilt is Akhlat[32]. Since blood (dam), phlegm (balgham), Yellow bile (safra) and Black bile (sawda) are mixed in blood vessels, they are called Akhlat (humours). This collection is referred to as blood because blood is dominant over the other humours, and the colour of this mixture is bright red.

Hippocrates laid the foundation of the humoral theory and attributed humour imbalance as the origin of diseases. According to Hippocrates, the human body is composed of three main components: (1) solid, (2) fluid, and (3) pneumas (ruh), and consists of components that are surrounding and components that are surrounded.

Hippocrates divided fluids into four coloured humours: (1) Red (Blood humour), (2) White (Phlegm humour), (3) Yellow (Yellow bile humour), and (4) Black (Black bile humour). The right combination and proportions of these four fluids create health, while incorrect proportions and irregular combinations cause disease.

In Unani medicine, the principle of concoction and elimination (Usool-e-Nuzj wa Istaferagh) is crucial. This principle is one of the most successful in treating all physical and humoural disorders. The treatment is based on identifying which humour is dominant and which is corrupted. The process involves eliminating excess or corrupted humours and replenishing the necessary fluids to restore balance.

The definition of humour

The definition of humour has been given by Abu Sahl Masihi[33] in his book 'Book of the Hundred chapters' (al maa fil sanaa);

'Humour is that liquid substance which is trapped in sinuses and vessels that prevents its flow.'

Abu Sahl Masihi has divided all the body fluids (Rutubat-i-Badan [including humours]) into three types according to their location:

1. Vascular Fluids (Rutubat-i-Uruqia) are the fluids that are found inside the vessels.

---

[31] خلط

[32] اخلاط

[33] Abu Sahl 'Isa ibn Yahya al-Masihi al-Jurjani (died 1010) was a renowned Christian Persian physician who lived during the Islamic Golden Age. He is known for his pioneering contributions to the field of medicine. Among his many achievements, he authored a seminal work entitled 'al-maa fi-l-sanaa al-tabiiyyah,' an encyclopaedic treatise on medicine comprising one hundred chapters. He wrote other treatises on measles, the plague, the pulse, etc. Ibn Sina was one of his notable students.

2. Interstitial Fluids (Rutubat-i-Tajawif or Rutubat-i-Talliyya) are fluid that are filtered by the vessels (capillaries) and are found in the cavities of the organs.
3. Intercellular fluid or protoplasm (Rutubat-i-Ustuqussiyya/Rutubat-i-Joharia/Ansaria/Rutubat-i-Ghariza). This is the fluid that is found inside the cells. This fluid is not included in the humours because it is the essence of the organ to which the functions and benefits of the organs are associated.

Ibn Sina defined humour as follows:

'Humour is that liquid substance that originated from food.'

(The Canon of Medicine - Al-Qanun fi al-Tibb)

According to the definition given by Ibn Sina, the humours are divided into two groups:

Primary Fluid (Rutubat-i-Ula):

Which is obtained in the liver after metabolism of food and enters the bloodstream.

Secondary Fluid (Rutubat-i-Thaniya):

The secondary fluids are also obtained from humours. These accumulate in the cavities of the organs after passing and filtering through the blood vessels or enter the blood from the organs and glands, such as the secretions of the endocrine glands that enter the blood.

The creation of humours

The variety of foods that a person consumes starts digesting starting from the mouth. Further changes occur in the stomach and intestines with the help of heat and digestive juices until the food becomes a solution, which is called Kaylus (chyle). This solution is then absorbed into the vessels and travels to the liver and then to other organs where, after various changes, different types of fluids are produced, which are called Akhlat (humours).

Most of the components of the digested food enter the stomach and intestines through their specific vessels (Mesenteric vessels), enter the liver and then are metabolized to form Akhlat (humours). Other than that, some moistures are absorbed through diffusion by vessels and reach the blood.

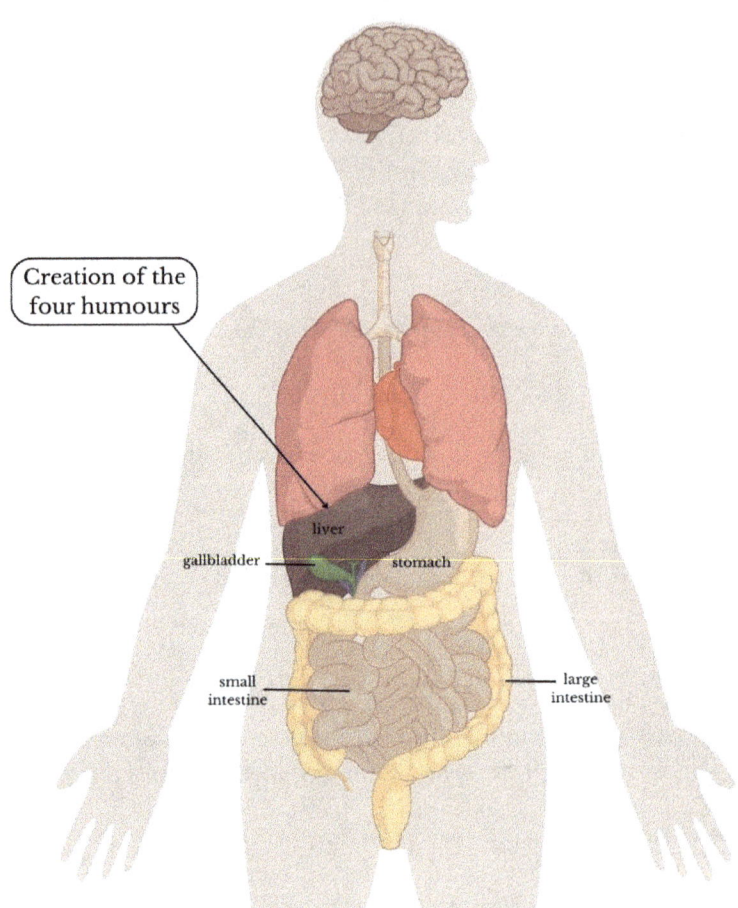

The absorption of the humours into the organs

Humour from blood capillaries seeps out and enters the cavities of the organ structures. This secretion of humours is similar to dew. The organs possess an absorptive faculty (Quwwat Jadhiba), which absorbs these humours. The digestive faculty (Quwwat Mughayyira) then changes them to adjust their temperament, consistency and colour accordingly. This is how the humours take the form of organs.

The evidence for Components of Humour

The classification of humours into four types can be proven through observation. For instance, if blood is taken out through venesection (Fasd) and kept open in a container, the components can be seen. The yellow foam floating upwards is khilt safra (yellow bile humour), while the frozen red lump is the khilt Dam (blood humour). If the blood is taken in a container containing hot water, two other components can be observed: a white component that appears like egg white is khilt balgham (phlegm humour), and the other black component that sits at the bottom is khilt Sawda (black bile humour).

Kilit Dam (blood humour), khilt Balgham (phlegm humour), khilt Safra (yellow bile humour), and khilt Sawda (black bile humour) are four humours that include different types of moistures. For example, phlegm is a type that includes all the white fluids that differ in nature, temperament, properties, and composition. The mucoid fluid is filtered from the mucous membrane, the lymphatic fluid flows in the lymphatic vessels, and the gastric and intestinal fluid is found inside the stomach and intestines. Although these white fluids have different functions and properties, they are included under phlegm due to their cold and moist nature and colour.

Similarly, yellow bile is another humour that includes bile in the liver and what is excreted in the urine and other hot and dry fluids.

Blood Humour (Khilt Dam[34])

Mizaj (Temperament)
Harr Ratb (Hot and moist)

Importance

It nourishes the body, that is, replaces the dissolved components in the body, which keeps the body safe and healthy. Also, the blood warms the body, which maintains the strength of all the organs and ensures their proper actions.

There are two types of blood humour.

1. Normal blood humour (Dam Tabi'i/Khun Tabi'i)
2. Abnormal blood (Dam Ghayr Tabi'i/ Khun Ghayr Tabi'i)

Normal blood humour

This is the blood in which air (oxygen - ruh: pneuma) is dissolved in. It is red and odourless. It is moderate in consistency (neither too thick nor too thin), and the taste is sweet. Other Khilt (humours), along with blood humour, i.e., phlegm and yellow bile, are also present in blood in suitable quality and quantity.

Abnormal blood humour

This is the blood whose characteristics are devoid of its normal qualities[35].

---

[34] It is important to understand that humours are essential to blood, which sets it apart from other nutrients. Therefore, it's crucial to differentiate between blood humour and blood itself because the latter contains humours and several other vital nutrients.

[35] Changes in temperament, such as experiencing hot or cold temperatures or being exposed to external or internal factors that affect the blood humour, can cause the blood to produce abnormal yellow and black bile. This happens when a part of the blood putrefies, with the lighter portion becoming yellow bile and the heavier portion becoming black bile.

Colour of normal blood

The arterial blood is bright red, whereas the colour of the veins is blackish red. In the case of anaemia, the colour of the blood becomes lighter as the number of red blood cells decreases.

Release of blood with odour

When there is an infection (Ufuniyya) in the blood, an odour is created in it. The smell of blood is an infection – this idea was introduced by Ibn al-Nafis. Similarly, acidification (Tarshi) of blood has also been included in infections. This is because an infection produces acidification in the same way as it produces fermentation (Khamir).

Moderate consistency of blood

Blood must have a moderate consistency. In anaemia, the consistency of the blood decreases, and the benefits of blood are lost, whereas in food poisoning, the consistency of the blood becomes thick, causing it to not infiltrate the small vessels, which leads to death.

The sweetening of blood

Sweet ingredients are found in large quantities in the composition of blood, but they contain salted ingredients as well, which make the taste of blood salty.

The benefits of blood salts are as follows:

1. Salt does not allow the phlegm to freeze.
2. Prevents dirt and infection.

Clotting/coagulation of blood

The nature of the vessel is the protector of the blood inside the vessel. When the blood seeps out of the vessel, it clots. This is because when the blood comes out of the vessel, it takes the form of a clotted substance which contains fibres. Clotting can also be caused by damage to the inner surface of the vessel.

Phlegm Humour (Khilt Balgham)

Mizaj (Temperament)
Barid Ratb (Cold and moist)

There is a difference of opinion among physicians about the temperament of phlegm. Some say that phlegm is cold and moist, but others have said it is hot and moist. Ibn Sina believed that normal phlegm is a type of sweet phlegm that is not too cold; instead, it has some heat compared to blood but is colder than yellow bile.

Types

Normal phlegm is a category which includes different types of white fluids that are types of phlegm; thus, the temperament of phlegm is different.

Normal phlegm humour (Balgham Tabi'i):

According to Galen, normal phlegm is similar to blood and is needed by all organs. That is why phlegm flows with the blood. If necessary, phlegm can also transform into the blood to fulfil the organs' requirements.

Abnormal phlegm humour (Balgham Ghayr Tabi'i or Balgham Mutaghayyir):

This is the phlegm whose physical attributes, such as taste and consistency, change, as well as its temperament and smell.

There are five types of abnormal phlegm humour in terms of taste

1. Saline Phlegm (Balgham Malih/Balgham Shor): This is saline or alkaline in taste and is inclined towards hotness and dryness.
2. Sour phlegm (Balgham Hamid/Balgham Tursh): It is sour in taste and inclined towards coldness and dryness.
3. Tasteless phlegm (Balgham Tafih or Balgham Masikh): It is tasteless, immature and quite cold.
4. Astringent Phlegm (Balgham Afis): This type of phlegm has a dry, astringent taste, similar to unripe fruit or tea. It is characterised by its cold and dry qualities.
5. Sweet phlegm (Balgham Hulw): It is sweet in taste and inclined towards hotness and moistness.

There are four types of abnormal phlegm in terms of consistency

1. Watery phlegm (Balgham Ma'i): Phlegm that is very thin and watery.
2. Calcareous phlegm (Balgham Jassi): Phlegm that has a thicker consistency, is very impure, and is similar to white lime.
3. Mucoid Phlegm (Balgham Mukhati): Its consistency is as thin as liquid mucus.
4. Vitreous Phlegm (Balgham Zujaji): This type is gelatinous and sticky, akin to the consistency of melted glass or thick syrup.

Based on smell, abnormal phlegm has a single type that is called Balgham Muntin (foul-smelling phlegm). It is the phlegm in which odour is produced by sepsis/ infection/ putrefaction.

Importance of phlegm humour

1. The first benefit of phlegm humour is that it becomes blood; that is, when it is dissolved in the body, phlegm converts into blood. Among the changes and

transformations that take place within it is that the white cells convert to red cells.
2. Phlegm humour keeps the organs wet and hydrated and does not allow them to dry, which facilitates the function of the organs. This type of humour lines the passages of the gut from the oesophagus, stomach, intestines, larynx, urinary bladder, uterus, etc. and is a membrane that keeps the organs fresh and nourished.
3. Provides food and nourishment to the organs, especially to 'white' organs, such as nerves (A'sab), ligaments (Ribatat), bones, etc.

Physicians like Galen believed that the phlegm humour that normally flows with the blood in the vessels is very similar to blood. This phlegm is present in vessels, and it concocts and becomes food for the organs. Since every part of the body contains digestive faculties, when the components of phlegm pass close to the organs, they change and become food for the organs, even taking on the organs' form.

During times of nutritional scarcity, such as fasting or starvation, the body's natural abilities come into play. The innate natural faculty (Quwwat Tabi'yyah[36]) and inherent heat (Hararat Ghariziyya) inside the body work together to break down the stored phlegm, using it to provide the body with the necessary nutrients. This process results in the consumption of stored phlegm and fat, reducing body mass.

Phlegmatic Ailments

Physicians have described the following diseases as phlegm diseases, which also makes it clear which fluids are included in phlegm.

1. Catarrh (Nazla[37]): This is a phlegm disease characterized by a flow of catarrhal fluids from the brain towards the throat and chest.
2. Swelling (Tahaiiyaj): This is a mild inflammation that develops on the face, hands and feet. Physicians call this inflammatory substance diluted phlegm.
3. Phlegmatic vomiting (Qay Balghami): A morbid state characterized by expulsion of phlegmatic material through vomiting, decreased thirst and sour, salty or sweet taste, borborygmi and increased salivation.
4. Phlegm diarrhoea (Ishal Balghami): This is a disease in which phlegm is excreted with faeces.
5. Soft tumour (Sal'a 'Asaliyya): This a tumour whose content is similar to diluted honey.
6. Vitiligo (Baras): This disease is also caused by the discharge of phlegm, which causes the skin, flesh and, finally, the blood of these structures to turn white.

---

[36] Faculty serves the functions of nutrition, growth, reproduction, and evacuation of waste products from the body to preserve the individual and the species.
[37] A disease characterized by a flow of catarrhal fluids from the brain towards the throat and chest.

Yellow Bile Humour (Khilt Safra)

Mizaj (Temperament)
Harr Yabis (Hot and Dry)

There are two types of Yellow bile:

1. Normal Yellow bile (Safra Tabi'i)
2. Abnormal Yellow bile (Safra Ghayr Tabi'i)

Normal Yellow Bile (Safra Tabi'i)

Normal Yellow Bile can be observed as yellowish-red froth in blood. The taste of Yellow bile is bitter, its colour is yellow, and its consistency is diluted.

Ibn Al-Nafis has stated that pure bile is yellowish, resembling the colour of saffron. However, due to excessive consumption of legumes, the colour of Yellow bile can change to green. The lightness of Yellow bile implies that it weighs less than blood.

Importance of Yellow Bile

1. Blood dilution: When the blood is diluted, it becomes less concentrated, which helps it flow more easily through narrow vessels.
2. Organ nutrition: All humours are involved in organ nutrition. Therefore, yellow bile is also used to nourish organs. Some organs have more or less yellow fibres in their structures, the existence of which indicates that Yellow bile is also responsible for their nutrition. The organs that have yellow fibres in their structure are the lungs, gastrointestinal tract, tongue, blood vessels and some yellow connecting structures.
3. The movement and washing of the intestines: The movement and washing of the intestines is related to the Yellow bile. This bile travels from the liver to the gall bladder and then to the intestine. The Yellow bile that goes from the gall bladder to the intestine has two functions. Firstly, it washes the wastes and laced phlegm of the intestines. Secondly, it creates a hot sensation in the muscles of the abdomen, which leads to the urge to defecate. When the Yellow bile is depleted, it can result in a disease like colic. The decrease in Yellow bile causes the yellow colour of the faeces to turn grey. Yellow bile is a natural purgative (Mushil) that washes and cleanses the intestines.
4. Intestinal worms: Ibn Al-Nafis writes that Yellow bile is very hot, and its heat and dryness, as well as its bitterness and sharpness, kills intestinal worms; on this basis, physicians prescribe bitter medicines such as Baobarang (Embelia Ribes - False black pepper) to kill worms.
5. Yellow bile prevents infection: According to Ibn Al-Nafis, yellow bile can prevent decay in the upper intestines, resulting in faeces free from putrefaction. However, as it moves towards the lower intestine, its effectiveness decreases, leading to

putrefaction in the stool, particularly in the rectum, where the weakened yellow bile results in greater putrefaction.
6. Yellow bile produces heat in the stomach: Ibn Al-Nafis writes that yellow bile clears phlegm and digests it, thus helping in the digestion of food.

Abnormal Yellow Bile (Safra Ghayr Tabi'i)

It has two forms.

1. Becomes abnormal due to the addition of extraneous material.
2. Alteration in its own composition, i.e., its consistency, colour, smell, etc., changes.

Abnormal Yellow Bile types

1. Vitelline Yellow Bile (Safra Muhhiya): It is bile produced by the admixture of thick phlegm.
2. Serous Yellow Bile (Mirra Safra): It is the bile produced by the admixture of thin phlegm.
3. Burnt Yellow Bile (Safra Muhtariqa): It is the bile produced by the admixture of burnt black bile in which oxidation occurs and increases its intensity and irritation.
4. Leek green yellow bile (Safra Kurrathi): Produced by the combustion of ordinary yellow bile, resulting in the development of a leek green colour due to the mixing of the burnt material with the original yellow bile.
5. Verdigris green yellow bile (Safra Zanjari): The hottest and the most harmful of all abnormal types of yellow bile, produced due to extreme combustion of leek green bile

Yellow Bile Ailments

To understand the nature of bile in medicine, it is also important to understand the diseases caused by bile. Some of the biliary diseases are as follows.

a. Jaundice (Yarqan Safra)
b. Yellow bile related obstruction (Sabur Safrawiyya): cause of obstruction with high burning and hotness.
c. Hepatic calculi (Hasa al-Kabid): Biliary calculi/gallstones in the liver.
d. Decreased size of liver due to yellow bile (Sighar al-Kabid Safrawiyya).
e. Bilious vomiting (Qay Safrawi): Vomiting in which a large amount of bile is expelled.
f. Bilious Diarrhoea (Ishal Kabidi Safrawi): Diarrhoea due to involvement of the liver in which there is the passage of bilious matter not mixed with stool as a result of the accumulation of morbid matter in the liver. These biliary rings are more yellow and cause high irritation/burning.
g. Yellow urine (Bawl Asfar): Yellowing of urine.

    h. Bilious fever (Hummayat Safra): It is characterized by bilious vomiting, intense burning and headache.
    i. Bilious large intestinal colic (Qulanj Safrawi): Characterized by severe pain of the colon with burning sensation, excessive thirst, sleeplessness, bitter taste, bilious vomiting, and loose motions.

Black Bile Humour (Khilt Sawda)

Mizaj (Temperament)
Barid Yabis (Cold and Dry)

According to Ibn Sina, black bile is a component which includes many types, and their temperaments may vary.

Types of Black Bile

1. Normal Black Bile (Sawda Tabi'i)
2. Abnormal Black Bile (Sawda Ghayr Tabi'i)

Normal Black Bile (Sawda Tabi'i):

This is the black bile that mixes with the blood and provides nutrition to the organs, for example, to black organs like hairs, strong organs like the bones, or the nerves.

Abnormal Black bile (Sawda Ghayr Tabi'i):

This is that black bile that arises from the combustion/oxidation (Ihtiraq[38]) of every humour, even from the oxidation of the black bile itself, and is not a cause of nourishment but a cause of corruption resulting in various kinds of black bile related diseases.

Oxidation is a process in which the black bile in the body changes abnormally (Ghayr Tabi'i Taghayyur), causing the fluids (humours) in the body to turn black. According to modern research, when blood is exposed to the open air for some time, the blood component haemoglobin converts into haematin, which further turns into melanin, a black substance. Physicians consider this black substance as abnormal black bile produced from the oxidation of blood.

There are four types of abnormal black bile:

1. Sanguineous (blood) black bile (Sawda Damwi/Dam Aswad): Abnormal black bile produced by the combustion of blood.
2. Bilious black bile (Sawda Safrawi/ Marar Aswad): Abnormal black bile produced by the combustion of yellow bile.

---

[38] 'Ihtiraq' literally describes burning due to the charring of bodily fluids and humours. This process is commonly caused by excessive heat, resulting in the charring of the fluids.

3. Phlegmatic black bile (Sawda Balghami): Abnormal black bile produced by the combustion of phlegm.
4. Melancholic black bile (Corrupted black bile) (Sawda Sawdawi): Abnormal black bile produced by the combustion of black bile itself.

Importance of Black Bile

   a. It thickens the consistency of the blood: The more the amount of black bile in the blood, the thicker its consistency.
   b. Included in the diet of organs: Black bile is a vital component in the diet of the human body's organs. When mixed with other humours, it provides nourishment to the organs. It is worth noting that black bile is more abundant in specific organs, particularly those that are black or have black parts, such as the retina of the eye, black hairs, skin, and moles. Once modified, it can also enter organs such as bone, cartilage, or ligament, contributing to their density and hardness.

Black Bile Ailments

The following are some common Unani black bile diseases:

1. Yarqan Suddi (Obstructive jaundice): In which the colour of the body and urine becomes black. Similarly, in some diseases, the mucous membranes, gastrointestinal tract, ligaments, and even heart fibres become black.
2. Sawdawiti Jildiyya (Black bile skin): A disease in which the amount of black bile increases in the skin. Due to this, the skin becomes black and thus dry.
3. Sal'a Sawdawiyya (Black bile Tumours): These tumours contain black matter. When they are small, they are called saccule; when they grow, they are called tumours.

Saratan Sawdawiyya (black bile carcinoma): Malignant black bilious tumour (cancer) caused by oxidation of black bile, which can occur anywhere in the body; spreads very rapidly, and the roots of the swelling are deep; sometimes appears due to accumulation of burnt yellow bile and phlegm.

GENERAL FACTORS OF THE EXISTENCE | 59

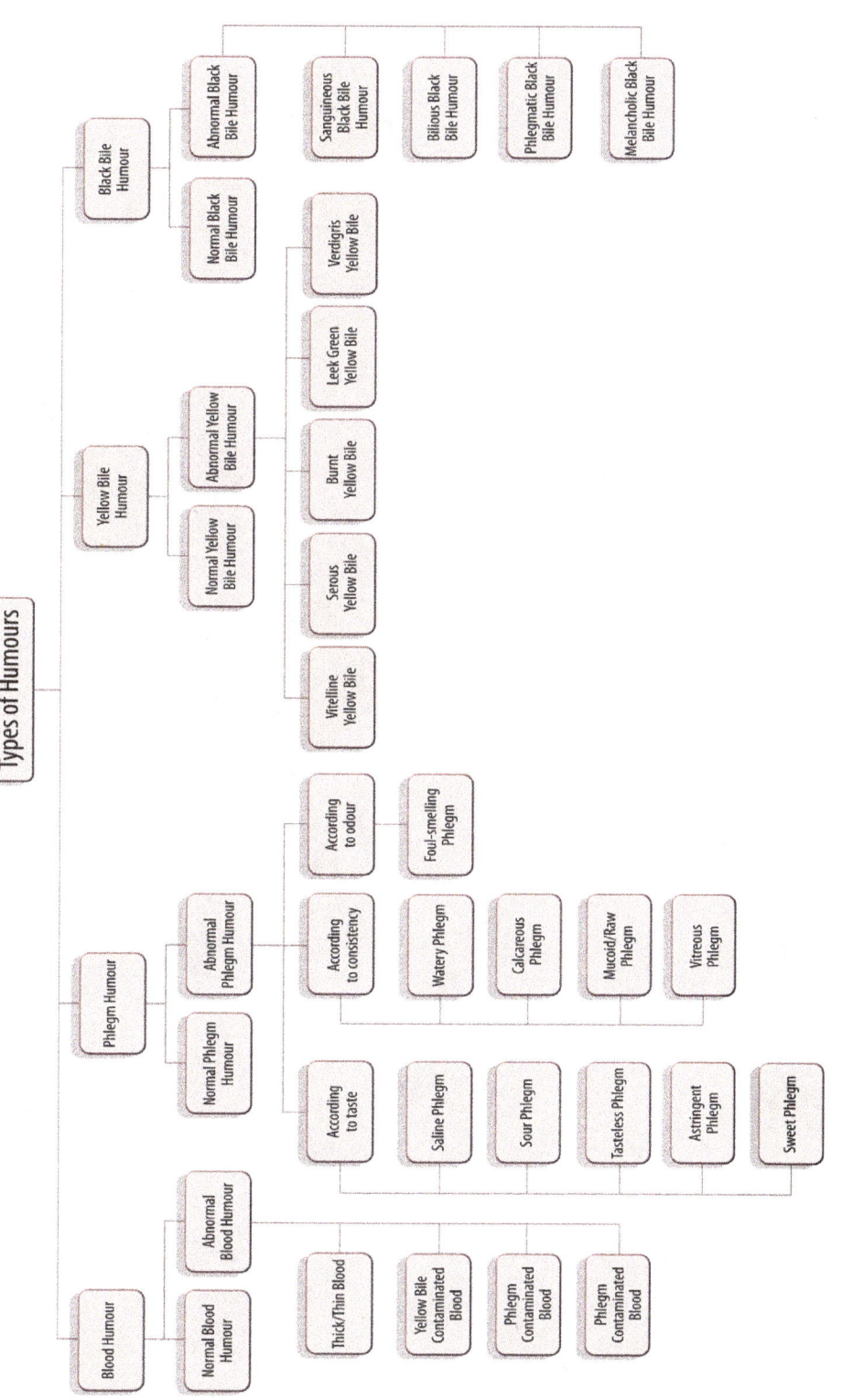

HUMOURS IN UNANI MEDICINE

Types of Humours

- Blood Humour
  - Normal Blood Humour
  - Abnormal Blood Humour
    - Thick/Thin Blood
    - Yellow Bile Contaminated Blood
    - Phlegm Contaminated Blood
    - Phlegm Contaminated Blood

- Phlegm Humour
  - Normal Phlegm Humour
  - Abnormal Phlegm Humour
    - According to taste
      - Saline Phlegm
      - Sour Phlegm
      - Tasteless Phlegm
      - Astringent Phlegm
      - Sweet Phlegm
    - According to consistency
      - Watery Phlegm
      - Calcareous Phlegm
      - Mucoid/Raw Phlegm
      - Vitreous Phlegm
    - According to odour
      - Foul-smelling Phlegm

- Yellow Bile Humour
  - Normal Yellow Bile Humour
  - Abnormal Yellow Bile Humour
    - Vitelline Yellow Bile
    - Serous Yellow Bile
    - Burnt Yellow Bile
    - Leek Green Yellow Bile
    - Verdigris Yellow Bile

- Black Bile Humour
  - Normal Black Bile Humour
  - Abnormal Black Bile Humour
    - Sanguineous Black Bile Humour
    - Bilious Black Bile Humour
    - Phlegmatic Black Bile Humour
    - Melancholic Black Bile Humour

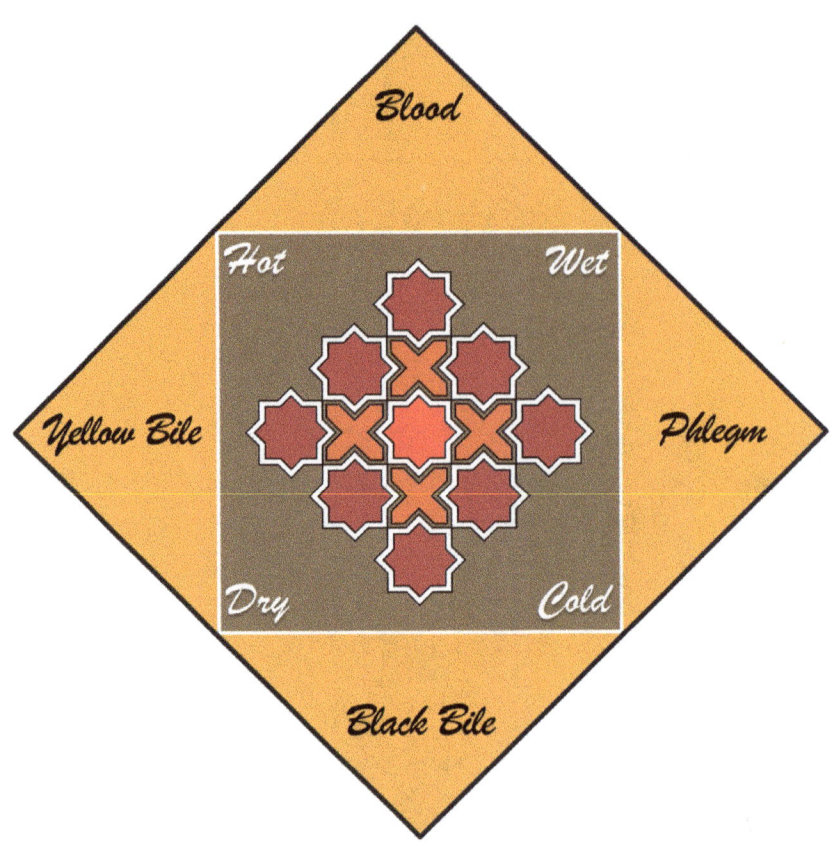

The four humours

Organs (Udw[39])

The solid parts of the body are called organs. They are stable and are derived primarily from humours. They do not flow like fluids, nor do they spread like air.

Organs are divided into two major types:

1. Simple organs/ homogenous organs (A'da' Mufrada)
2. Compound organs (A'da' Murakkaba)

Simple organs

Simple organs are those whose components have a unique, simple or similar appearance. These are also known as simple or homogenous organs (A'da' Basita) because a part or the entire organ is the same, such as flesh. A single organ can also be referred to as tissue (Nasij).

The simple organs are as follows:

1. Bone 2. Cartilage 3. Ligament 4. Tendon 5. Membrane 6. Nerve 7. Fat 8. Flesh 9. Arteries 10. Veins

Some physicians also included marrow, nails and hair as simple organs.

Compound Organs

Compound organs are composed of simple organs, such as the liver, lungs, and heart.

Compound organs

Classification of Compound organs

They can be divided into five types.

1. In terms of composition
2. In terms of system
3. In terms of power
4. In terms of facilities
5. In terms of reproduction

---

[39] A'da' singular اعضاء

1. Classification of Compound organs in terms of composition

Classification of Compound organs in terms of composition

1. Compound organs Type I or Primary type (A'da' Murakkaba ba Tarkib Awwali): Compound organs are composed of only simple organs, e.g., muscle, which is composed of flesh, fat, etc.
2. Compound organs Type II or Secondary type (A'da' Murakkaba ba Tarkib Thanwi): Compound organs composed of a compound organ type I with other organs, e.g., eye, which is composed of muscle (a compound organ type I), fluids and seven layers.
3. Compound organs Type III or Tertiary type (A'da' Murakkaba ba Tarkib Thalithi); Compound organs composed of a compound organ type II with other organs, e.g., a face which is composed of an eye (a compound organ type II), nose, mouth, cheeks, etc.
4. Compound organs Type IV or Quaternary type (A'da' Murakkaba ba Tarkib Rabi'i): Compound organs composed of a compound organ type III with other organs, e.g., head which is composed of a face (a compound organ type III), ear, brain, etc.

The term 'primary type' refers to organs that are made up of simple components without any compound organs. For instance, muscle tissue is composed of flesh, nerves, ligaments, and membranes, all of which are simple organs. On the other hand, the 'secondary type' refers to organs made up of a combination of primary-type components and other elements. For example, the eye is a secondary type organ, as it contains a primary type component, the muscles of the eye.

2. Classification of Compound organs in terms of systems

The human body can be viewed as a collection of systems, each with a principal or vital organ (Udw Ra'isa) at its centre. All other organs in the system are referred to as subservient organs (A'da Khadima).

According to the different systems of the body, there are four vital organs: three in terms of survival of race and one in terms of survival of species. In terms of survival of the race, the three types of vital organs are:

1. **Brain:** One of the vital organs with a cold and moist temperament; it is the seat of mental faculties, sensations, and movement. It is located in the head and is the centre of the nervous system. The nerves are its subservient organs.
2. **Heart:** One of the vital organs with a hot and moist temperament, which is the seat of the vital faculty. It is located in the thorax and is the centre of the vascular system. The vessels are their subservient organs.
3. **Liver:** One of the vital organs with a hot and moist temperament, which is the seat of the nutritive and vegetative faculties. It is located in the abdomen and is

the centre of the mesenteric vessels. The mesenteric vessels are their subservient organs.

In terms of survival of the species, the vital organ in males is the testes, where primitive/seminal fluid and sperm are produced, and the ovaries are in females. Its subservient organs are the vessels that transport blood, ejaculate seminal fluid and all other reproductive organs.

Subservient organs are those organs which indirectly serve the principal organs or assist in their functions.

3. Classification of Compound organs in terms of faculties

Organs are divided into four categories according to their faculty because four forms of faculties are found in the body.

1. Psychic faculty /Mental faculty (Quwwat Nafsaniyya[40])
2. Vital faculty (Quwwat Haywaniyya[41])
3. Physical or Natural faculty (Quwwat Tabi'iyya[42])
4. Reproductive faculty (Quwwat Tanasuliyya[43])

The organs within which these powers are found are named after them, that is, the organs of the nervous system (A'da' Nafsaniyya), vital organs (A'da' Haywaniyya), digestive organs (A'da' Tabi'iyya) and reproductive organs (A'da' Tanasul).

a. Organs of the nervous system:
These are the organs of sensation and movement. The principal organ of this group is the brain, and the nerves and the sensory organs are its subservient organs.

b. Vital organs:
Vital organs are the source of primary faculties in the body and are indispensable for the existence of the individual or the species. The principal organ of this group is the heart, and the heart vessels are its subservient organs.

c. Digestive organs:
They are the organs that digest and metabolize food. The principal organ of this group is the liver, and its subservient organs are the stomach and intestines.

d. Reproductive organs:
These are the organs of reproduction, and the principal organs of this group are the testes and ovaries.

---

[40] Faculty which is furnished in an individual for sensory/perceptive and motor/motive function of the body; it controls nervous tissues to perform the functions of sensation/perception and regulates the nervous system for motor activity.

[41] Faculty, which is essential for life, reaches from heart to body, organs through arteries, and keeps them alive.

[42] Faculty serves the functions of nutrition, growth, reproduction, and evacuation of waste products from the body to preserve the individual and the species.

[43] Primary physical faculties are provided to an individual to preserve its species.

4. Classification of Compound organs in terms of facilities

There are two types of service:

1. Pre-serving facilities
2. Post serving facilities

Pre-serving facilities:

The helping organ acts before the principal organ in the execution of a particular function and prepares the organs for its function.

Post serving facilities:

The organ which serves after the act of the principal organ in accomplishing the needs of a function.

Classification of organs of the nervous system in terms of facilities:

The brain is the primary organ of the nervous system, while the sensory nerves act as the organs that help preserve it. These nerves stimulate the brain, which then generates a response. On the other hand, the motor nerves act as the post-serving organs that transfer the motor response from the brain to the muscles.

The eye, ear, nose, tongue and skin are the five senses that help preserve the brain and are therefore subservient to it. All the senses of the body reach the brain through the nerves. These organs are also commonly referred to as the senses of the brain.

Classification of vital organs in terms of facilities:

The heart is the principal organ of vital organs. It receives the necessary resources like nutrients and oxygen through the vessels that carry blood to the heart. Similarly, the vessels that carry blood and oxygen from the heart to other organs perform the necessary functions for the heart. Ibn Sina included lungs in the pre-serving organs of the heart as they have a crucial role in the heart's functioning.

Classification of digestive organs in terms of facilities:

Among these organs, the liver is the principal organ for which the stomach, intestines, vessels, mesenteries, etc., are pre-serving organs, and the post-serving organs are the vessels that carry humour (nutrients) to the blood after metabolism. Similarly, the bile duct carries bile from the liver to the gallbladder and intestines.

From the digestive organs, the urinary organs are also included in the post-serving organs for the liver because they filter out the components of urine before excretion.

Classification of reproductive organs in terms of facilities:

The testes, along with the ovaries, are the primary reproductive organs. They receive oxygenated blood through vessels that serve as pre-serving facilities. Post-serving facilities are provided by the spermatic vessels, which also act as storage organs for sperm.

5. Classification of Compound organs in terms of reproduction

There are two theories on how organs are classified in terms of reproduction. The first theory suggests that simple organs are initially nourished by semen and later by blood. Reproductive facilities form the body of the foetus and absorb specific ingredients of semen separately to form the flesh and gut. In this way, all the organs are created by the separation of the specific components of semen.

The second theory suggests that all the components of simple organs are made from semen, except fats and flesh, which are made from the components of thick blood and not from semen.

Ibn Nafis writes that the meaning of this statement is not that the simple organs are entirely made of components of semen, but it means that these components are initially made from semen and later develop by obtaining nutrients from the blood.

Therefore, in terms of reproduction, the organs are divided into two parts

1. Essential organs[44]
2. Secondary organs/Haematogenic organs[45]

According to the first theory, since all the organs are made from semen initially, these simple organs are called essential organs.

According to the second theory, since fats and flesh develop by getting nutrients from blood, these organs are called secondary/haematogenic organs.

And then, finally, from the combination of the simple organs, the compound organs are formed, and from the compound organs, the human body is formed.

Serving and Receiving Organs

Serving organ

The organ that serves the power/function of other organs, e.g., the heart, is a serving organ for the blood vessels.

---

[44] Organs that originate from semen and cannot regenerate once damaged.
[45] Organs which are produced by the humours and can be regenerated.

Receiving organ

An organ that receives power from other organs, e.g., blood vessels receive blood from the heart, and nerves receive commands/ interpretations from the brain.

Natural faculty of the organ

Ibn Sina also wrote in the Canon:

> *'In the cell of every organ, there is an innate faculty through which the nourishment continues.'*

Nutrition

Nutrition refers to the process of absorbing food, storing it in organs, digesting it, converting it into the organ's structure, and excreting waste products.

Tabari[46] referred to this process as the inner faculty, which is present in every organ of the body. This faculty converts food into the substance of the corresponding organ. Therefore, all the organs in the body act as both receiving and serving organs. They accept materials and, at the same time, provide materials for other organs.

---

[46] Abu al-Hasan Ali ibn Sahl Rabban al-Tabari (c. 838 – c. 870 CE) was a Persian physician and psychologist. He wrote the first encyclopaedic work on medicine and discovered that pulmonary tuberculosis is contagious.

GENERAL FACTORS OF THE EXISTENCE | 67

ORGANS IN UNANI MEDICINE

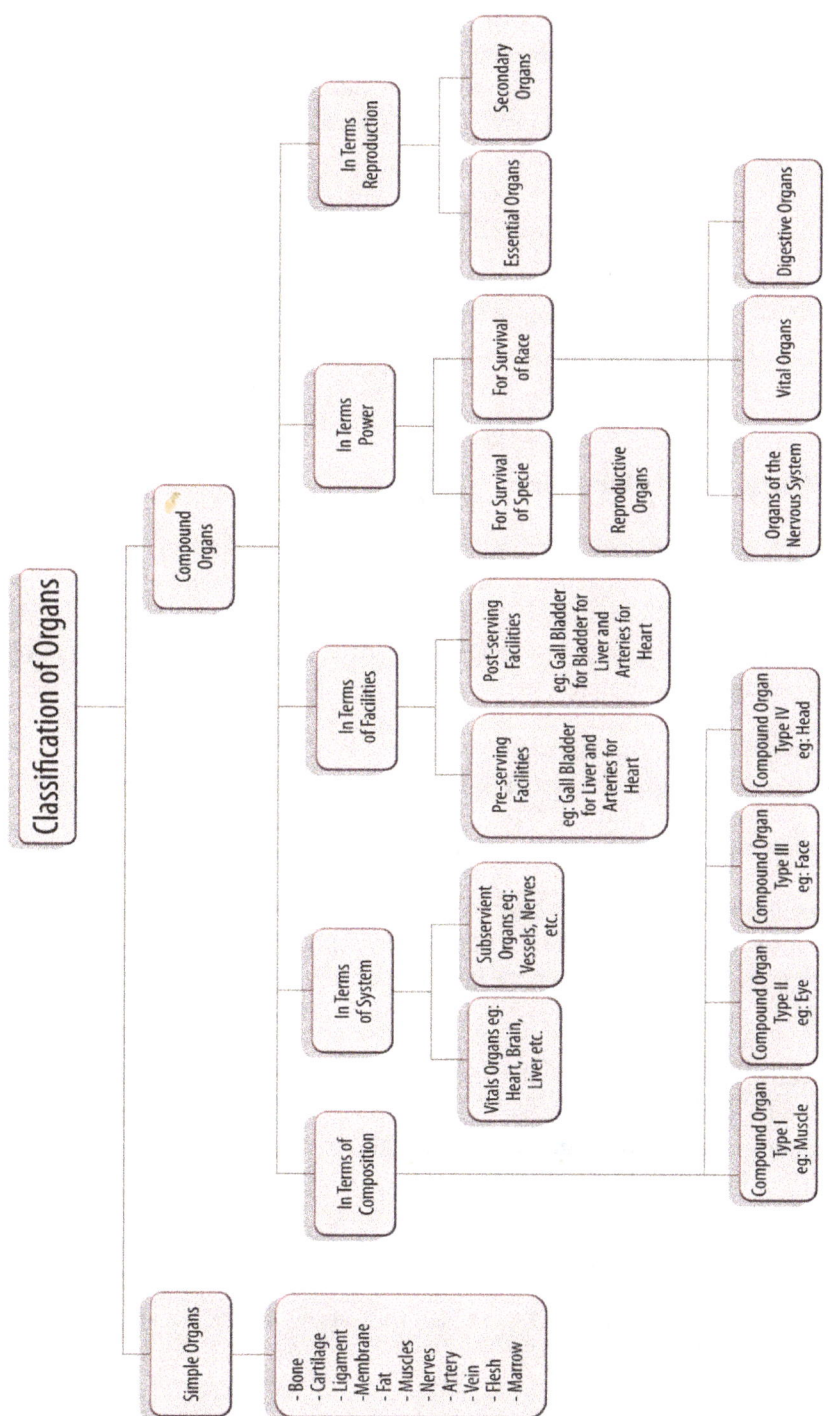

Pneumas (Arwah[47])

Definition of Ruh (pneuma)

Unani scholars say ruh (pneuma or vital energy) in medicine is not 'ruh', which is commonly understood as the soul in Arabic. Rather, it is a light and gaseous substance which is produced from easily diffusible humours (Latif Akhlat[48]), just as organs are produced from coarse humours (Khatifa Akhlat[49]). Since these easily diffusible elements are in gaseous form, they are called Arwah (pneumas).

The benefits of pneumas are as follows:

1. The pneuma causes movement in the organs.
2. The natural innate heat of the body is maintained due to pneuma.
3. Pneumas sustain life and power in the organs. If the link between pneumas and organs is disrupted, then the organs will become cold with no sensation and movement and will eventually die.

The nature of the Ruh (pneuma)

Pneuma is a light gaseous substance that is an essential component of the human body. It is referred to as a light substance because it is not visible due to its lightness and is also known as a gas. Ancient physicians believed that the organs and fluids of the human body contained light gaseous substances that performed important functions for life. The absence of these substances can cause the death of an organ.

Although the pneuma is a vapour and gaseous body, it is dissolved in the blood and fluids just like air is mixed in external water.

The active substance of the Ruh (pneuma)

Ibn Sina writes that the air around us is an element for our body and pneuma, constantly supporting and improving them. However, this atmospheric air does not become pneuma but rather reaches the lungs through respiration, where it helps the pneuma through its essence.

Essentially, the substance of the pneuma is made up of two things: easily diffusible humours and atmospheric air. This is similar to how the lighter component of the humours is involved in the formation of the pneuma.

---

[47] روح/ارواح singular Ruh - Light gaseous substance obtained from the interaction of inspired air with subtle humours found in organs and fluids of the body and help faculties in their functions (not the same as Ruh in pharmacy)
[48] لطيف اخلاط
[49] كثيف اخلاط

Masihi also agrees that the substance of the pneuma is obtained from the air inhaled by the lungs. This air is not the pneuma itself but rather the material from which it is obtained. The essence of the air enters the lungs through respiration and then reaches the heart, where it becomes a source of heat.

It is only when the lungs absorb the specific essential substance of the air, and it enters the blood, becoming a part of the body, that it is called pneuma. The essence of the air is not called the pneuma until it becomes a part of the body, as the pneumas are components of the factors of existence, which are part of the body.

So, when the air is outside the body, it is an unrecognized component, but when it enters and becomes a part of the body, it is referred to as Ruh (pneuma).

Blood is the carrier of Ruh (pneuma)

When the external air reaches the lungs, the specific component of the air, i.e., Nasim[50] (subtle air), is absorbed and reaches the blood, and so this Nasim goes where the blood flows. Although Nasim is found dissolved in all bodily fluids, however, the red component among the four humours, which is called haemoglobin, has the highest ability to absorb Nasim, and so, it can be stated that khilt Dam (blood humour) is the carrier of ruh (pneuma).

When the Tabi'at (medicatrix naturae) wants to send the ruh towards the diseased part of the body, the blood flows towards it because, without the blood, the pneuma alone cannot reach there.

Locations and routes of Ruh (pneuma)

The pneuma is more or less present in every part of an organ because, without the pneuma, no part of any organ can survive. However, the amount of pneuma varies from place to place.

When the active substance in the air reaches the lung cavities, certain components in the blood attract specific components in the air, which are then absorbed and enter the lung capillaries. From there, these pneumatic components travel wherever the blood flows.

Thus, from the capillaries of the lungs to the pulmonary arteries, which opens in the left atrium, it traverses from the left atrium to the left ventricle of the heart and then through the aorta and its branches, it enters the capillaries in the structures of the organ. Since oxidation occurs there, these pneumatic components are utilized there, and waste gases are produced, readily absorbed by the capillaries and enter the veins. Then, through these veins, it drains into the vena cava and enters the right atrium. It then passes by the right

---

[50] نسیم Nasim is that part of the air which is subtle or is subtle air, which through lungs enters the blood and then to the heart to become Ruh Haywaniyya (Vital pneuma), giving life to the whole body.

ventricle and enters the lungs through pulmonary arteries, where these waste gases are expelled. This relation of blood or pneuma continues for life.

It is important to note that the Ruh is more important than the blood, and for this reason, the vessels in which the pneuma is abundant were named arteries, the name of which was coined by Erasistratus[51].

If the food produces fuel in the organs, then the air produces the pneuma, and just as the burning of fuel produces smoke, the oxidation in the human body produces waste gases, which are called wastes of pneuma. And are excreted from the body through exhaled respiration. And just as smoke is produced in the atmosphere as a result of combustion, so is smoke produced in our body, which is called waste gases.

Types of pneuma

There are three types of pneumas types according to location and its function:

1. **Psychic pneuma (Ruh Nafsaniyya):**
   The pneuma found in the organs of the psychic faculty whose centre is brain and helps psychic faculty to perform its functions.
2. **Vital pneuma (Ruh Haywaniyya):**
   The pneuma found in the organs of the vital faculty whose centre is heart and helps vital faculty to perform its functions.
3. **Physical pneuma (Ruh Ṭabiʻiyya):**
   The pneuma found in the organs of the physical faculty whose centre is liver and helps physical faculty to perform its functions.

Faculties/power (Quwwa[52])

Definition of faculty

The term 'faculty' denotes the capacity of an organ to perform an action or serve as the source of an action. The presence of a faculty is indispensable for any function to take place. According to Ibn Sina, the faculty is inherent to the function, and the function is inherent to the faculty. The two are intertwined, with every function originating from some faculty and every faculty being the source of some form of function.

Division of Faculty

Faculty is divided into three categories.

    a.   Mental faculty /Psychic power (Quwwat Nafsaniyah[53])

---

[51] a Greek anatomist and royal physician (died 250 BC).
[52] قوّت/قوی - Quwwat (Plural)/Quwa (Singular) faculty(ies)/power(s).
[53] قوّت نفسانیه

    b. Vital faculty (Quwwat Haywanniya[54])
    c. Natural/Physical faculty (Quwwat Tabi'iyya[55])

In terms of survival of the race, some consider there is a fourth type called reproductive faculties (Quwwat Tanasuliyya[56]).

Mental faculty (Quwwat Nafsaniyah)

The mental faculty refers to a person's ability to perform sensory and motor functions within their own body. It manages the nervous tissues that allow for sensations and perceptions while also controlling the nervous system for motor activities. The brain is the primary organ responsible for this faculty.

There are two types of mental faculty:

    a. Motor faculty/power (Quwwat Muharrika[57])
    b. Receptive faculty/power[58] (Quwwat Mudrika[59])

1. Motor faculty (Quwwat Muharrika)

Type of psychic and mental faculty which regulates motor activities in the body; the motor faculty contracts and relaxes the tendons, through which the organs and the joints extend and flex; the movement of muscles is due to the motor faculty.

2. Receptive faculty (Quwwat Mudrika)

It is a faculty that is related to perception and sensation, it is either receptive or aids in perception.

Types of motor faculty

There are two types of motor faculties:

    a. motivating faculty/preparatory faculty (Quwwat Shawqiyya[60])
    b. stimulating power/efficient faculty (Quwwat Fa'ila)

1. Motivating faculty[61] (Quwwat Shawqiyya):

The faculty that prepares the mind to do something either in favour or against the will.

---

[54] قوت حیوانیه
[55] قوت طبیعیه
[56] Primary physical faculties provided to an individual for preservation of its species.
[57] Also called Quwwat Harakiyya.
[58] Or sensory faculty/perceptive power.
[59] Also known as Quwwat-i-Idrak /Quwwat Hissiyya.
[60] Or Quwwat Nuzū'iyya /Quwwat Isti'dādiyya.
[61] preparatory faculty

There are two sub serving powers of Quwwat Shawqiyya:

1. desiring faculty (Quwwat Shahwaniyya) - motivating faculty, which directs the mind to obtain things perceived to be useful.
2. protective faculty/raging power (Quwwat Ghadabiyya) - directs the mind for a reaction against a threat or an event comprehended to be harmful.

2. Stimulating power/efficient faculty (Quwwat Fa'ila):

The faculty that causes an action or function and is composed of the following faculties.

1. Faculty of imagination (Quwwat-i-Khayal) preserves knowledge perceived by the faculty of composite sense and the knowledge or sense with which new sensory experiences of the same or similar types can be compared.
2. Faculty of imagination with interpretation (Quwwat Wahima); interprets the meanings of those particular forms perceived by faculty of composite sense and decides what is in favour of an individual and what is against him or her.
3. Faculty of composite sense (Hiss Mushtarak) which receives all sensations, composes them into precepts and enables proper sensory appreciations.
4. Faculty of memory (Quwwat Hafiza[62]); preserves the meanings derived by the faculty of imagination with interpretation; the memory may be instantaneous, short-term or long-term.
5. Faculty of modification/administration (Quwwat Mutasarrifa[63]) modifies various sensory information in various ways and gives new dimensions to preserved knowledge.

Carriers of Motor faculties

The carrier of motor faculties are the nerves, which are connected to the brain and spinal cord on one end and the muscles on the other. The motor faculty travels from the centre of motion to the muscles directly through the nerves, and these nerves are called the carriers of sensation and motion.

Varieties of motor faculty

Motor function is a broad category that encompasses a wide range of functions that are linked to different types of muscles. Each muscle has a specific type of function and nature. This is why muscles differ in colour, shape, and consistency, why the effects of toxic drugs and substances on different muscles vary, and why organs like the heart, stomach, uterus, testicles, etc., perform different functions. Therefore, it is evident from these facts that different types of muscles have distinct natures and functions.

---

[62] Or Quwwat Dhakira
[63] Or Quwwat Mufakkira/ Quwwat Mutakhayyila)

The ten senses or the receptive faculty (Quwwat Mudrika)

There are ten types of receptive faculties; known as the five external senses (Hawas Khamsa Zahira[64]) or external receptive faculty[65] (Quwwat Mudrika Zahira) and the five internal senses (Hawas Khamsa Batina[66]) or the internal receptive faculty[67] (Quwwat Mudrika Batina).

Five external senses (Hawas Khamsa Zahira)

They are dependent on the five external faculties:

- A. The power/sense of vision (Quwwat Basira)
- B. The power of hearing (Quwwat Sami'a)
- C. The power of the smell (Quwwat shamma)
- D. The power of taste (Quwwat Dha'iqa)
- E. The power of touch (Quwwat Lamisa)

Five internal senses

There are also five:

(1) Faculty of composite sense (Hiss Mushtarak)
(2) Faculty of imagination (Quwwat Khayal)
(3) Faculty of modification/administration (Quwwat Mutasarrifa[68])
(4) Faculty of imagination with interpretation (Quwwat Wahima)
(5) Faculty of memory/cognitive faculty/ memorising power (Quwwat Hafiza[69])

Faculty of composite sense (Hiss[70] Mushtarak)

It is the faculty that perceives the sensations of symptoms, signs, and images of the body, and it is associated with the external senses. That is, the senses which are perceived through the external senses are absorbed by the composite sense, and through the composite sense, the effect of these sensations reaches the other internal senses. Signs and symptoms which are perceived separately by the external senses are all brought together by a single faculty.

---

[64] حواس خمسہ ظاہرہ
[65] One of the sensory faculties, which help to interpret the outer sensations of the body
[66] حواس خمسہ باطنہ
[67] One of the sensory faculties recognises, receives, and collects the sensations forwarded by external senses; this faculty has its centre/seat inside the brain.
[68] Or Quwwat Mufakkira/Quwwat Mutakhayyila
[69] Or Quwwat Dhakira
[70] حس (Hiss) means sense

Existence of composite sense and its need:

Ibn al-Nafis presented the notion of composite sense and its significance through these points:

a) When observing a falling drop, we perceive it as a straight line despite its non-existence externally. This line is a composite sense that our vision cannot detect. Another faculty collects the continuous images of the falling drop and transforms them into a line, enabling us to perceive it as such.
b) Our brain possesses a faculty that perceives all senses simultaneously. Without it, we would not be confident in asserting that something we touch is both hard and colourful. Every external sense can only perceive the senses of its corresponding organ.
c) Even in our sleep, we experience various forms, sounds, and objects in our dreams. The power that perceives these senses remains active in our dreams. The shapes, forms, and sounds we encounter in our dreams are collected by this power and perceived as dreams.

Faculty of Imagination (Quwwat Khayal)

The Faculty of Imagination is responsible for preserving the knowledge we gain through our senses. It works by comparing new sensory experiences with previous ones, and even after the external objects disappear from sight, their information remains stored in our minds for some time. This faculty is the storage of common sense, which preserves multiple information and helps us recall previous information. Additionally, it serves as the source of our imagination.

Without the Faculty of Imagination, we would not be able to recognize someone whom we have met previously.

Faculty of modification/administration (Quwwat Mutasarrifa)

The faculty of modification/administration is responsible for interpreting sensory information and assigning meaning to it. This faculty performs two functions: combination and separation.

Forms of combinations include:

a) Combining different forms to create new combinations, such as imagining a man with wings instead of hands.
b) Associating certain meanings with other meanings, like associating enmity with a person based on their appearance.

Forms of separation include:

a) Separating certain structures from other structures, such as imagining a man without his hands.
b) Separating certain meanings from other meanings, such as imagining a person without their desire for friendship.
c) Separating certain meanings from certain structures, like thinking about a friend in a way that forgets their friendship.

These mental imaginations and perceptions can be related to or against events.

The faculty of modification is like a lawyer who presents all matters to the judge but does not have the power to decide. Similarly, this faculty interprets sensory information and presents it to the faculty of imagination, which then decides how to proceed.

Faculty of Imagination with Interpretation (Quwwat Wahima)

The Faculty of Imagination with Interpretation interprets sensory information and decodes its meanings. This faculty helps us perceive partial meanings related to certain forms. For instance, it enables us to guess a person's emotions, such as hostility or love, merely by looking at their face. When we see a person, our brain first recognizes their face and then processes their qualities and habits.

The faculty of imagination with interpretation is regarded as the most powerful as it dominates over sensory faculties. It is responsible for perceiving meaning as a whole by combining or separating other faculties. This decoding of meaning is solely done by the faculty of imagination and interpretation, as other faculties of the brain do not contribute to it.

Faculty of Memory (Quwwat Hafiza)

The Faculty of Memory is responsible for preserving and storing the meanings derived by the faculty of imagination with interpretation (Quwwat Wahima). Its relationship with Quwwat Khayal (faculty of imagination) is similar to that between the Quwwat Khayal and Hiss Mushtarak (composite sense). Quwwat Hafiza is also known as memorising power[71] (Quwwat Dhakira[72]), as when we remember or mention (dhakir[73]) something, we verbalise our thoughts.

Dhakir (Mentioning/Remembering) is composed of two things.

a) To perceive something that has been realised previously.

---

[71] Or literally remembering/mentioning power/ability.
[72] قوت ذاکره
[73] ذکر is to remember/repeat/mention – by doing so, you are vocalising your thoughts.

b) To store something in the mind after perceiving so that it can be remembered at a later.

Three things are needed when mentioning or remembering something (Dhakir):

a) To imagine the things saved in mind and present them to the Quwwat Wahima (faculty of imagination with interpretation) to decode their meaning.
b) To perceive the meanings of things is the work of the faculty of apprehension.
c) To preserve those meanings, this is done by Quwwat Hafiza (faculty of memory).

Vital faculty (Quwwat Haywanniya)

The vital faculty is responsible for sustaining life, with its centre located in the heart. It spreads through the arteries and reaches all the organs in the body, providing them with the energy they need to function properly.

The arteries carry blood substances that nourish the organs and generate heat. The vital power of the heart pumps oxygenated blood through the arteries, providing life-sustaining power to all organs. When this system fails, the life of the organs comes to an end, and the motor and sensory faculties that reach that organ also cease to exist.

The proof of the existence of the vital power is that even if a limb is paralysed, it continues to survive, and the signs of life persist in it. If there were no life, the organ would undergo putrefaction, which only happens after death.

Types of vital power

Vital power is based on two forms:

1. Stimulating power (Quwwat Fa'ila):

It is the faculty that causes the heart and arteries to contract and expand, which is detected through the pulse.

2. Passive power (Quwwat Munafila):

It is the faculty that produces factors affecting psychic faculty, such as sadness, anger, pain and happiness, fear and panic, etc.

Natural/Physical faculty (Quwwat Tabi'iyya)

Ibn Sina divides the Natural/Physical faculty (Quwwat Tabi'iyya) into two faculties:

1. Reproductive faculty (Quwawat Tanasuliyah)
2. Personal faculty (Quwwat Shaksiyya)

Reproductive faculty (Quwawat Tanasuliyah): Primary physical faculties provided to an individual for preservation of its species.

Personal faculty (Quwwat Shaksiyya): Primary physical faculty making alteration in the food for the preservation of the individual. There are two types:

1. **Faculty of growth (Quwwat Namiya[74])**: It is the power that develops the organs in the required form and size and integrates the nutrient material to complete individual development.
2. **Nutritive faculty (Quwwat Ghadhiya[75])**: It is the power that is related to digestion.

Nutritive faculty (Quwwat Ghadhiya)

Nutritive faculty alters the digested food in such a manner that it becomes temperamentally similar to the body and suitable to replace daily wear and tear. This process is known as Badal Ma Yatahallal (replacement of fluids and energy).

To provide nutrition to the body, the nutritive faculty first replaces the dissolved components with an active component (Jawhar), i.e., blood in this case. This blood can form organs in place of the dissolved components.

Next, the active component attaches to the organ and becomes a part of it until it is similar to the organ in terms of components, consistency, and temperament. The nutritive faculty involves three faculties in this process.

1. **Collecting faculty** (Quwwat Muhassila): Selects and collects the matter for digestion.
2. **Adhesive faculty** (Quwwat Mulassiqa): Attaches digested matter to the organs for their nutrition.
3. **Faculty of assimilation** (Quwwat Mushabbiha): Transforms the matter attached to the organ by the adhesive faculty in such a way that it resembles the nourished organ in all respects and becomes a part of that organ.

The action of Nutritive faculty can be disrupted due to various reasons:

1. Disruption in the first act of nutritive faculty, i.e., the act of absorption, as is the case with atrophy (Huzal) disease.
2. Disruption in the second act of the nutritive faculty, i.e., the act of attachment, as happens in oedema (Istisqa).
3. Disruption in the third act of the nutritive faculty, i.e., the act of assimilation, as happens in vitiligo (Bars) and pityriasis alba[76] (Bahaq Abyad), etc.
4. Improper diet to the organ due to famine or scarcity or due to any disease.

Requirements for nutrition

---

[74] قوت نامیہ
[75] قوت غاذیہ
[76] Hypopigmented patches on skin.

There are two requirements for nutrition.

1. The appropriate temperament and composition of the organ to be nourished.
2. The quality and quantity of the food should be appropriate.

Both of these conditions can be met when the vital organs, heart, liver and brain, are healthy.

Stages of action of nutritive faculty

1. Sometimes, the nutritive faculty takes more food for dissolution, as it does in the growing age.
2. Sometimes, the nutritive faculty takes equal food to dissolution, as it does in adulthood, in which the volume of the organs is maintained.
3. Sometimes, the nutritive faculty takes less food for dissolution, as it does in advanced age, in which the organs shrink and weaken.

Therefore, the nutritive faculty is stronger in the growing age, moderate in adulthood and weaker in advanced age.

During the growing age, the functions of the nutritive faculty and power of growth tend to be faster, resulting in a higher innate heat. However, as one ages and enters a period of decline, these functions tend to slow down, leading to a decrease in the innate heat.

Transformative faculty (Quwwat Mughayyira)

According to Ibn Sina, the transformative faculty (Quwwat Mughayyira[77],[78]) can be found in each organ according to its temperament. This power alters the dietary substance and transforms it similarly to the nourished organ. The transformative power continues the metabolism in every part of the body so that useful components can become a part of the body and the useless waste components can be eliminated.

The transformative faculty is not a single power but innumerable powers of various kinds that alter dietary components. This power starts functioning when the dietary components change the shape and structure of the organ, and the waste substances are expelled from the body.

Some organs have double transformative faculties, one that aids nutrition and the other that helps them to function. For example, the stomach and the liver have double transformative faculties. One helps in the production of gastric juice and bile, and the other aids in digestion. Adult females' breasts (mammary glands) also have double transformative faculties. One of them nourishes the breast, and the other produces milk.

---

[77] قوت مغيّره
[78] Or Quwwat Hadima/Hazima

Digestion of food

Digestion and transformation is constantly occurring inside the organs of the body. All the digestion occurring in the body are divided by physicians into four:

1. First digestion/alimentary digestion/chyme formation[79] (Hadm Mi'di[80])
2. Hepatic digestion/chyle formation[81] (Hadm Kabidi[82])
3. Tertiary digestion/vascular digestion[83] (Hadm Uruqi[84])
4. Fourth digestion/organic digestion[85] (Hadm Udwi[86])

Sub serving powers of nutritive faculty

These are four powers and they are assigned for the service of the faculties and the digestion of food.

(1) Absorptive faculty (Quwwat Jhadiba[87])
(2) Retentive faculty (Quwwat Masika[88])
(3) Digestive faculty (Quwwat Hadima[89])
(4) Expulsive faculty (Quwwat Dafi'a[90])

1. **Absorptive faculty:** serves the nutritive faculty by absorbing beneficial materials into the body.
2. **Retentive faculty**: supports the nutritive faculty and holds onto the food until the digestive process is complete. It keeps the dietary material in place while the digestive process occurs, breaking down and transforming the nutrients into substances the body can use.
3. **Digestive faculty:** serves the nutritive faculty and digests the dietary material to make it part of an organ.
4. **Expulsive faculty**: assists the nutritive faculty in removing waste products from the body. This is because not all components of the food we eat are beneficial or harmful to our body. If these constituents accumulate and are not expelled from the body, they can decay and result in various health problems and diseases.

Absorptive faculty (Quwwat Jhadiba)

---

[79] occurring in the alimentary canal to form chyme
[80] بضم معدی
[81] taking place in the liver to form chyle
[82] بضم کبدی
[83] It takes place in the vessels and helps to assimilate food to make it part of the organs.
[84] بضم عروقی
[85] takes place in the organs
[86] بضم عضوی
[87] قوت جاذبہ or written as quwwat jaziba
[88] قوت ماسکہ
[89] قوت ہاضمہ
[90] قوت دافعہ

The absorptive faculty of each organ of our body attracts those components from the blood that are suitable and similar to it. Substances are also drawn due to the vacuum created, just as the substance is drawn in an injection. The Tabi'at (medicatrix naturae) tries to fill the created vacuum with some fluid; thus, the substance is drawn into the organs. Fluid is absorbed into the organs because of heat in the organ as the light of a lamp draws out oil.

Digestive faculty (Quwwat Hadima)

a) Digestion and concoction (Hadima wa Nudj):

The digestive faculty digests the food, makes it a part of the body, transforms food components into waste that cannot be digested, and induces such changes in them, which makes the waste easily expelled. This function of the digestive faculty is called Indaj[91] (concoction).

Although digestion (Hadima) and concoction are synonyms, if the digestive system fails to remove certain waste materials, the body will isolate the waste to prevent it from decaying.

The process of digestion is characterised by a series of transformations that resemble those that occur during the degradation of a substance. More specifically, the essential prerequisites for digestion are analogous to those that underpin the putrefaction of a substance, namely heat and moisture.

b) Four stages of digestion:

Many changes occur in the food from the time it enters the stomach till its active components (Jawhar) are converted into the organs, but generally, they are divided into four categories: alimentary digestion, hepatic digestion, vascular digestion and organic digestion.

1. **Alimentary digestion (Hadima Mi'di[92]):** It refers to the digestion that occurs in the mouth, stomach and intestine (digestive tract).

    Digestion in the mouth: The process of digestion of food in the mouth is when saliva, which has the power of lubrication and digestion, is mixed with the food. Also, chewing digests the food, too, and thus, they change their condition and temperament to some extent.

    Digestion in the stomach: is completed through the rotatory movement of the stomach, which also secretes gastric juice.

---

[91] Process by which morbid matter/humour matures and is made easily evacuable from body

[92] بضم معدی

Abu Sahl Masihi says that food does not cook in the stomach in the same way as it cooks in the oven because the heat, according to the function found in the stomach, cannot heat anything enough. Therefore, the food does not boil or cook in the stomach, but the nature of digestion in the stomach is such that the essence of something transforms into something new, and this is called metabolism. The substance obtained from digestion in the stomach is called chyle.

Digestion in the intestine: The intestines have two functions: Absorption of chyle and absorption of bile. In the absorption of chyle, Abu Sahl Masihi, writes that the food extract that travels from the stomach to the liver is absorbed into the liver by the mesenteric plexus. In the absorption of bile, the bile is absorbed in the first part of the small intestine (duodenum), which has three important functions: helps in digestion, stimulates the expulsive faculty and aids in the absorption of food.

Three things are required for digestion in the intestine: digestion in the stomach, heat, fluids and rotatory movement.

Just as gastric juice is secreted from the inner layers of the stomach, intestinal juice is also secreted from the innermost layers of the intestine.

In addition to the absorption process, there is also a digestive faculty in the intestines, which induces changes in the digested food so that it can be absorbed into the mesenteric vessels, i.e., enter the bloodstream. When this digested food reaches the liver, it undergoes further digestion till it takes the form of humours. Bile, secreted in the intestines, stimulates the digestive faculty and helps move nutrients and excrete wastes. In the upper part of the small intestine, the digestive faculty, digestion, and the expulsive faculty are faster than in the large intestine as these faculties slowdown in the large intestine.

Digestion in mesenteries: The gastric glands fill the empty spaces between the mesenteric vessels and help in the digestion and metabolism of food in the intestine. That is, after digestion in the stomach and intestine, the nutrients, when passing through vessels and absorptive glands, undergo further digestion, which is called supplement of gastric digestion.

2. **Hepatic digestion (**Hadm Kabidi[93]**)**
The liver contains vessels that are spread throughout its muscles, with some of them serving as the origin points for the porta hepatis and vena cava. These vessels divide into smaller branches that spread to the liver cells and communicate with each other. This allows the liver to absorb substances from the stomach and intestines and transform them

---

[93] بضم كبدى

into the four humours, which are then sent to the entire body through the bloodstream via the vena cava.

How nutrients transform in the liver and what they produce is still unclear, however, the main functions of the liver are:
(1) Production of humours   (2) Production of bile
(3) Production of urinary substance   (4) Treatment of toxic substance

Production of the four humours: Ibn Sina writes that the liver is the organ that produces and completes the four humours, and the digestive faculty found in the liver performs a very wide and useful process that benefits the whole body.

Production of bile: Part of the bile produced in the liver enters the blood, and a part of it goes to the gallbladder and intestine.

Production of urinary substance: Urinary fluid is formed by the action of the liver's digestive faculty, which is then filtered by the kidney and passed to the bladder.

Treatment of toxic substance: The way the digestive faculty of the liver changes some component's colour and some's nature, it similarly treats the waste substances.

3. **Vascular digestion (Hadm Uruqi[94]):** The digestion that takes place in the vessels and helping in assimilation of food to make it part of the organs.

4. **Organic digestion (Hadm Udwi[95]):** the digestion that occurs inside the structure of the organs is included in organic digestion.

Expulsive faculty (Quwwat Dafi'a)

The human body has an expulsive faculty that eliminates waste materials that cannot be used as nutrients.

Urine, which contains a significant amount of water and other waste materials, is one of the ways in which the body excretes waste. This process helps with the diffusion of nutrients into small vessels, digestion and metabolism, and the dissolving of waste materials from different structures in the body. In addition to urine, the body also excretes water and waste materials through sweat from the skin.

The body produces substances that are later expelled after nourishing its organs. Examples include milk produced by the breasts and semen produced by the testicles. These substances are not waste materials but serve specific purposes before they are expelled from the body. The liver also produces components that enter the bloodstream, such as

---

[94] بضم عروقی
[95] بضم عضوی

humours that nourish other organs and secretions of endocrine glands, which are beneficial to the body.

There are two types of waste material in the body (Fudlat). Suitable waste material aids in the growth of the organ and can be assimilated into the body. On the other hand, unsuitable waste material cannot be assimilated into the body. If it accumulates in any structure and is not excreted, it can cause various diseases.

If the body excretes suitable waste material in higher quantities, it can lead to weakness in the body. This is why they are called suitable waste materials.

Waste material routes (Masalik Fudlat)

The human body has specific routes for excreting waste material. Urine is expelled towards the bladder and exits through the urethra, while faeces are excreted towards the rectum and exit through the anus. When no such routes exist, the body repels the waste material from the donor organ towards the inferior organ or from the hard to the soft organs. The body tries to maintain the natural direction of excreta as much as possible. However, sometimes, due to certain conditions and barriers, the body's natural functions are diverted, causing a change in the excretion routes. For instance, in cases where the contents of the stomach and intestines are expelled through emesis, putrid food is excreted from the stomach instead of entering the intestine.

Sometimes, the flow of waste material increases on one side and decreases on the other side. During increased defecation, the urination may stop because fluids start excreting through faeces, as in the case of food poisoning. Similarly, when perspiration increases, urination decreases, as happens in summer, and when perspiration decreases, urination increases, as in winter.

84 | THE FOUNDATIONS OF UNANI MEDICINE

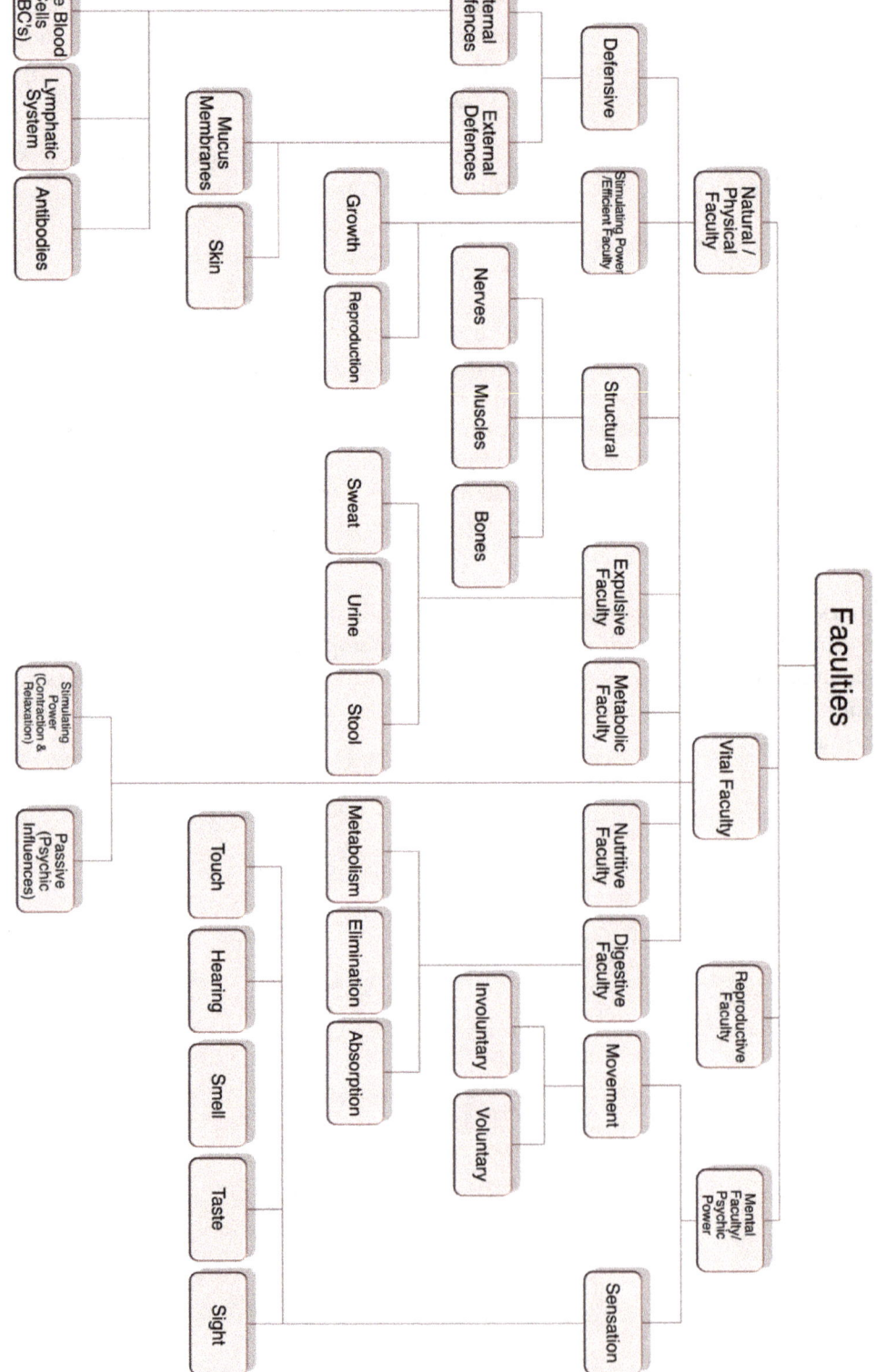

FACULTIES IN UNANI MEDICINE

Functions (Af'al)

An inextricable link exists between faculties (Quwwa) and function (Af'al[96]). That is, if faculties are the cause, then functions are their effects. This is why the existence of a faculty is evident from the observation of its functions. Therefore, the definition of function is the same as that of faculty and has the same number of types.

From a medical point of view, the importance of faculties is due to their functions because the faculties cannot be observed directly, whereas functions can be observed. When a physician discusses a person's health and illness, they look at their functions in both cases.

If the functions are balanced, the person is healthy, but if they are not, the person suffers from some illness. The types of functions in terms of faculties are Mental or psychic (Nafsaniyya), Vital (Haywaniyya) and Physical/Natural (Tabi'iyya).

Mental or psychic functions (Af'al Nafsaniyya[97])

Functions controlled by the psychic faculty. Their types are, Intellect function (Af'al Mudabbira[98]), Sensory function (Af'al Hissiya[99]) and Motor functions (Af'al Muharrika[100]).

There are two types of sensory functions: internal sensory (intellect functions) and external sensory functions.

Internal Sensory Functions:

There are five internal sensory functions:

   a. Composite sense function (af'al Hiss Mushtarak)
   b. Imagination function (af'al mutakkhayyul)
   c. Imagination with interpretation function (Af'al Wahima)
   d. Memory function (Af'al hafiza)
   e. Modification function (Af'al Mutasarrifa)

External Sensory Functions:

There are five external sensory functions:

   1. Act of sight/vision
   2. Act of smell
   3. Act of taste
   4. Act of hearing

---

[96] افعال
[97] افعال نفسانیہ
[98] افعال مدبره
[99] افعال حسیہ
[100] افعال محرکہ

5. Act of touch

Vital functions (Af'al Haywaniyya[101])

Functions which are indispensable for survival and are performed by the vital faculties through the vital organs.

Physical/Natural functions (Af'al Tabi'iyya[102])

Functions which are essential to energize all powers and develop the organs and are of three types; nourishment (Ightidha[103]), growth (Numu[104]) and reproduction (Tawlid[105]). A fourth, act of desire (Af'al Shahwat[106]) has also been included in the vital functions.

Some physicians have described assimilation based on four functions.

    a. Act of absorption (Af'al Jazb[107])
    b. Act of retention (Af'al Imsak[108])
    c. Act of digestion (Af'al Hadm[109])
    d. Act of expulsion (Af'al Dafa[110])

Types of functions according to composition

There are two types of functions in terms of composition:

    a. Single function (Af'al Mufrad[111])
    b. Compound function (Af'al Murakkab[112])

Single functions

These functions are accomplished by a single faculty. An example of a single function in psychic functions is the sensation that is achieved by different sensory organs individually; for example, the visual function is performed by the power of vision and the act of smell by the power of smell.

An example of a single function in vital functions is the contraction or expansion of the heart and arteries. In the natural function, the single functions, such as the act of

---

101 افعال حیوانیہ
102 افعال طبیعیہ
103 اغتذا
104 نمو
105 تولید
106 فعل شہوت
107 فعل جذب
108 فعل امساک
109 فعل ہضم
110 فعل دفع
111 افعال مفردہ
112 افعال مرکبہ

absorption, are performed by the absorptive faculty, and the expulsive faculty performs the act of expulsion.

Compound Functions

Compound functions are those that involve two or more faculties working together. For instance, in psychic functions, thinking and reflecting are examples of compound functions which involve faculties such as awareness and apprehension.

In vital functions, respiration is an example of a compound function performed by the power of contraction and expansion of the thorax muscles.

In natural functions, swallowing is an example of a compound function involving two functions: sensory and absorptive. For instance, during hunger, the sensory faculty of the stomach stimulates the sensory nerve, compelling a person to eat food, and then the absorptive faculty aids in swallowing. Ibn Sina has linked this stimulation with the function of absorptive vessels.

The act of swallowing is compound and is completed by two faculties because bitter drugs are difficult to swallow due to the absorptive faculty's inability to absorb it because of its bitterness, whereas the expulsive faculty spews it out.

Body movements such as walking are clear examples of compound functions.

88 | THE FOUNDATIONS OF UNANI MEDICINE

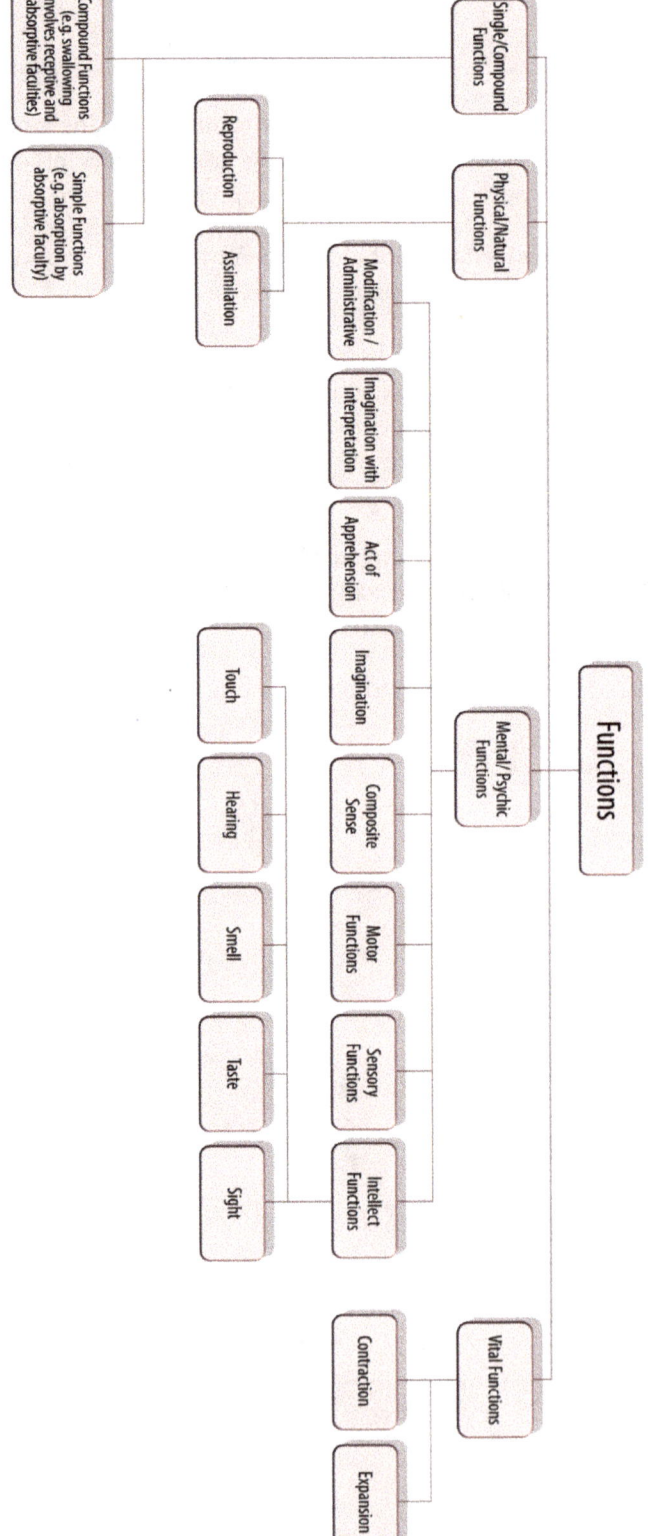

FUNCTIONS IN UNANI MEDICINE

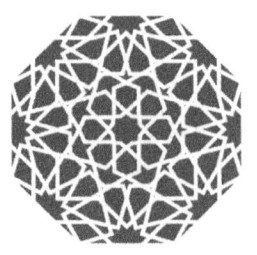

SECTION 2

DISEASES, CAUSES AND SIGNS

'The physician is only nature's assistant'.

- Galen

States Of The Human Body

States, properties and complications

In medicine, the three states of the human body are:

1. Health (Sihhat)
2. Disease (Marad/Marz[113])
3. Intermediate state (Halat Thalitha[114])

Intermediate state is considered to be in between health and disease (such as congenital blindness).

However, according to Ibn Sina, two states are present in the human body throughout life:

1. Health
2. Disease

Galen says there is a difference in comparison between health and diseases, and so an intermediate form of Intermediate state exists.

Health (Sihhat)

Galen and Ibn Sina had different views on the human body's appearance. According to Galen, the body's appearance is normal when all its functions are executed correctly, depending on the temperament and composition of the body. However, Ibn Sina's definition doesn't include the word 'all,' indicating that he doesn't believe in an intermediate state. In other words, the body is either healthy or diseased, and there is no partial state.

Disease (Marad[115])

Pain, ache, sickness, and disease are common conditions in which the body's normal functioning is disrupted.

According to Ibn Sina, disease is an abnormal appearance of the human body in which a crisis occurs in the functions of the body, either directly or indirectly. Therefore, disease is an abnormal temperament or composition. The term 'individually' differentiates

---

[113] مرض
[114] حالت ثالث
[115] Or Marz

between disease and symptoms because symptoms do not cause any condition. The term 'indirectly' is used to exclude the cause from the disease because the cause does not indirectly affect the function, but the disease directly affects the functions of the body.

Disease is of three types:

1. Su-e-Mizaj[116] (Impaired temperament[117])

Impaired temperament is a condition where the heat, cold, moisture or dryness in the body or a specific organ exceeds the normal moderate level. This abnormality can result in the organ being unable to perform its functions to its full potential, thus causing disruption in the body. It is essentially a disease that affects the organ's ability to function correctly.

2. Amrad Su-e-Tarkib[118] (Structural Diseases)

The disruption in the structure of the diseased organ.

3. Tafarruq Ittisal[119] (Loss of continuity[120])

Loss of continuity refers to any interruption or disruption in the connection among the components of a simple or complex organ. This condition may occur due to an external cause, like an abrasion or a tear on an organ, or an internal cause, like inflammation or swelling of an organ.

Psychological and emotional illness

Psychological and emotional illnesses are conditions related to the mind, such as dementia, anger, admiration, arrogance, oppression, jealousy, and cunningness.

Diseased condition

This is the state in which the human body in which some or all functions related to it are not working. That is, all organs or some cannot perform their functions. It is an abnormal condition of the body.

---

[116] Change in four physical properties occurs, i.e., hotness, coldness, dryness and wetness/moistness.
[117] dyscrasia/immoderate temperament.
[118] امراض سوء التركيب
[119] تفرّق اتصال
[120] Loss of continuity of any organ or part of the body.

Intermediate state

The intermediate state, i.e., the state between health and disease, is when neither complete health nor complete disease is present, such as during recovery after disease, congenital blindness, or old age. However, some physicians do not believe in an intermediate state.

The intermediate state is the state in which some of the functions of the human body are healthy, and some are diseased. This condition is often present after recovery from disease in weak and debilitated people. According to Galen, the condition of the human body is that some organs are healthy and some are diseased; that is, the body is not completely healthy nor completely in a state of disease. This condition is termed an intermediate state or condition of incomplete health or disease. Galen has termed the following states as Intermediate states.

1. People who do not have full health or disease.
2. People in which health and disease occupy the same organ, which has two forms:
    a. The state of health and disease are present in separate organs, for example, blind, disabled persons, etc.
    b. In which the healthy and diseased states are present in the same organ, even if they are present in different categories. For example, a person who is healthy in terms of temperament but is ill in terms of composition is included in the Intermediate state, like an increase in head size in proportion to the body's, or six digits in hands or feet, etc.

1. Condition of children and old people:

The faculties of children are weak in comparison to those of adults. Similarly, the faculty of old people is reduced due to age. Therefore, according to Galen, children and old people cannot be considered completely healthy or completely sick.

2. Blind and disabled person:

Since the disease is in the eyes, legs or hands and the rest of the body is healthy, in this state, the whole body cannot be called healthy, nor can it be termed as diseased.

3. Asthmatic and epileptic patients:

These people are healthy between the episodes, although they have asthma and epilepsy, and occasionally, they experience the symptoms. Therefore, they cannot be called completely healthy or ill.

4. People recovering from a disease:

After recovering from a disease, a person does not immediately achieve full health. It takes some time for the body to fully heal. During this intermediate state between recovery and full health, the body is neither completely healthy nor sick. Galen referred to this condition as an intermediate state.

However according to Ibn Sina and modern physicians believe two states of the body:

1. Health
2. Disease

Diseases[121]

The causes and symptoms are also included with the diseases; therefore, to understand a disease, it is necessary to first understand its causes and symptoms.

Cause

The cause is a pre-existing condition whose presence in the body gives rise to a new health or disease condition or it provides stability to previous states.

Disease

It is that abnormal condition of the body which indirectly or individually describes the function of the body. So, the disease is either a Su-e-Mizaj (impaired temperament) or an abnormal composition.

Symptom

Symptoms are abnormal conditions that coexist with a disease. Although a symptom indicates an abnormality, it may be harmful in itself, such as the pain of colic, or harmless, such as the flushing of cheeks in pneumonia.

An example of a cause is putrefaction. The disease that follows is often characterised by fever. Accompanying symptoms of this fever may include thirst and headache.

The symptom is called a sign when the physician identifies the presentation and diagnoses the disease through it.

Sometimes, a symptom can also become a cause; for example, severe colicky pain can become the cause of syncope disease. Sometimes, the symptom becomes the disease; for example, a headache due to a fever becomes constant even after it subsides and turns into a disease.

Sometimes, a simple condition itself, either previously or later on, becomes a disease, symptom or cause. For example, low fever itself is a disease that can cause pulmonary

---

[121] In Western medicine, a disease is generally defined as a particular pathological process that manifests with a specific set of symptoms. However, Ibn Sina considers a disease to be an abnormal condition that disturbs normal bodily functions. The severity of the illness is determined by the degree to which these natural processes are impeded.

ulcers, weakness and impairment, and so, in this way, the cause keeps transforming in the three forms of the disease.

Types of diseases

There are two types of diseases

1. Simple diseases (Amrad[122] Mufrad)
2. Compound diseases (Amrad Murakab)

---

[122] امراض - also transliterated as Amraz

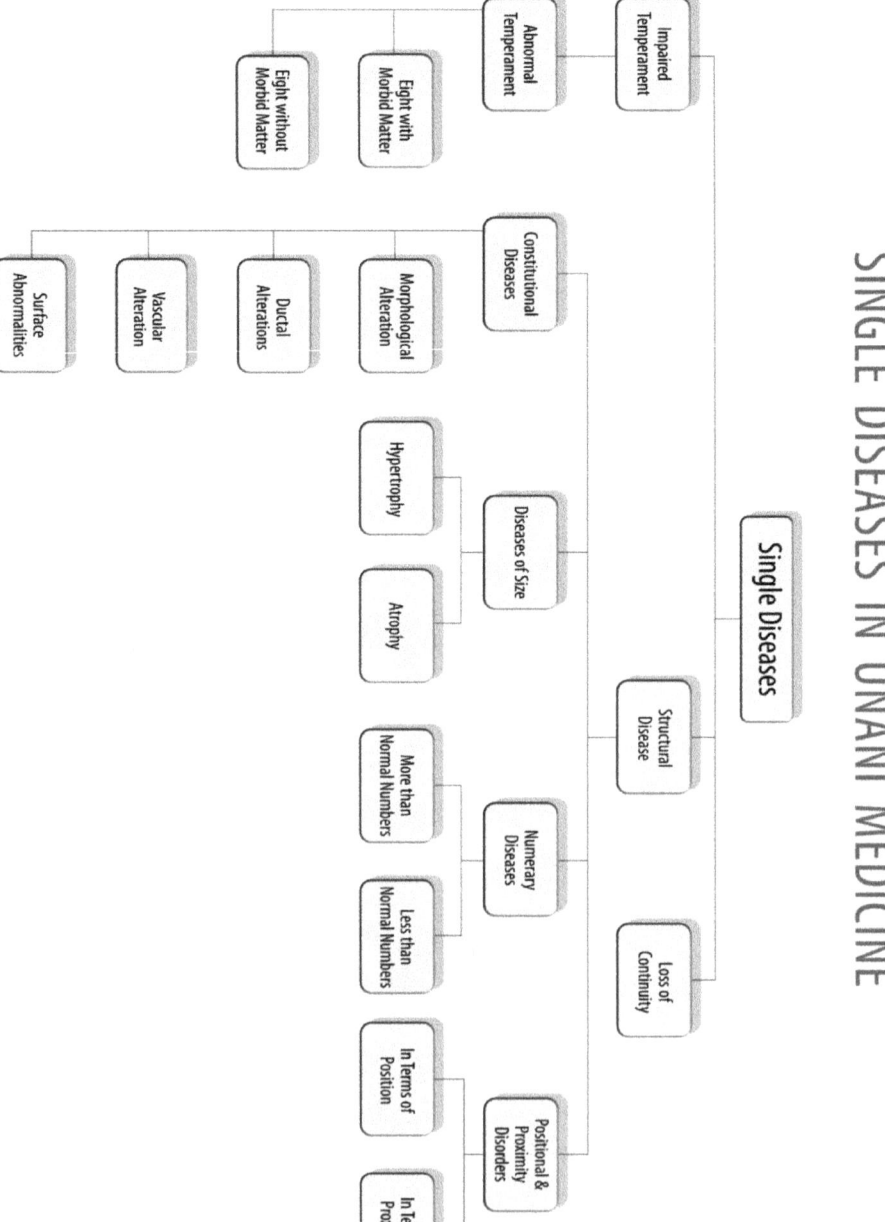

Simple diseases are single diseases that are not a combination of multiple diseases, such as fever. Simple diseases refer to those states in which either Su-e-Mizaj (impaired temperament), Amrad Su-e-Tarkib (Structural Diseases), or Tafarruq Ittisal (Loss of continuity) is present. This means that if the temperament is impaired, then only one type of temperament impairment will be found. Similarly, if a structural disease is present, only one of its types will be found. If there is a loss of continuity, only a simple type of discontinuity will be found.

Compound diseases (Amrad[123] Murakab)

Compound illnesses arise from the combination of diseases and are given a single name. For example, diseases with specific names and treatments, such as inflammation, result from the combination of Su-e-Mizaj (impaired temperament), Tafarruq Ittisal (loss of continuity), and Amrad Su-e-Tarkib (structural diseases). These combined conditions are referred to by a single name, such as inflammation. In contrast, if a few diseases coexist in the body or a particular organ without a specific name or treatment, it is not called Marad Murakkab (compound disease) but simply a combination of diseases (Amrad Mujtam'a[124]), for example, fever, cough, and oedema.

When a person experiences a cough along with other symptoms like diarrhoea, it is not considered a compound disease. Compound diseases refer to the combination of two or more types of Su-e-Mizaj (impaired temperament), Amrad Su-e-Tarkib (structural diseases), Tafarruq Ittisal (loss of continuity) or their types, which, when combined, become a single disease. The diagnosis and treatment principles for this disease would be unified. For instance, inflammation includes all three types: Su-e-Mizaj (impaired temperament), Amrad Su-e-Tarkib (structural diseases), and Tafarruq Ittisal (loss of continuity).

Types of Simple Diseases

As mentioned, there are three types of simple diseases:

1. Su-e-Mizaj (Impaired temperament)
2. Amrad Su-e-Tarkib (Structural Diseases)
3. Tafarruq Ittisal (Loss of continuity)

---

[123] Marad – singular i.e., disease
[124] مراض مجتمعه

Impaired temperament (Su-e-Mizaj)

This abnormal condition occurs in the body or any specific organ due to the dominance of heat, cold, moisture or dryness, which makes the body or organ unable to perform its function according to its ability.

It refers to diseases that occur directly in simple organs and compound organs via simple organs. It has sixteen types: eight single and compound Sada (plain, i.e., without morbid matter) and eight single and compound Maddi (with morbid matter).

We will now discuss the sixteen types of Su-e-Mizaj.

1. **Su-e-Mizaj Sada** [125] **(simple morbid temperament)** this is an abnormal temperament that is not associated with a madda[126] (substance/matter) and it has eight types:
    a. **Su-e-Mizaj Sada Mufrad** [127] **(single, simple morbid temperament)**
    That abnormal temperament in which one of the following four states dominates:

    i. Su-e-Mizaj Harr (morbid hot temperament)
    ii. Su-e-Mizaj barid (morbid cold temperament)
    iii. Su-e-Mizaj Ratb (morbid moist temperament)
    iv. Su-e-Mizaj Yabis (morbid dry temperament)

    b. **Su-e-Mizaj Sada Murakkab** [128] **(compound, simple morbid temperament)**
    That simple abnormal temperament in which compound of two states are predominant:

    i. Su-e-Mizaj Harr Ratb (morbid hot and moist temperament)
    ii. Su-e-Mizaj Harr Yabis (morbid hot and dry temperament)
    iii. Su-e-Mizaj Barid Ratb (morbid cold and moist temperament)
    iv. Su-e-Mizaj Barid Yabis (morbid cold and dry temperament)

2. **Su-e-Mizaj Maddi**[129] **(morbid temperament associated with substance)**
    Morbid temperament is a change in four physical properties, i.e., hotness, coldness, dryness and wetness/moistness, that takes place with the associated madda (substance/matter), and this also has eight types.
    a. **Su-e-Mizaj Mufrad Maddi** [130] **(morbid simple temperament with substance):**

---

[125] سوء مزاج ساده
[126] مادّی / مادّه (maddi) – Generally, the term refers to any substance or matter, but in this context, we are talking about the humours that have become corrupted or altered, which can lead to illness. Removing these corrupted substances is necessary to prevent such illnesses.
[127] سوء مزاج ساده مفرد
[128] سوء مزاج ساده مرکب
[129] سوء مزاج مادّی
[130] سوء مزاج مفرد مادّی

That abnormal temperament with a substance in which one condition dominates and has four types:
    i. Su-e-Mizaj Harr Maddi (morbid hot temperament with substance)
    ii. Su-e-Mizaj Barid Maddi (morbid cold temperament with substance)
    iii. Su-e-Mizaj Ratb Maddi (morbid moist temperament with substance)
    iv. Su-e-Mizaj Yabis Maddi (morbid dry temperament with substance)

b. Su-e-Mizaj Murakkab Maddi[131] (morbid compound temperament with substance):

The abnormal temperament with a substance in which two states are predominant. It has four types:
    i. Su-e-Mizaj Harr Ratb Maddi (morbid hot and moist temperament associated with predominance of hot and wet substances)
    ii. Su-e-Mizaj Harr Yabis Maddi (morbid hot and dry temperament associated with predominance of hot and dry substances)
    iii. Su-e-Mizaj Barid Ratb Maddi (morbid cold and moist temperament associated with predominance of cold and moist substances)
    iv. Su-e-Mizaj Barid Yabis Maddi (morbid cold and dry temperament associated with predominance of cold and dry substances)

---

[131] سوء مزاج مرکب مادی

For example, to illustrate Su-e-Mizaj Barid Ratb Maddi (morbid cold and moist temperament associated with predominance of cold and moist substances) with an example:

Scenario: Let's imagine an individual living in a predominantly cold and damp environment, such as a coastal region during winter. They have a diet rich in cold and moist foods like melons, dairy products, and certain seafood. Additionally, their daily activities are minimal, resulting in low physical exertion and reduced metabolic heat.

Development of Su-e-Mizaj Barid Ratb Maddi:

Accumulation: Due to their diet and environmental conditions combined with a sedentary lifestyle, there's an excessive accumulation of cold and moist qualities in the body, leading to a material imbalance.

Manifestation: They might frequently feel cold and might have cold extremities (hands and feet).

Their digestion could become slow and sluggish, with potential bloating or a feeling of heaviness in the stomach.

There might be increased mucus production, leading to symptoms like a runny nose or productive cough.

They could feel lethargic, with a decreased desire for physical activity.

Fluid retention might be evident, leading to symptoms like oedema or puffiness.

Further Complications: If this condition remains unaddressed, it can make the individual more susceptible to diseases related to cold and wet imbalances, such as respiratory tract infections, sinusitis, or even certain types of arthritis characterized by dampness in the joints.

Structural Diseases (Amrad Su-e-Tarkib)

Those simple diseases first appear in compound organs, such as dislocation. Any abnormality in the composition and structure of the organ is termed abnormal structure (Su-e-Tarkib).

This has four types

1. Constitutional diseases/malformations/organic diseases (Amrad-i-Khilqat[132])
2. Diseases of size (Amrad-i-Miqdar[133])
3. Numerary diseases (Amrad-i-Adad[134])
4. Proximity disorders / diseases of position (Amrad-i-Wad'[135])

1. Constitutional diseases:

Diseases in which the original shape of an organ is changed. It has four types

a. morphological alterations (Amrad-i-Shakl[136])
b. diseases of tracts (Amrad-i-Majari[137])
c. vascular diseases / cavitational disorders (Amrad-i-Aw'iyya[138])
d. surface abnormalities (Amrad-i-Safa'ih[139])

Morphological alterations refer to diseases that cause changes in the shape or structure of an organ, which can disrupt its function. For example, rickets can cause the bending of a straight organ, while other diseases can cause the flattening of a round organ.

Diseases of tracts result from abnormalities in the ducts and canals of the body. There are three forms: dilation, constriction, and occlusion. Dilation occurs in conditions like varicose veins or piles, while constriction occurs in conditions like asthma. Occlusion happens when there is a blockage in a duct or canal, such as with thromboembolism or intestinal obstruction.

Vascular diseases or cavitational disorders affect hollow organs and can either narrow or dilate their cavities. There are three forms: narrowing of the cavity, expansion of the cavity, and occlusion of the cavity. Spasms of the stomach and intestine can cause narrowing, while dilatation of the heart is an example of expansion. Occlusion of the bladder due to urine retention is an example of cavity occlusion.

---

[132] امراض خلقت
[133] امراض مقدار
[134] امراض عدد
[135] امراض وضع
[136] امراض شکل
[137] امراض مجاری
[138] امراض اوعیہ
[139] امراض صفائح

Surface abnormalities come in two forms: roughness of a smooth surface and smoothness of a rough surface. Irritation of the throat is an example of the roughness of a smooth surface, while lienteric diarrhoea is an example of the smoothness of a rough surface.

2. Diseases of size

One of the types of disease of constitution concerning pathological changes in the size/weight of body viscera/organs. It has two types.

1. Hypertrophy
2. Atrophy

Hypertrophy: means that the volume of the organ increases. It has two forms:

a. Generalized hypertrophy, such as obesity.
b. Localised hypertrophy, for example, cardiomegaly, splenomegaly.

Atrophy: It also has two forms.

1. Generalized atrophy, such as emaciation.
2. Localized atrophy, for example, atrophy of liver.

3. Numerary diseases

Diseases affecting the number of organs of the body are one of the types of diseases of the constitution that are associated with congenital or acquired numerical abnormality of viscera or body organs. It has two forms.

1. More than normal numbers
2. Less than normal numbers

More than normal numbers: It also has two types:

a. Normal/natural increase: It refers to an increase in the number of organs at birth. For example, polydactyly or increased hair growth.
b. Abnormal/unnatural increases: It means an increase in the number of organs after birth. For example, fistula.

Less than normal numbers: It has two types:

a. Normal/natural decrease: For example, both kidneys joined as one.
b. Abnormal/unnatural decrease: For example, amputation of a hand or leg after an accident.

DISEASES, CAUSES AND SIGNS

4. Proximity disorders/diseases of position

    a. In terms of position
    b. In terms of proximity

There are four types of diseases in terms of position.

    i. Complete displacement of an organ from its place. For example, dislocation.
    ii. Incomplete displacement of an organ from its place. For example, hernia.
    iii. Abnormal movement of an organ in its place. For example, tremors.
    iv. Inability of an organ to move from its place. For example, ankylosis.

Proximity refers to the disruption in structures that are positioned between organs. For instance, when an organ stops moving towards another organ, like in the case of fingers affected by indolent ulcers. The other condition is when an organ cannot move away from another organ, which happens in ptosis.

Loss of continuity (Tafarruq Ittisal)

This refers to diseases that affect individual organs directly and separately, whether they are simple or compound. Such diseases can occur in various organs, and physicians have designated different names for them according to their type, length, breadth and depth.

For instance, a scratch on the skin or internal organs is known as surface discontinuity or abrasion. A wound can also be a kind of discontinuity on the flesh, but if pus accumulates, it becomes an ulcer (Qarha). A discontinuity in a bone is called a fracture (Kasr).

When the layers of arteries become loose, and blood collects in them, it results in an aneurysm (Umm al-Dam [140]). Similarly, if an artery or vein ruptures, it is called a haemorrhage, which can happen in cases of hemiplegia. Finally, a hernia refers to discontinuity in a membrane.

---

[140] ام الدم

104 | THE FOUNDATIONS OF UNANI MEDICINE

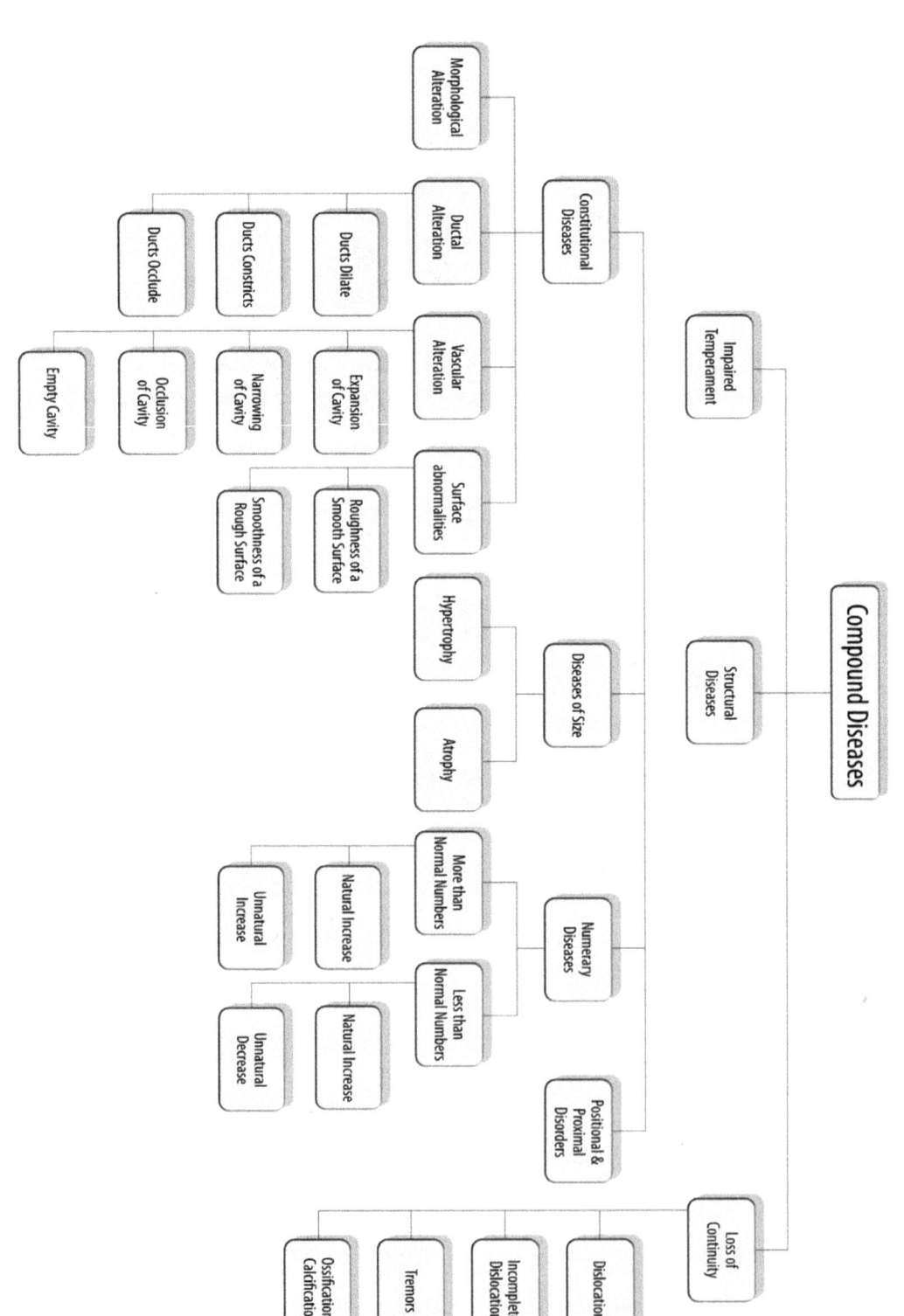

COMPOUND DISEASES IN UNANI MEDICINE

Compound Diseases (Amrad Murakkab)

Compound diseases refer to the combination of simple diseases that present themselves collectively. For instance, swelling is considered a compound disease since it involves three types of simple diseases, namely Su-e-Mizaj (impaired temperament), Amrad Su-e-Tarkib (structural diseases), and Tafarruq Ittisal (loss of continuity) at the same time.

Inflammation or swelling (Waram) is only produced when there is Su-e-Mizaj Maddi (morbid temperament with substance). Structural diseases (Amrad Su-e-Tarkib) occur because the form of the swelling remains unclear unless there are changes in morphology, volume, and position. Loss of continuity (Tafarruq Ittisal) is also present because space is necessary for the accumulation of the swelling substance, which requires discontinuity in the structure of an organ where the excess substance can be collected. Therefore, swelling is a compound disease as it contains these three types of diseases.

In Unani Medicine, swelling encompasses any abnormal swelling that results from inflammation or organ abnormalities such as tumours, gases, or oedema.

Swellings (Awram)

Swelling (Awram[141]) is the growth of any part of an organ or the entire organ due to an abnormal substance (madda). During normal growth, organs also grow, but the substance of growth is normal, and it grows in all three dimensions - length, width, and height - in normal measures. In contrast, swellings occur due to Su-e-Mizaj Maddi (morbid temperament with substance), where abnormal substances accumulate in the spaces and gaps of an organ, causing an increase in the organ's size, deformity in shape, and discontinuity in the organ's structure. As a result, all three types of Simple Diseases (Amrad Mufrada) are found in swellings, i.e. Su-e-Mizaj (impaired temperament), Amrad Su-e-Tarkib (Structural Diseases), and Tafarruq Ittisal (Loss of continuity), since swelling cannot occur without morbid temperament with substance. Structural disease causes abnormality in morphology and size, and the accumulation of inflamed substances causes discontinuity.

Before Ibn Sina, physicians believed that swelling could only occur in soft organs and not in hard organs such as bones, but Ibn Sina denied this theory and was the first to accept that swelling can occur in bones. Although swelling is usually found in soft organs, it can also occur in hard organs like bones since bones can absorb abnormal substances and become swollen, just as they absorb nutrients and grow.

Swelling is not always caused by external factors; it can also occur due to internal body causes. For example, when one organ expels its substance towards another organ, and the second organ accepts this substance, it becomes swollen. Often, abnormal substances

---

[141] Awaran (اورام) plural - singular Waram (ورم)

from outer organs move towards inner organs and cause swelling. This transference of substances is analogous to the condition of coryza[142].

Ibn Sina also stated that sometimes toxic substances are present in the body but are kept at bay by beneficial substances. If, due to some reason, these beneficial substances are lost, for example, due to bodily evacuations, these toxic substances become active, and the medicatrix naturae works to expel them from the body. The route of the expulsion of the substance is towards the skin, and due to this, skin eruptions are more common in some diseases. Therefore, skin diseases are often present in some diseases.

Types of swellings

Swellings have been divided into a number of different forms.

The first division is done based on the type of madda (substance) that causes swelling. Swelling is divided into six types based on the madda (substance).

1. Waram Safrawi (Bilious Khilt (humour) swelling): Related to bile and the gallbladder.

2. Waram Balghami (Phlegm Khilt (humour) swelling): Related to phlegm.

3. Waram Damawi (Blood Khilt (humour) swelling): Related to blood.

4. Waram Sawdawi (black bile Khilt (humour) swelling): Related to black bile.

5. Waram Ma'i (Watery swelling): Related to the accumulation of water.

6. Waram Reeh[143] (Air (gaseous matter) related swelling: Emphysema): Airy swelling that is caused by the collection of air in an organ. In these types of swelling, the air accumulates in the spaces and gaps between the cell membranes.

Swelling and Kayfiyat (qualities): Another way of looking at swellings (Waram) is through its properties/qualities (Kayfiyat), and these are either Waram Harr (hot swelling/acute swelling) or Waram Barid (cold swelling /chronic swelling).

Waram Harr (hot swelling/acute swelling)

These are swellings produced not only by blood Khilt (humour) and yellow bile humour but also by any substance whose essence is hot or substances in which heat is present due to infection. For example, because of the corruption of madda (substance) waram harr (acute swelling) is created from waram damawai (blood humour swelling) and is called phlegmon [144] and from pure bilious humour swelling Muhamra [145] (Erysipelas) is

---

[142] inflammation of the mucous membrane of the nose, with discharge of mucus.
[143] Reeh = air, which is a matter in a gaseous state.
[144] From Greek phlegmone, an inflammation of soft tissue that spreads under the skin or inside the body.
[145] Literal meaning – redness. Although this disease can occur in any part of the body, it often occurs on the face, in which case it is called facial erysipelas.

produced. Their compound form is called damawai waram muhamra (blood humour erysipelas swelling) and is an abscess (Khuraj[146]) if it becomes purulent[147].

There are four stages of Waram Harr (hot swelling/acute swelling):

1. Initial stage: In this stage, the Khilt (humour) or substance accumulates at the site of swelling, and the swelling appears.
2. Progressive stage: The volume of the swelling increases in this stage because the substance is being transferred.
3. Late-stage: This stage is also called the static phase because in this stage, the swelling reaches its end-stage and stops.
4. Degenerative stage: This is the phase in which the swelling degenerates and reduces.

Result of Waram Harr (hot swelling/acute swelling):

Acute swellings may result in one of the three states.

1. The substance concocts and resolves.
2. The substance becomes purulent.
3. It converts to a hard swelling.

Waram Barid (cold swelling/ chronic swelling)

These includes four types of swelling:

1. Awram[148] Sawdawiyya (Melancholic/Black bile swellings)
2. Awram Balghamiya (Phlegmatic swellings)
3. Awram Maiya (Watery swellings)
4. Awram Reeh (Gaseous swellings – Emphysema)

Awram Sawdawiyya (Black bile swellings)

Awram Sawdawiyya (Black bile swellings) are produced from Sawdawi madda (Melancholic/Black bile substances) and are hard, with hardness being one of their specific signs. These swellings are usually Sawdawi (Black bile), but occasionally, they arise from other non-black bile substances and then become Sawdawi waram (Black bile swelling). For example, if Awram Damawi (blood humour swellings) hardens and converts to Sawda (Black bile), it is referred to as Waram Sawdawiyya Damawi (Black bile-blood humour swelling). Similarly, if Awram Balghami (phlegmatic swellings) hardens, this substance changes into Sawdawi (Black bile), and it is known as Waram

---

[146] خُراج
[147] An inflammatory swelling filled with pus and accompanied by redness and pain.
[148] Awram (اورام) plural of Waram (ورم)

Sawdawiyya Balghami (Black bile-Phlegmatic swelling). There are three types of Awram Sawdawiyya (Black bile swellings):

    a. Waram Sulb (hard Black bile swelling - Scleroma)
This swelling is of three types: one in which the substance is only Black bile, two in which the substance is phlegmatic and the third in which the substance is the complex of Black bile and phlegm.
    b. Waram Saratan (Carcinoma swelling)
This is a very dangerous form of swelling or tumour which is often fatal.
    c. Gudad (Glands) and Sal'at (tumours)[149]

a. Waram Sulb (Hard Black bile swelling - Scleroma/scirrhous)

Scleromas, or hard black bile swellings, are fibrous growths that develop due to an imbalance of black bile. These growths are firmly attached to the surrounding tissues, making them immobile and difficult to move without displacing the adjacent structures. Scleromas are typically painless and insensitive to pressure, and they exhibit clear boundaries that distinguish them as distinct pathological entities.

b. Waram Saratan[150] (Carcinoma swelling)

Swelling in the body that is connected to a structure, but it has a tendency to move and grow quickly. It has roots that penetrate into nearby structures. The swelling can cause pain, and sometimes it can damage the surrounding structures, resulting in a loss of sensation in that area.

c. Gudad Sal'at (Glandular tumours)

They are separated from the surrounding structures and can be easily felt to move away from the surrounding structures on palpation, such as simple glandular swelling.

Awram Balghamiya (Phlegmatic swellings)

Phlegmatic swellings are produced from phlegmatic substances and are of two types:

    a. Waram Rikhw (soft swelling/Oedema)
    b. Sal'at Rikhw (Soft/transudative tumour)

The phlegmatic substance in Oedema (Waram Rikhw) accumulates in the spaces and gaps of an organ, due to which it is difficult to establish its boundaries, but in contrast,

---

[149] سلعات Movable swellings of varying sizes, ranging from gram seed to watermelon.
[150] In Unani, carcinoma is understood as a malignant black bilious tumour which can occur anywhere in the body; it spreads very rapidly, and the roots of the swelling are deep; it sometimes appears due to burnt yellow bile and phlegm accumulation.

transudative tumours (Sal'at Rikhw) are limited to their sheath and are separated from the adjacent structures.

Most swellings in cold weather are phlegmatic, and sometimes the signs of Waram Harr (hot swelling/acute swelling) may be similar to the Awram Balghamiya (Phlegmatic swellings).

Phlegmatic swellings may be different in terms of the concentration and dilution of the madda (substances); often, the swelling that results from the thick phlegmatic substance is mistaken for black bile swelling. Sometimes, the swellings that are produced from the thin phlegm can be thin and soft, like those that are produced from watery swelling or emphysema. So, in this aspect, the phlegmatic swelling can be soft and hard.

Awram Ma'iya (Watery swellings)

Watery swellings are those in which a water-like fluid accumulates in the cavity of an organ and causes swelling. For example, the matter found in ascites, hydrocephalus and fluid pleurisy is a watery, concentrated fluid that diffuses out from blood vessels; physicians call these swellings Awram Ma'iya (Watery swellings).

Awram Reeh (Gaseous swellings)

Awram Reeh is produced as a result of the accumulation of Reeh (flatus/gas) in any organ and are of two types:

    a. Tahabbuj[151] (soft gaseous swelling)
    b. Apara[152] (Swollen/Bloating)

a. Tahabbuj (soft gaseous swelling)

In Tahabbuj (soft gaseous swelling), the air is mixed with the essence of the organ in the gaps and spaces of organs. That site of oedema is soft to the touch and depresses when pressure is applied, which then returns to its original state after some time.

b. Apara (Swollen/Bloating)

Here, air accumulates in the cavity and causes compression and pressure. The site of distension is found to be hard on compression.

---

151 تَهَبُّج
152 اپھارہ

Buthur[153] (Eruptions)

Eruptions are small swellings and, therefore, are also compound diseases. Like swelling, eruptions also have six types based on the madda (substance).

1. **Buthur Damawi (Blood Khilt (humour) eruptions, pimples):**
   Contains blood humour madda (substance) such as in smallpox.
2. **Buthur Safrawi (Bilious eruptions):**
   Examples are small itchy eruptions on the body such as hives, urticarial. Also, small millet grain like eruptions that causes extreme itching. Causes of both of these are yellow bile.
3. **Buthur Sawdawi (Black bile eruptions):**
   Such as warts, i.e., black coloured moles.
4. **Buthur Balghami (Phlegmatic eruptions):**
   For example small white coloured eruptions on the face that have large heads and small roots.
5. **Buthur Ma'iy (Watery eruptions):**
   E.g., blisters
6. **Buthur Reeh (Gaseous eruptions):**
   For example, small blisters that contain gases.

Other conditions that are included with the subject of diseases:

Cosmetology

Cosmetology factors are generally not included in the above section on diseases but present hidden diseases and, therefore, are included below:

The diseases of cosmetology are related to four things:

   a. Hair
   b. Colour of body/skin
   c. Odour
   d. Physique

A. Hair-related diseases

There are various hair-related diseases, including hair loss due to illness, poor quality or thinning, excess hair growth, premature greying, or other changes in hair colour.

B. Body colour

There are four types of diseases based on body colour.

---

[153] بثور

a) Change in colour of the body due to Su-e-Mizaj (impaired temperament). This can be due to either due to Su-e-Mizaj Maddi (morbid temperament with substance), such as jaundice or due to Su-e-Mizaj Sada (simple morbid temperament), e.g., Su-e-Mizaj barid (morbid cold temperament) in which the body appears lime white in colour.
b) Body colour changes due to external factors such as during hot air, cold or different types of winds.
c) Abnormal skin spots include pityriasis, leucoderma/vitiligo, moles, blackheads, naevus, freckles, lentigo, and melasma.
d) Those marks that remain on the skin after the resolution of wounds or Tafarruq Ittisal (Loss of continuity), such as marks of smallpox and other wounds.

C. Smell

Different malodours are included in the diseases of smell, which come from different body parts, such as smell from mouth, nose, ear or bromidrosis.

D. Physique

Emaciation and obesity are included in these diseases.

Stages of Disease

Every disease follows a pattern of four stages or periods. A variable disease affects a healthy person and resolves in that person's life. It is not a disease that someone is born with. If a person is born with the disease in its late stage, its initial and progressive stages will remain unknown. Similarly, if a person dies during the progressive stage, then the disease will not go through the late and degenerative stages. Therefore, it cannot be called a variable disease.

Most diseases have four periods or stages:

1. Initial period: This is the period when the disease starts, but its clinical presentation is not yet evident. During this phase, the extent of the disease is also not known.

2. Progressive period: This is the growing stage of the disease. During this period, the disease gradually advances.

3. Late period: In this stage, the disease reaches its end and stops progressing. Neither progression nor regression occurs.

4. Degenerative period: This is the final stage of the disease. During this period, the disease slowly regresses and ultimately dies out.

Amrad Zahira[154] Wa Amrad Batina[155] (External and Internal diseases)

Galen believed that there are two types of diseases: external and internal. External diseases, such as swelling and eruptions on the skin, can be identified through inspection and palpation. On the other hand, internal diseases can be either easily or difficultly diagnosed. For example, pain in the lungs and obstruction can be easily diagnosed, while diseases of the ducts, lungs, and liver are often diagnosed through estimation. Similarly, diseases of the urethra can be difficult to diagnose.

Amrad Khassa[156] (Specific diseases)

Certain medical afflictions are associated with specific organs, such as visual impairment in the eyes and hearing loss in the ears.

Amrad Shirka[157] (Secondary diseases)

It is important to differentiate between primary and secondary diseases when it comes to treatment. A primary disease is the one that should be treated first, as it can be more harmful than a secondary disease. Secondary diseases occur when one organ is affected by the disease of another interconnected organ. For example, the brain and stomach are interconnected through nerves, and a disease in one can affect the other. The secondary disease persists with the primary disease and grows and declines with it, making it essential to treat the primary disease effectively. Sometimes, the two types of diseases can be mistaken due to two causes: when the sensation of the primary organ is slow, and the secondary organ is rapid, or when the primary disease is weak, but the secondary disease is dominant.

There are different reasons why secondary diseases occur:

a) Both organs are naturally connected through some other organ. For example, the stomach and brain are connected through the Vagus nerve.
b) One organ is the pathway for another organ. For example, the glands of the thigh become inflamed in any pain of the legs.
c) Both the organs are adjacent. For example, throat and larynx. Specifically, if one is weaker and accepts the waste of another organ easily, like the larynx, it becomes easily inflamed when the throat becomes inflamed. Similarly, the glands of the axillae near the arm easily accept the effects and substances of diseases of the arms.
d) One organ is the source of the function of another organ. For example, the movement of the lungs is secondary to the movement of the diaphragm. If the

---

154 امراض ظاہرہ
155 امراض باطنہ
156 امراض خاصّہ
157 امراض شرکیہ

diaphragm is affected by a disease that alters the function or movement of the diaphragm, then the functions of the lungs will also be affected.

e) An organ is a subservient of another organ. For example, nerves are subservient to the brain, so if the brain is affected by some disease, then the related nerves are also affected. Similarly, vessels are subservient to the heart.

f) Both organs are related to each other through a third organ, either anatomically or physiologically. For example, the brain is linked to the kidney in a way that if the kidney does not excrete the urinary waste, then it may poison the blood and affect the functions of the brain.

g) Sometimes, the reason is that one organ's secretion is related to another organ's function. For example, the functions of the liver and stomach are related to the secretion of bile.

Complex and Simple Disease Classifications

There are two main types of diseases: Simple and Complex. Simple diseases are relatively easy to manage as they do not present complications during treatment. However, complex diseases are much more challenging to treat because they come with complications that can interfere with the treatment process. For instance, imagine a patient with oedema who also develops a fever. In this case, treating the oedema with hot medication, which typically reduces swelling and improves circulation, may inadvertently cause the fever to rise. On the other hand, using cold medication to lower the fever might worsen the oedema.

Amrad Hadda[158] (Acute diseases) and Amrad Muzmina[159] (Chronic diseases)

Diseases can be categorized into two types based on their extent and severity. Acute diseases are those that have a short duration but severe symptoms that can be life-threatening, such as food poisoning, pneumonia, meningitis, etc. They can be classified into four types: Full acute (maximum duration of 14 days), moderate acute (7 days), absolute acute (13 days), and transferred acute (21-40 days), during which the person either recovers or dies. On the other hand, chronic diseases are those that persist for a longer duration and have mild, tolerable symptoms that can be fatal or non-fatal. Examples include leprosy, elephantiasis, etc.

Intiqal Amrad[160] (disease transfer[161])

Disease transfer is a phenomenon in which a diseased substance is presented differently. In some cases, this transfer can be beneficial and can help cure other diseases. For instance, quartan fever can sometimes relieve epilepsy, gout, varicose veins, polyarthritis, and spasms. Similarly, some diarrhoeal diseases can provide relief from conjunctivitis and

---

[158] امراض حاده
[159] امراض مزمنہ
[160] انتقال امراض
[161] The transfer of disease from one organ to another; metastasis.

pleurisy, and in cases of obstruction of vessels in the anus, such as in piles, a cure for black bile diseases, buttock pain, kidney disease, uterus disease, and other diseases can be observed.

Grades of health and diseases found in the human body

1. Extremely healthy body.
2. The body is well but health is not up to its full potential.
3. Body that is neither healthy nor diseased.
4. Body which has the ability and capacity to easily accept any disease.
5. The body is slightly ill.
6. Diseased body in which the disease is dominant over the whole body.

Study of Causations (Ilm al-asbab[162])

'The acquisition of complete knowledge of anything requires understanding its causes since all things have causes.'

- Ibn Sina

Definition and classification of causes

Sabab[163] refers to the source, root, origin, or reason for something. In medicine, it stands for the factor that comes before and triggers one of the primary states of the human body, namely health, disease, or an intermediate state. This factor is known as Asbab Fa'iliyya[164] (acting causes/ efficient causes). If the cause is aimed at maintaining any of the said states, be it health, disease, or intermediate state, it is referred to as Asbab Hafiza (maintaining causes).

Definition of causes

The term Sabab refers to the state before the onset of a disease, which either produces a new condition in the human body or maintains the previous one. When the human body is in a moderate normal state, it remains healthy; however, if it becomes abnormal, it can result in disease. Just as poor air and diet can lead to diseases, good diet, air, and freshwater can reduce diseases and promote health in the body. If appropriate measures are not taken, the disease can persist, or it can be the result of some other cause.

A cause can be either bodily, such as temperamental conditions or structural or humoural substances, or external, such as food, hot or cold conditions, or any psychic conditions like sorrow, anger, and factors affecting the psychic faculty.

For a new condition to arise due to a cause, the following states must be present:

a) The Sabab (cause) must be strong. If the cause is weak, it usually does not produce a prominent effect. For example, lukewarm water does not affect the body.
b) The body being affected by the cause can accept it. Those people who are not affected by that particular cause do not become sick.
c) The cause needs appropriate time to show its effects; otherwise, no changes occur.

---

[162] علم الاسباب
[163] سبب Singular – plural اسباب Asbab
[164] اسباب فاعليه

Cause (Sabab)

As discussed, the cause is defined as the thing that is present first, and its presence in the body produces a new condition or it maintains the previous condition. Causes are divided into two categories:

1. Asbab Badaniyya[165] (bodily causes)
2. Asbab-i-Sihhat-o-Marad (causes/means of health and disease)

1. Asbab badan (Bodily causes)

The human body depends on the following four factors.:

1. **Material causes (Asbab Maddiyya[166]):**
   Those causes which are related to organs and their Ruh[167] (pneuma)[168] and also Ikhlat (humours) and elements.
2. **Efficient causes (Asbab Fa'ila[169]):**
   Those causes produce either health, disease or Intermediate state in the body or maintain the state of the body irrespective of whether it is normal or abnormal. That is, those causes that produce changes in the human body or maintain them and are (a) various types of air and associated factors, (b) food, water and other drinks, etc.; (c) evacuation and retention; (d) habitat and residence, etc.; (e) physiological and psychological rest and activity; (f) sleep and wakefulness; (g) various phases of life and variations therein; (h) male and female differences; (i) occupations; (j) habits; and (k) favourable and unfavourable agents affecting the human body by contact.
3. **Formal causes (Asbab Suriyya[170]):**
   Factors of structure and temperament and those related to it. For example, temperament and faculty.
4. **Final causes (Asbab Tammiyya[171]):**
   The causes that complete the body or any condition of the body. For example, functions.

---

[165] اسباب بدنیہ

[166] اسباب مادیہ

[167] روح

[168] Light gaseous substance obtained from the interaction of inspired air with subtle humours found in organs and fluids of the body and help faculties in their functions

[169] اسباب فاعلہ

[170] اسباب صوریہ

[171] اسباب تمامیہ

2. Asbab-i-Sihhat-o-Marad[172] (Causes/means of health and disease)

The causes of health and diseases are divided into the following types based on their effects.

1. **Predisposing causes (Asbab Sabiqa[173])**
   Those causes, whether temperamental, structural, or humoral, that directly produce or maintain a condition. For example, fever cannot occur without congestion of a substance.

2. **Interdependent causes/immediate causes (Asbab wasila[174])**
   Those causes are present in the body and create a condition in the body without any other cause. For example, infection without any other cause produces septic fever.

3. **External causes (Asbab Badia[175]):**
   External causes such as fire, sunlight, and cold can have an impact on the human body. These non-bodily causes can directly or indirectly create or sustain a certain bodily condition. For instance, heat, cold, pathogens, psychological factors, food and drinks, and injuries are some of the external factors that can affect the body.

4. **Internal causes (Asbab Badaniyya[176]):**
   They are the internal or bodily causes such as abnormal temperament or abnormal structure.

Note that:

Predisposing and immediate causes: both are body causes.

Interdependent and external causes: interdependent causes always affect indirectly, and external causes occasionally affect indirectly.

External and predisposing causes: external causes occasionally affect directly, and the predisposing causes always affect directly.

On the other hand:

Predisposing and immediate causes: predisposing causes always affect directly, and immediate causes always affect indirectly.

---

[172] اسباب صحت و مرض
[173] اسباب سابقہ
[174] اسباب واصلہ
[175] اسباب بادیہ
[176] اسباب بدنیہ

Interdependent and external causes: interdependent causes are body causes and always affect indirectly, whereas external causes are outside the body causes and always affect directly.

External and predisposing causes: external causes outside the body cause and occasionally affects indirectly, whereas predisposing causes are related to the body and always affect directly.

Three states are necessary for a cause to produce an effect.

1. The quwwat fa'ila (stimulating power/ efficient faculty) of the cause is strong.

2. The body has the facility or capacity for the cause.

3. The link between the cause and body is maintained till cause effects appear.

What happens when the causes have been removed?

It is not uncommon for effects to persist after removing their causative factors. However, it is worth noting that this phenomenon is not universal. In some cases, eliminating causal factors results in the cessation of their corresponding effects.

Causes can be explained with the following analogy:

*Wood is needed to make a throne (**Material cause**), a carpenter is needed to make the throne (**Efficient cause**), and then the specific form of the throne is formed (**Formal cause**). It is then used for the purpose of sitting (**Final cause**).*

Different effects can be produced by a single cause simultaneously, depending on their impact on different people or at different times. This is because the effects of causes vary among people based on their ability and capacity. For instance, the effects of a cause on a strong person differ from its effects on a weak person. Moreover, the effects of a cause are different in more sensitive people than in less sensitive people.

The causes are divided based on different factors.

The following are the types of causes based on their effects.

Asbab Hafiza (Maintaining causes): the causes that maintain and protect the body's condition.

Asbab Mughayyara (Modifying causes): the causes that maintain and protect the body's condition.

Those causes that produce changes in the body's condition.

Another division of the causes is in terms of essential (Asbab Dharruriyya[177]) and non-essential factors (Asbab Ghayr Dharruriyya[178]).

Essential factors: Six factors are essential for human life. These factors are so important that human life would not be sustained without them. In other words, if any of these six factors were to cease to exist, human life would also cease to exist. These factors are

Non-essential factors: are those that are not necessary for human life but can be beneficial or harmful. For example, the use of medicine is beneficial, while burns and drowning can be harmful.

The Six Essential Factors (Asbab Sitta Dharruriyya)

They are the six essential factors for maintaining physical, mental, social and spiritual health that are necessary for human life and life cannot exist without them. These are:

1. Hawa[179] (Air)
2. Makulat-o-Mashrubat[180] (Food and drinks)
3. Harkat-wa-Sukun-e-Badani[181] (Physical movement and rest)
4. Harkat-wa-Sakoon-e-Nafsani[182] (Mental activity and rest)
5. Ihtebas-wa-Istefragh[183] (Retention and evacuation)
6. Nawm wa Yaqza[184] (Sleep and wakefulness)

Air

We breathe the air that surrounds us for us to live; therefore, air is one of the necessary elements for our body and Ruh (pneuma). That is, just as the air is involved in the structure and composition of the organ, similarly, it is also involved in the production of Ruh. Air is a constant and continuous help for the Ruh and reaches it through the act of respiration and is also involved in the modification of Ruh.

The modification that occurs in our Ruh through the air is through two functions: Tarwih[185] (moderation) and Tanqiya[186] (Purify).

---

[177] اسباب ضروریہ
[178] اسباب غیر ضروریہ
[179] ہوا
[180] ماکولات و مشروبات
[181] حرکت و سکون بدنی
[182] حرکت و سکون نفسانی
[183] احتباس و استفراغ
[184] نوم و یقظہ
[185] ترویح
[186] تنقیہ

Tarwih (moderation)

Tarwih (moderation) refers to the moderation in the hot temperament of the Ruh (pneuma), that is, to provide coolness to reduce its heat which increases due to hyperaemia or some other cause such as exercise or anger.

The modification refers to removing excess heat from Ruh and bringing it to its original temperament, which is naturally moderate. Ruh's natural temperament is warm but should not become too hot.

There are two routes for modifications:

a. through lungs
b. pores of the skin.

Ambient air (Hawa Muhit) is much colder than the normal temperament of Ruh (the vital spirit). When this cold air mixes with Ruh, it prevents the Ruh from weakening since the mizaj (temperament) of Ruh is not naturally as hot due to hyperaemia. Without this protective effect, two things may occur as a result of excessive heat. Firstly, Su-e-Mizaj Harr (morbid hot temperament) may occur in the Ruh, which affects the Quwwat Nafsaniyya (mental faculties), including Quwwat Hissiyya (sensory functions) and Quwwat Ḥarakat (motor functions), which are vital for sustaining life. Secondly, the excess heat may cause the essence of Ruh, which is gaseous, to dissolve, leading to death.

Tanqiya[187] (Purify/Purification)

Tanqiya (purification) is a process that modifies the Ruh (pneuma/the vital spirit). When we breathe out, we expel the Bukharat (vapours), which are the waste products of Ruh. These waste products are harmful and have no useful function in the body. Just like Khilt Fadil[188] (superfluous humour), these wastes must be purified and eliminated from the body.

Purification is necessary because the air we breathe in is only useful until it gets warmed up by our body and modifies the vital spirit. When this happens, it becomes harmful and must be expelled from the body so that the inspired air can take its place. Failure to do so can lead to hyperaemia, which can increase toxicity in the vital spirit and even become fatal.

Moderation and purification occur in the tissues through the blood. The blood absorbs the cold air and takes it to the tissues for moderation. Then, it absorbs the warm air from the tissues and takes it to the lungs.

---

187 تنقیہ
188 خلط فاضل

Seasons

Four seasons and their qualities[189] (Fusul Arba'a Kayfiyat)

Spring season

According to Unani physicians, the Spring season is moderate; either it is moderate according to the heat and coldness, or it is moderate according to our body and blood.

Summer season

The temperament of this season is hot and dry because the sun's rays fall vertically, causing the temperature to rise. Moisture resolves due to a rise in temperature, and the essence of the air becomes porous, so, in this season, warm air is blown, which increases dryness. In this season, the days are longer, and the nights are shorter, which also causes the temperature to increase.

Autumn season

In autumn, the temperament is inclined more towards dryness. Because the summer season dries the air, and then in the autumn season, there is nothing in the atmosphere to help humidify the air (according to the principles of Unani medicine, a hot object can lose heat and become cold, but a dry object cannot become moist. Also, heat can produce dryness, but coldness is unable to produce moisture).

So, we can see in the seasons that there is a difference in how the moisture from the winter season changes in the spring season and what happens to the dryness of the summer season when moving into the autumn season; these two are not the same situations. Winter season's moisture decreases very quickly in the spring season, but the summer season's dryness remains for a long time into autumn.

The autumn season is not moderate in terms of heat and coldness because, due to autumn dryness, this season does not have the capacity to balance between hot and cold. On the contrary, the spring season is near to moderate in heat and coldness, as unlike autumn, spring air does not quickly move between hot and cold.

Winter season

The temperament of this season is cold and moist. There is an excess of water vapours in the air, due to which it becomes dense, and its nature resembles the nature of water, so resolution in this season decreases.

---

[189] Or properties /qualities

Characters of the four seasons

Spring season

The temperament of the spring season is perfect for the Ruh (pneuma) and blood. Spring changes the colour of the body to red because it causes blood to be absorbed in moderation more towards the skin surface, and its hotness does not reach the extent to resolve the blood as it does in the summer season.

The spring season is especially beneficial for children and those that have a temperament similar to the temperament of a child (i.e., hot and moist). Chronic diseases enter the state of crisis in the spring season because in this season, those Ikhlat (humours) that were static in winter become active with some warmth, and so, this season produces an active state in humours. The body also prepares itself against the diseases produced by the dietary substances that are formed from the intake of food and lack of exercise during winter as the spring season activates such substances.

Spring diseases: Epistaxis, bloody diarrhoea, haemorrhage, hemiplegia, polyarthritis, black bile.

There are two causes of diseases in the spring season.

a) Excess body or mental activity
b) Musakhkhinat[190] (heat-producing causes[191]) i.e., excessive use of hot foods.

Prevention: Following measures are therapeutic for the diseases produced in the spring season.

a) Fasd (Venesection)
b) Istifragh[192] (Evacuation)
c) Decrease in food and drink intake
d) Decrease in intake of stimulants such as tea, coffee, etc.

Summer season

During this season, the Ruh (pneuma) and Akhlat[193] (humours) in the body dissolve, which causes a weakening of the Quwa (faculty) and Af'al (functions). The Dam (blood humour) and Balgham (phlegm humour) decrease, resulting in an increase of Safra (yellow bile). This makes this season's Kayfiyat (quality) more favourable for Safra, allowing it to increase and activate, which can cause issues such as nausea, vomiting, and

---

[190] مسخنات (singular مسخّن Musakhkhin)
[191] Agents/substances or procedures which increase the metabolism of the body due to their hot temperament or heat-producing property
[192] استفراغ
[193] اخلاط

so on. Towards the end of the season, there is an excess of Sawda (black bile) and a decrease in Dam (blood humour).

The duration of diseases also reduces during this season because of the warmer air and water, which helps Nudj[194] (concoct) substances more easily. This aids Tahlil[195] (dissolve) of any morbid matter found in diseased conditions. However, if the body's faculty is reduced, then the summer heat will increase weakness and further domination of the disease. If the summer season is extremely hot and dry, then the disease reaches its end quickly. But if it rains and this season becomes wet, then the duration of the disease will increase. Hence, some wounds in this season heal more slowly and are sometimes converted into wounds that can damage the organs.

Summer diseases: Summer diseases are those caused by extreme heat. Examples include continuous fever, burning fever, conjunctivitis, and bilious eruptions. Excessive perspiration dries out and roughens the skin. Measles, smallpox, and other diseases are also prevalent during this season. Lienteric diarrhoea and oedema can also occur, and diarrhoea becomes more common during this season. People with the yellow bile temperament (Safra mizaj) are particularly vulnerable to acute and chronic fevers in this season. The burning of yellow bile produces black bile (Sawda), which can cause black bile diseases.

Autumn season

The temperament of this season is cold and dry, and in terms of the effect on health, it is the worst season and has the highest prevalence of diseases, and this is due to the following reasons:

a) Exposure to the wide fluctuation of heat and cold during this season.
b) Weakness from the preceding summer carried on to this season.
c) In this season, the excessive consumption of fruits putrefies Ikhlat (humours).
d) The thin components of the humours resolve in autumn, but the thick components don't, which then oxidize and cause diseases.
e) Blood is scanty during autumn because this season is contrary in temperament to the blood; hence, it fails to replace the blood dissipated during summer.
f) The burnt humours
g) Produced during summer are cooled during autumn and become Sawda (black bile).
h) The earlier part of autumn is somewhat beneficial for elderly persons, but towards the end, it becomes highly injurious for them.

Autumn diseases: Scabies, pruritus, dermatophytosis, ulcers, polyarthritis, dysuria, dribbling of urine, lienteric diarrhoea, sciatica, tonsillitis, back pain, worms.

---

194 نضج
195 تحليل

Winter season

The temperament of this season is cold and moist. Winter aids digestion, and in this season:

a) Cold traps the innate heat and makes it more concentrated and less prone to dispersion.
b) During this season, people tend to engage in more exercise and physical activities that generate more heat.
c) Winter is the ideal season to reduce bile as it is colder with shorter days and longer nights.
d) Since winter has a greater tendency to stagnate morbid matter, there is a greater need for liquefying and resolving foods.
e) This season is troublesome for old and debilitated persons, but it is beneficial for the young and healthy.

Winter diseases: During winter, diseases such as catarrh, coryza, pleurisy, pneumonia, and pains are common, all caused by phlegmatic substances. Additionally, the cold brought by autumn winds can increase the prevalence of flu and other similar illnesses. Those who are old, weak or have a similar temperament may face greater difficulties during this season. It's important to note that the quality of seasons can vary depending on the region of the earth.

Abnormal changes in Ambient air

Air quality changes can cause the air to become hotter or colder, which can affect human living conditions. There are various earthly and celestial factors that can lead to abnormal changes in the air.

Celestial factors

The change that is produced due to celestial factors is related to stars. When huge, bright stars gather together in line with the sun, then there is heat, and when they disperse, this hotness decreases.

Earthly factors

There are various factors that can cause changes to occur on Earth. The quality of seasons differs in various regions of the world. For instance, summer seasons in arid lands of the Indian Subcontinent can be extremely hot, while in mountainous areas, they are not too hot, and the temperature is moderate on beaches. The reasons behind these differences are as follows:

1. **Distance from the equator (changes due to latitude)**
   Regions located closer to the equator experience higher temperatures, while those located farther away tend to be colder. This is because the sun's rays hit the Earth at

a perpendicular angle for most of the year in equatorial regions, while in regions farther from the equator, they hit the Earth at a steep angle.

2. **Higher ground and sea level**

   The higher the altitude, the colder the temperature. This is because air, which is a mixture of various gases, does not directly absorb heat from the sun's rays. Instead, the sun's rays fall on the Earth's surface and heat the land, which then reflects heat, warming the air. Therefore, the air at lower elevations, like near the sea level, is warmer compared to air at higher elevations, such as in the mountains, which are colder.

   The second reason for the colder temperatures in higher elevations is due to the fewer gaseous and dust particles in the air. Near the ground, there are more gaseous and dust particles that absorb more heat from the sun's rays. In contrast, the air in the mountains has fewer of these particles, which results in colder temperatures.

3. **Distance of land from the sea**

   The climate of a place is also affected by its distance from the sea. Places that are closer to the sea tend to have an oceanic climate which means that they are less hot in the summer and less cold in the winter. This is because water heats up or cools down at a slower rate than land.

4. **Direction from mountains**

   When the mountains' face is parallel to the wind, the wind passes through without any rain. This can cause the area to become arid. However, if the mountains' face is opposite to the winds, then the moist winds will strike the mountains, resulting in rainfall. But the opposite face of the mountains will remain dry.

5. **Direction of winds**

   The winds blowing from the sea carry vapours, which result in rainfall. For instance, the western monsoon causes heavy rainfall in the mountains from June to August because they originate from the sea. However, the north-eastern monsoon, which originates from land, does not cause any rain.

6. **Cyclone**

   In some regions, cyclones move at a high speed and can cause monsoons. For instance, cyclones are responsible for summer rainfall in the plains of Punjab.

7. **Forests**

   Heavy rainfall in areas with dense forests, such as the Congo in Africa, is due to the abundance of water in the forest, which creates a cold and wet environment.

8. **Oceanic streams**

   Winds passing over the warm surface of the sea become heated, leading to increased conversion of water into vapours. These vapours ultimately result in rainfall. Due to the impact of the Gulf Stream, Western Europe experiences greater rainfall. However, if the winds pass over cooler surfaces, the amount of rainfall will decrease.

9. **Difference in sand/land**

   The areas where the land absorbs more water are colder, and the places where the land absorbs less water are hotter.

The effects of living in different locations and habitats

1. **Hot areas:**
   Living in hot areas can lead to faster ageing, weakened digestion, and changes in physical appearance, such as darker skin and curled hair due to the dissolving of moisture and lowered body humidity.
2. **Cold areas:**
   People living in colder regions are usually hardy and brave. They tend to have good digestion. In areas with high humidity, the inhabitants tend to be fleshy and fatty, with sunken joints and healthy skin. Their veins are not prominent.
3. **Humid areas:**
   People living in humid areas may experience health problems such as chronic fevers, diarrhoea, menorrhagia, and haemorrhoids. They may also be more susceptible to wounds and infections.
4. **Dry areas:**
   The inhabitants of arid regions tend to have dry skin and a prevalence of dryness in their organs and brains. Extreme temperatures also characterize these regions.
5. **Uphill areas:**
   People who live in hilly regions tend to be tall and have longer lifespans.
6. **Low areas:**
   People living in areas with low elevation often have a higher likelihood of experiencing health problems. This is because of the prevalence of lukewarm, stagnant, cloudy, or salty water sources in their vicinity, which can cause physical responses that result in feelings of weakness, a weakened immune system, and sadness.
7. **Rocky and stony areas:**
   Rocky and stony areas are regions characterized by rocky terrains and lack of exposure. The extreme temperatures in these areas cause their inhabitants to develop hard and solid bodies, more hair on their skin, strong and prominent joints, and predominantly dry skin.
8. **Coastal areas:**
   Individuals residing in coastal areas are subjected to a moderate climate in terms of temperature but tend to experience high levels of moisture. If the habitat is located north of the sea, it has a moderate temperature, but if it is situated in the south, the climate is colder.
9. **Areas below mountain areas:**
   a. Eastward areas: These regions are not covered by mountains from the east but by mountains from the west. The climate of such areas is usually good because the sun purifies the air as it rises, which protects the area from the extremes of daytime.
   b. Westward areas: These are the areas that are covered from the east and open from the west by the mountain. The sun's rays do not reach these areas at sunrise, which is why the air remains thick and wet, and so these areas are more susceptible to western winds. The health benefits of

eastern areas are absent here. The significant issue in this area is that the sun's rays reach it when the sun is at its peak, and the sun's rays fall perpendicularly, making the area hot. Therefore, the climate here is not always suitable for health, and there are usually more colds. Even the voices of the inhabitants were raspier.

Wind Direction and its effects

Northerly Winds

Quality: Northern winds are cold as they originate from snowy mountains.
Characteristics: The air that blows from north to south has cold and dry properties, which may vary depending on the geographical location. The northern winds can strengthen, tighten, prevent superficial secretions, clog skin pores, improve digestion, produce constipation, act as a diuretic, and correct putrefactive and epidemic air. However, the moisture in the northern winds can sometimes enter the body and cause vessel bleeding. That is why people in areas affected by northern winds complain of substances flowing from their heads. Chest diseases such as catarrh, cough, and chest pain are common in such areas, along with polyarthritis, uterus and bladder pain, etc.

Southerly Winds

Quality: Southern winds are hot and wet as they flow from seas and oceans.
Characteristics: Generally, they have a relaxing effect on the body, open skin pores, and move Ikhlat (humours) to excrete them out. Wounds heal slowly, and itching and different types of wounds are prevalent in this wind.

Easterly Winds

Quality: They are usually hot and dry but become cold and wet at night.
Characteristics: Morning easterly winds are soft due to the sun's rays, which decrease their moisture.

Westerly Winds

Quality: They are somewhat wet as they are not much affected by the sun's rays.
Characteristics: In the morning, they are thick and dense as they are not affected by the sun's rays. However, if they blow at night, they are light and soft.

Please note that the rules and principles described by Ibn Sina were specific to Persia during his time. In other countries like England, these principles would be different. For instance, the 17th-century English Physician Culpeper[196], who also practised the four-humour medicine (Unani medicine), describes winds differently:[197]

'The East wind is hot, dry, and blasting…

Winds from the West are cold and moist…

The South wind is hot and moist…

The North wind is cold and dry….'

In India, the eastern wind is very wet because it blows from the sea to the east of India and carries vapours unaffected by the sun's rays. This wind can cause breaks in organs, such as polyarthritis, and delay wound healing due to an increase in the substance of the wound and an increase in the frequency of wet swellings and diseases. When this wind blows, the water in pitchers and pots does not cool rapidly.

As you can see, the characteristics of western winds are very different from those of eastern winds.

Effects of different types of air:

Hot air

This type of air is known to dissolve moisture and increase thirst. It can also dissolve the vital facility or pneuma (Ruh) and reduce strength (Quwa). It dissipates the innate heat (Hararat Ghariziyya), which weakens digestion. It also dissolves the humours (Akhla[198]) that cause redness in the body, leading to an increase in yellow bile (Safra) and a yellowish colour. This air can cause abnormal contractions in the heart, increasing the flow of humours, which can affect weak organs and cause abnormalities. However, this air can benefit those suffering from hemiplegia, catarrh, cold, ligament spasms, oedema, and other conditions.

Cold air

Cold air has several effects on the body. It can trap heat within the body, stop the flow of substances, and close the pores of structures. It is harmful to those suffering from flu-like diseases and weak nerves. However, it can strengthen digestion and increase hunger, making it more beneficial than hot air for healthy individuals. On the other hand, cold air can harm all the functions related to nerves.

---

[196] Nicholas Culpeper (1616 – 1654) was, Physician, botanist and herbalist.
[197] Summarised from Culpeper's Medicine: A Practice of Western Holistic Medicine, Graeme Tobyn 1997, Element books. Ltd
[198] اخلاط

Moist air

Moist air benefits most skin types as it moisturizes and opens pores but can also harbour infections.

Dry air

Dry air differs significantly from moist air and produces opposite effects.

Turbid air

Produces abnormality in pneuma which causes difficulty in breathing. It stimulates the humours.

Food and Drinks

Water

Water is an essential component of the human body and serves as a source of nutrition by diluting and dissolving nutrients, which are then carried through narrow vessels and expelled. However, while water enters the body, its quality does not change, and it does not become a permanent part of the body. Instead, it is a compound that helps to diffuse and eliminate nutrients.

Types of water

Spring water:

Best quality water is from springs in an unpolluted area free from stony soil or soil decay. Water from clay soils is preferable to that from stony soils. Running water that is exposed to the sun and wind is considered of the highest quality. Stagnant water may be of lower quality because of exposure, but this can be prevented by keeping it below the surface. If a spring is not flowing, it should be enclosed from all sides to protect it from toxic substances. Furthermore, directing the water flow towards the sun, particularly towards the east during the summer when the sun rises, can enhance the water quality.

Properties of spring water:

Spring water is tasteless and odourless. A small quantity of this water reduces the acidity of alcohol. Due to its softness, it is more affected by heat or cold. It quickly passes down through the stomach and does not stay for a long duration. Food is readily cooked in this water.

Rainwater:

Rainwater is a good source of water, especially the water that comes from summer rain accompanied by thunder but without strong winds. However, this type of water is easily contaminated because it is thin and soft, making it vulnerable to land and air infections.

Once it is contaminated, it can become a source of infection for the body's humours, which can harm health.

The water of wells, canals and tap water:

The quality of well and canal water is not as good as that of spring water because it is stored for an extended period and exposed to earth materials, which can lead to putrefaction. Water transported through lead pipes is the most harmful as it can absorb some of the lead's properties and cause stomach and intestine ulcers.

Marsh water:

Water found in wetlands is considered inferior in quality to well water due to its long stagnation in sodden ground and among herbaceous plants and is more susceptible to contamination.

Glacier water:

Glacier water, while thick in consistency, is effective in alleviating thirst. However, it may provoke nervous pain in some individuals. Fortunately, boiling the water is an effective method of eliminating its potentially harmful effects.

Turbid water:

It is important to note that turbid water can lead to the formation of kidney stones and blockages. In such cases, it is advisable to use a diuretic to help alleviate the issue. If someone is experiencing diarrhoea, they can benefit from consuming thick and heavy water as it is retained in the stomach and released slowly. In constipation caused by turbid water, consuming fats and sweets can be helpful.

Stagnant water:

This type of water is commonly found in forests that are surrounded by reeds, bamboo, and bushes and are covered by algae. This type of water is usually dirty and contains many toxic substances that can harm our health. Using stagnant water can cause various health issues such as spleen diseases, ascites, abdominal distension due to accumulated gaseous matter, and a weakened liver. Additionally, women may face difficulties during childbirth if they are exposed to stagnant water.

Mineral water:

Water that contains different minerals or salts.

   a) Salty water weakens the body and produces dryness in the body. Causes diarrhoea due to its expulsive faculty (Quwwat Dafi'a) but then later causes constipation. Also causes scabies and pruritus.

b) Ammonia water is specific for the stomach; it can be taken orally or used in a bath or enema.
c) Alum water is beneficial in haemoptysis, piles, menorrhagia, and eye washing. It also stops haemorrhage.
d) Iron and copper water water which contains iron or copper. It is beneficial for the spleen, treats the liver and is useful in ascites.

Hot and cold water:

Medium cold water is useful in diarrhoea, strengthens the stomach, increases hunger and relieves thirst. It harms those who have inflammation in membranes or suffer from flu-like illnesses.

Hot water causes nausea, but if it is taken early in the morning in sips, it relieves constipation. But this type of water weakens the stomach and digestion and does not relieve thirst.

Effects food and drinks

Foods and drinks affect the body in three ways:

Affects due to their Kefiyat (quality/properties):

That is due to its heating nature, which warms the body, or due to its cooling nature, it cools the body. So, producing either warmth or coolness without becoming part of the body. So, for example, consuming mint or applying mint oil can introduce a cooling sensation.

Affects due to their anasir (elements/composition):

That is, the effects of the substance; after entering the human body, the substance changes and becomes similar to the organs of the human body. Ibn Sina explains, 'For example, the lettuce has a cold temperament that is colder than that of humans and cools down the blood, while garlic has an opposite warming of the blood effect'.

Affects due to their Jawhar (nature/essence):

The specific action that produces effects by its essence and Surat Naw'iyya[199] (specific form or structure) and not from the Kefiyat (quality/properties) nor its composition as mentioned above. Refers to the inherent substance or essence of the food or drink. For example, mint's inherent essence, such as menthol, gives it its characteristic aroma and cooling effect. The effects could be favourable (peony, which helps with epilepsy) or unfavourable (poisonous effect of aconite).

---

[199] صورت نوعیہ

The effects of food and drinks when they enter the human body

The interaction between food and drinks when they enter the body and the organs of the body are of three ways:

a. The dietary substance that enters the body changes but does not cause any change in the body.
b. The dietary substance that enters the body changes and also produces a change within the body.
c. The dietary substance that enters the body does not change but does produce a change within the body.

A. The dietary substance that enters the body changes but does not cause any change in the body has two forms.

1. The dietary substance which is assimilated by the body and does not produce any qualitative change, such as heat, cold, etc., is an absolute dietary (Ghidha' Mutlaq[200]) substance.
2. But if the dietary substance does not become part of the body or cause any changes, then this is a balanced or a moderate drug (Dawa' Mu'tadil[201]).

B. The dietary substance that enters the body changes and also produces a change within the body has two forms:

1. The substance has the ability to be assimilated into the body.
2. The substance does not have the ability to be assimilated into the body.

If the ability to become part of the body is present, then it is called a dietary drug (Dawa Ghidhai'[202]). If it acts on the body by its properties or qualities and is not assimilated into the body and excreted, then it is called a pure drug (Dawa Mutlaq[203]). If the entering substance itself changes and produces changes in the body, and these changes continue and do not regress, then this is called a toxic drug / poisonous drug (Dawa sammi[204]).

C. If the substance entering the body does not change but produces a change in the body to the extent that it causes putrefaction, it is called absolute or pure poison (Samm Mutlaq[205]). Antidotes or theriac (tiryaq[206]) and virucides (fad zeher[207]) which are also included in this category.

---

200 غذاء مطلق
201 دواءِ معتدل
202 دواءِ غذائی
203 دواءِ مطلق
204 دوا سمی
205 سمّ مطلق
206 تریاق
207 فاد زبر

In Summary, the substances that enter the body and their interaction with the body functions are of six types:

1. Absolute diet (Ghidha' Mutlaq)
2. Moderate drug (Dawa' Mu'tadil)
3. Dietary drug (Dawa Ghidhai')
4. Pure drug (Dawa Mutlaq)
5. Toxic drug (Dawa Sammi)
6. Absolute poison (Samm Mutlaq)

In Unani medicine, five substances are used when treating diseases.

Dawa (drug): A drug that does not become part of the body and can produce wanted or unwanted effects. The actions of a drug in Unani medicine are based on temperament, which can be correlated on a physiological level, not on a molecular basis.

Ghiza (Diet): These are substances that become part of the body's cells, tissues, or organs, contributing to their maintenance and function. They include essential nutrients like carbohydrates, proteins, lipids, vitamins, and minerals.

Ghidha Dawai (Food with Medicinal Properties): These substances are primarily used as a diet but also contain some therapeutic properties. Such substances have more dietary constituents than drug constituents, e.g., pumpkin, cucumber, musk melon, and watermelon.

Dawa Ghidhai (Drug with nutritional Value): These substances which are primarily used as drugs but have some nutritional values. e.g., mint, pepper, cardamom, ginger.

Zulkhassa (Specific drugs): These are substances used for their therapeutic effects, but their mechanisms of action are not fully understood.

Types of diet

There are three types of diet.

1. Ghidha Latif [208] (Light diet): Diet producing fine/thin consistency Ikhlat (humours).
2. Ghidha Kathif [209] / Ghidha Ghaliz [210] (Dense diet): Diet producing thick humour.
3. Ghidha Muʿtadil (Moderate diet): Moderate blood producing diet.

From these three diet types, the diet may be very nutritious or lightly/slightly nutritious, which produces light blood humour.

The following is a list of foods based on their nutritional and dietary value:

1. Light diets are very nutritious, such as meat soup, egg yolks, half-boiled eggs.
2. Light diets that are slightly nutritious, for example, legumes with moderate texture and quality, and fruits such as apples and pomegranates.

---

[208] غذا ء لطيف
[209] غذا ء كثيف
[210] غذا ء غليظ

3. Dense/heavy foods that are very nutritious, for example, boiled eggs and beef meat, produce thick blood.
4. Heavy food that is slightly nutritious, for example, cheese and dried meats.

From the mentioned food, some foods have either good or bad chyme.

1. Light diets that are very nutritious and have good chyme, for example, meat soup, egg yolk, and boiled egg.
2. Light diets that are very nutritious and have bad chyme, for example, liver and lungs.
3. Light diets that are slightly nutritious and have good chyme, for example, fruits like apples, pomegranates, etc.
4. Light diets that are slightly nutritious and have bad chyme, for example, spinach.
5. Heavy foods that are very nutritious and have good chyme, for example, boiled egg or lamb meat.
6. Heavy foods that are very nutritious and have bad chyme, for example, horse meat and duck meat.
7. Heavy food that is slightly nutritious and has good chyme, for example, buffalo's meat.
8. Heavy foods that are slightly nutritious and have bad chyme, for example, dried meat.

Meaning of Bad chyme - For example, while the liver has high nutritional value, eating food that contains bad chyme can lead to various health issues. Digestive problems like indigestion, bloating, constipation, or diarrhoea can occur due to difficulty in breaking down food. This also disrupts the balance of the four primary humours, causing systemic health problems and toxin accumulation.

Bodily Movement and Repose (Haraka wa Sukun Badani)

Haraka Badani (Bodily movement)

Physical activity affects the human body in various ways:

1. In terms of strength, i.e., weak and strong.
2. In terms of duration, i.e., the movement is short, long or moderate.
3. In terms of speed, i.e., movement is accompanied by rest or not.
4. In terms of work activity, such as a blacksmith working next to a furnace.

The intensity and duration of physical movements can have differing effects on the body, specifically in balancing heat and resolving imbalances. All types of movement produce heat but differ in their effects. Fast and short movements tend to provide immediate relief by alleviating symptoms or discomfort. However, they are less effective at resolving underlying issues, such as the accumulation or imbalance of madda (substances) or Ikhlat (humours) in the body, which is referred to as the resolution of matter (tahlil of madda).

The resolution of matter means breaking down and eliminating accumulated substances or humours that cause imbalance in the body.

The increased heat and metabolic activity from fast and short movements might provide immediate relief by promoting circulation or alleviating stiffness. However, compared to slower, more sustained activities (such as taking a long walk), they might be less effective in resolving deeper or more chronic imbalances of substances or humours in the body.

Activity and working in an environment where there is heat helps in the resolution of matter, and likewise, resolution is reduced when working in a moist environment. However, when there is excessive movement, innate heat (Hararat Ghariziyya) increases, causing natural moisture to dissolve, which leads to coldness and dryness in the body.

Sukun Badani (Bodily repose)

Rest (Sukun Badani) fosters both cooling (Mubarrid) and moisture (Murattib), preserving the environment within the body, which is essential for sustaining equilibrium and enhancing well-being. The cooling effect arises as rest inhibits the sustenance of heat and retains morbid matter (Mawad), thereby reducing internal heat. Concurrently, the state of rest prevents the excessive evacuation or resolution of bodily fluids and waste materials of the body (Fudlat[211]), increasing the body's overall moisture content

Mental Activity and Repose (Haraka wa Sukun Nafsaniyya)

In mental activity, both Dam (blood) and Ruh (pneuma) are drawn either outward or inward to the body, manifesting in five distinct forms:

1. A sudden outward movement, as seen in anger.
2. A gradual outward shift, as seen in states of happiness and pleasure.
3. An abrupt inward draw, characteristic of fear.
4. A slow inward transition when experiencing sadness and sorrow.
5. A simultaneous movement, both outward and inward, occurs when contrasting psychic states coexist. For instance, in guilt, the face might redden as the Dam (blood) and Ruh (pneuma) shift outward, while concurrently, due to sorrow, an inward movement might render the face pale.

In each of the aforementioned psychic movements, heat intensifies in the direction where Dam (blood) and Ruh (pneuma) are moving towards, while coldness prevails in the area they are leaving. This pronounced disparity between heat and cold can lead to imbalances, resulting in diseases. If such psychic movements reach extreme levels, they can be life-threatening. For instance, overwhelming joy can lead to a phenomenon known as 'death

---

[211] فضلات

from joy', while profound sorrow and sadness can result in a condition akin to shock or trauma, potentially proving fatal.

Sukun nafsaniyya (Mental repose)

Excess mental rest always leads to a cooling (Mubarrid) effect and a decrease in mental sharpness; this results in a rise in coldness and a slowing down of cognitive functions. Hence, individuals exhibiting these characteristics have a cold temperament.

Sleep And Wakefulness (Nawm wa Yaqza)

Nawm (Sleep)

Sleep bears a resemblance to rest due to the following reasons:

1. During sleep, both the Ruh (pneuma) and the organs are at rest, with the Ruh being inclined internally, akin to the state of rest.
2. Like rest, sleep sees a decrease in the resolution of madda (matter), resulting in an increase in bodily moisture.
3. Sleep alleviates the fatigue brought on by wakefulness, much in the same way that rest dispels the exhaustion caused by heat.
4. The efficacy of food digestion during sleep is comparable to that during rest.
5. Similar to the state of rest, the expulsion of substances is halted during sleep.

Yaqza (Wakefulness)

Wakefulness bears a significant resemblance to movement due to several reasons:

1. Similar to the heat generated during movement, wakefulness also induces heat production. This is because, in a state of alertness, the organs are active, generating heat. During this state, the pneuma (Ruh) and blood are channelled towards the external body.
2. Like movement, wakefulness increases dissolving (Tahlil) of matter, subsequently leading to dryness in the body.
3. Wakefulness holds the same importance to the psychic faculty as movement does to the body. In this regard, just as movement stimulates physical activity, wakefulness directs the pneuma (Ruh) outward from within.

Retention And Evacuation (Ihtibas Wa Istifragh)

Retention describes the condition when substances remain in the body, while evacuation refers to removing substances from the body. This removal can occur through various routes, such as urine, faeces, vomiting, sweat, epistaxis, menstruation, piles, and more. When substances are expelled in abnormally large amounts, it is termed abnormal evacuation.

Health is preserved when there is an equilibrium between retention and evacuation; any deviation from this balance can potentially result in diseases and illnesses.

Ihtibas ghayr tab'i (Abnormal retention)

Abnormal retention occurs when substances that should normally be expelled remain in the body. This condition can arise due to several reasons:

1. A weakening of the faculty or function responsible for expulsion.
2. Quwwat Masika (retentive faculty) becomes strong, preventing the release of substances.
3. Narrowing or obstruction of the ducts through which substances are expelled.
4. The substances meant for expulsion become overly thick and adhesive.
5. A weakening of the Quwwat Hadima (digestive faculty) causes digested substances to remain in the stomach for a long time.
6. An increase in the expulsion volume of substances overwhelmed the Quwwat Dafi'a (expulsive faculty).
7. A loss of expulsive senses.
8. A diversion of the Quwwat Tabi'iyya (physical or natural faculties) to other areas, such as during a crisis.

Diseases produced due to abnormal retention

1. Amrad Su-e-Mizaj (Impaired Temperament Diseases): This category includes ailments such as infections, congestion of innate heat, and increases or reductions in innate heat.
2. Amrad Su-e-Tarkib (Structural Diseases): These diseases relate to structural abnormalities such as obstructions or looseness in the nerves.
3. Amrad Tafarruq Ittisal (Loss of Continuity Diseases): Conditions falling under this classification include disruptions in continuity, such as ruptures of the ducts, as seen in hemiplegia.
4. Amrad Murakkab (Compound Diseases): This type includes complex diseases such as eruption swellings.

Istifragh ghayr tab'i (Abnormal evacuation)

Abnormal evacuation refers to where fluids and substances, which should ordinarily remain within the body, are expelled. This condition can arise due to several causes:

1. Quwwat Dafi'a (expulsive faculty) becomes too strong.
2. Quwwat Masika (retentive faculty) becomes weak.
3. When harmful or toxic substances are produced inside the body, either due to their large quantity or the presence of Riyahi (gases), they can provoke pressure, swelling, and burning, prompting evacuation.
4. A substance may flow out spontaneously when it becomes very thin.
5. Enlargement of the ducts can facilitate the expulsion of substances.

6. A rupture in the ducts will unavoidably lead to the leakage of substances.

Diseases produced due to abnormal evacuation

Diseases stemming from abnormal evacuation typically create coldness in the mizaj (temperament). However, temporary heat can occur when the expelled substances are Balgham (phlegm) or Dam (blood), as Sufra (yellow bile) predominates in such conditions. Likewise, abnormal evacuation can increase moisture when substances that induce dryness, such as sauda (black bile), are expelled. In this situation, innate heat diminishes, impairing the complete digestion of food and thus increasing the body's phlegm content.

Excessive evacuation can result in both coldness and dryness within the organs, thereby giving rise to diseases characterised by spasms in the affected organs.

Non-essential Factors (Asbab Ghayr Daruriyya)

These factors are not essential for maintaining life but are important in preserving and promoting health and preventing diseases. Unlike the Asbab Sitta Daruriyya (six essential factors), which are necessary for life, Asbab Ghayr Daruriyya (non-essential factors) are supplementary and contribute to the overall well-being of an individual, for example, Physical Exercise (Riyazat), Massage (Dalk) and Bathing (Hammam).

Hammam (Therapeutic bath / Turkish bath)

The function of Hammam

The function of Hammam lies in its dual capability, where the air induces warmth within the body while the water contributes moisture.

Specifications of Hammam

Ibn Sina says[212] that a Hammam is ideally housed within an older structure with well-ventilated rooms with optimal air quality, supplied with sweet water, and equipped with a furnace regulated to the human temperament. The environment transitions from moderate air in the first room to a hot and moist ambience in the second, culminating in hot, dry air in the third chamber.

Varied Effects of Hammam

Hammam provides warmth and moisture. Excessive exposure to its hot air can reduce innate heat, leading to a cooler mizaj (temperament) and a decrease in primary moisture,

---

[212] Cannon of medicine volume 1

thereby inducing dryness. When interacting with extremely hot water, the body may react by closing the skin pores, inhibiting the absorption of the Hammam's benefits and disrupting moisture balance.

Extremely hot water generates heat, while lukewarm water contributes to coolness and moisture. The heat experienced does not originate from the Hammam but from the body's reaction to cold water.

Digestive Heating & Diverse Baths

Hammam can also internally heat the body through the digestive process. When undigested food or cold Khilt (humour) is present, the bath's heat metabolizes it into blood, enhancing circulation, expelling waste, and increasing body heat. Techniques like a dry bath, where water is not applied, can induce body dryness, aiding in conditions such as irritation and oedema due to excessive moisture. Conversely, a moist bath adds moisture to the body.

Impact of Duration & Timing

Prolonged stays in Hammam can result in dryness due to extensive diaphoresis and resolution, while shorter durations contribute to moisture. The timing of Hammam, relative to meals, also plays a significant role; it can induce weakness when taken on an empty stomach and potentially cause obstruction if taken on a full stomach, but it proves beneficial and contributes to body fat when aligned with completed digestion.

Potential Side Effects

While Hammam serves various therapeutic purposes, being aware of potential side effects is crucial. The bath directs waste materials of the body (Fudlat) towards weaker organs, potentially weakening the body, resolving innate heat, desensitizing nerves, and potentially causing anaphrodisia.

Sunbathing

Engaging in strenuous activities under sunlight results in the resolution of waste materials in the body, increased perspiration, and potential weakening of the organs. However, sunbathing holds therapeutic value, particularly in addressing conditions like oedema and asthma. It exhibits a noticeable benefit for individuals with a cold temperament, providing relief from various forms of pain and chronic inflammation.

Prolonged exposure to sunlight leads to notable changes in the skin, characterised by increased thickness and darkening. This extensive exposure can cause a burning sensation on the skin and hinder the resolution of substances. Nevertheless, sunbathing is a valuable intervention in treating numerous skin conditions.

Splashing water

Splashing water, particularly on the face, holds therapeutic significance. This technique proves beneficial in alleviating conditions associated with pain, anxiety, and syncope. Enhancing the treatment with aromatic additions such as rose water or kewra water (a distillate from pandanus flowers) can amplify the benefits.

This method is not only limited to addressing common ailments but also plays a role in neonatal care. For instance, when a new born experiences difficulty establishing breath post-delivery, a balanced mixture of hot and cold water is gently splashed onto the infant's face and head. This stimulates a response, prompting the baby to initiate breathing and crying, indicating the commencement of independent respiration.

Oiling (Tadhin[213])

Lubrication through medicinal oils is used for therapeutics. This method involves utilising moderately hot or cold oil, depending on the ailment being addressed.

Olive oil can help alleviate nervine pain, tremors, phlegmatic diseases, and various types of pain. Olive oil can also help remedy the dryness of the skin and internal organs. Amla oil (Phyllanthus emblica) and rose oil are beneficial for mitigating headaches.

Cold oils such as pumpkin oil (roghan kadu) and lettuce seed oil (rogan Kahu) are preferred for conditions characterised by excessive heat and dryness. These oils are known for their cooling effects, making them especially effective for treating headaches arising from elevated internal heat.

Therapeutic massage (dalk)

Objectives of Therapeutic Massage (Dalk)

- Strengthening lax bodies and fortifying nerves.
- Modifying organ texture: hardening soft organs and softening hard ones.
- Regulating organ size and fat content: promoting growth, increasing or decreasing fat.
- Enhancing skin health: absorbing fats, expelling waste, and preventing diseases.

Massage that is done with dry hands or oil has the following types;
Therapeutic massages are done with either dry hands or oil, are categorized into the following types:

1. Dalk sulb (massage with firm pressure): A firm pressure with hands is exerted on the body parts. It strengthens the body by eliminating excessive moisture (Rutubat).

---

213 تدهين

2. Dalk layyin (massage with light pressure): This is done with gentle, slow hand movements, applying less pressure than a firm massage (Dalk Sulb). Its goal is to soften body parts by absorbing excess moisture.
3. Dalk kathir (prolonged massage): This massage is done for a more extended period. To make the body thin and lean by eliminating excess moisture from the body.
4. Dalk qalil (massage for a short duration): This massage is done for a shorter duration. It makes the body parts shiny and produces heat in the body.
5. Dalk mu'tadil (moderate massage): In this type of massage, body parts are manipulated with moderate force or pressure, which is qualitatively maintained between hard and smooth massage. This makes the body plumper and revitalized.

The above combinations produce nine compound (Murakab) types of massage:

1. Dalk Sulb Kathir: Firm massage for a prolonged duration
2. Dalk Sulb Qalil: Firm massage for a shorter duration
3. Dalk Sulb Mu'tadil: Firm massage for a moderate duration
4. Dalk Layyin Kathir: Smooth massage for a prolonged duration
5. Dalk Layyin Qalil: Smooth massage for shorter duration
6. Dalk Layyin Mu'tadil: Smooth massage for a moderate duration
7. Dalk Mu'tadil Kathir: Moderate massage for a prolonged duration
8. Dalk Mu'tadil Qalil: Moderate massage for shorter duration
9. Dalk Mu'tadil Mu'tadil: Moderate massage in both pressure and duration

Some other specific types of massage are as follows:

1. Dalk Khashin (Rough massage): a type of massage done with the help of a rough cloth. It draws the blood rapidly to the body's surface. It should not be done for a longer duration; otherwise, it will lead to an excessive elimination of moisture (Rutubat) from the body, which may further lead to dehydration.
2. Dalk Amlas (Gentle massage): This massage is done gently with the palm or a soft cloth. It draws and retains the blood slowly towards the treated area.
3. Dalk Isti'dad (Preparatory massage): A type of massage done before starting an exercise session. It is started in a gentle manner, which slowly and gradually increases and becomes vigorous towards the end, which heats the body after this exercise is started. Sometimes performed exclusively with hands and at other times incorporating oil, it aids in the quick expulsion of waste products.
4. Dalk Istirdad (Restoratory massage): This massage is done toward the end of the exercise, and it should be carried out gently and moderately, ideally with oil. It can dissolve and expel waste products generated during exercise, as their retention can induce fatigue.

Exercise (Riyadat)

Activities involving physical effort, due to which the breath becomes frequent and rapid, to maintain or enhance health.

Benefits of Exercise

1. Exercise enables rapid, long, and deep respiration, allowing for increased oxygen absorption and increasing the volume of blood in the system.
2. Regular physical activity enhances blood circulation, ensuring a consistent nutrient supply to every organ.
3. Exercise aids in expelling bodily waste, protecting against diseases arising from accumulated waste materials of the body (Fudlat).
4. Physical activity increases the body's primary heat (Hararat Asliyya), enhancing the overall function and competence of the organs.
5. Exercise optimises the organs' absorptive and digestive capabilities.
6. The thinning of bodily fluids through exercise facilitates their diffusion into the organs' essence, making the organs flexible and brisk.
7. Exercise leads to the dilation of pores, which aids in eliminating waste.
8. Regular physical activity strengthens the organs and the joints, promoting overall bodily strength.

Harmful effects of discontinuing exercise

There can be a detrimental effect on the body if exercising is stopped after regularly exercising. In this condition, the primary heat (Hararat Asliyya) is weakened, reducing the strength of various organs and making them more susceptible to diseases.

Types of exercises

Generally, there are two types of exercises:

1. Passive exercise
2. Intentional exercise

Passive exercise:

Exercise is not intentionally done but carried out as a part of a profession, e.g., farming or construction work.

Active exercise:

Exercise is done intentionally to get the benefits of exercise, and it has two types: Generalised exercise, whole-body exercise, and Localised exercise, which is the exercise of a specific organ or part of the body.

Different types of exercise:

Short-duration exercise: exercise done for a shorter duration.
Extensive or rigorous exercise: exercise that is rigorous and intense.
Light exercise: exercise done with gentle movements.
Rapid exercise: exercise done with rapid body movements.
Slow exercise: exercise done with slow body movements.
Rigorous and rapid exercise: exercise done with rapid and vigorous body movements.
Relaxing exercise: exercise which is done slowly and without much force.

Time of exercise

The best time for exercise is in the morning after ablutions, but many people prefer exercising in the evening. Therefore, exercise may be done at either of these two times.

Exercising on an empty stomach or immediately after a meal is harmful. The best time to exercise is when the food in the stomach and intestines has been digested, absorbed, and become part of the body.

Exercise should also not be done when the abdominal organs have fewer nutrients because, in this condition, the toxic substance and Khilt (humour) spread to the whole body and can cause diseases.

Intensity and timing of exercise

Everyone should exercise according to their energy capacity, and overall physical condition. The following factors should be considered:

- Exercise can be continued when the skin becomes red, indicating increased blood flow. However, if the skin turns pale, it signifies that the body is becoming fatigued, and exercise should be stopped.
- Exercise can be continued when the body's activities feel normal and comfortable. However, if movements become slow and the body feels fatigued, exercise should be stopped.
- When the organs keep swelling (indicating increased blood flow) and the sweat keeps drying, the exercise can be continued. However, when the organs stop swelling and the body starts sweating profusely, it is a sign that the body is overheating, and exercise should be stopped.

Instructions for exercise

- Avoid vigorous exercise on an empty stomach; consume light foods before exercising in summer, and some substantial meals should be included in winter.

- Exercise is more harmful on an empty stomach than on a full stomach.
- During exercise, the body should be moderate in terms of hotness and coldness.
- The person should relieve themselves with urination and defecation before exercising.
- Preparatory massage is essential before exercise to stimulate the innate heat and to open the pores of the body, and restoratory massage after exercise is essential to avoid fatigue.
- If an organ is weak or diseased, then exercise should be done in such a way that less pressure is applied to the diseased organ.
- Avoid continuous, extreme, and vigorous exercises; instead, incorporate short breaks intermittently.
- The exercise should change; after some days, some changes should be made from the previous sessions.
- Exercise should always be done in well-ventilated or open areas.
- Exercise should be gradually increased and done at a specific time.

Fatigue (I'ya'[214])

There are three original types of fatigue: Ulcerative (Quruh), Distension (Tamaddudi) and Inflammatory (Waram).

Ulcerative (Quruh) fatigue: This type occurs when the skin feels a pain similar to that of an ulcer or wound. Shivering is observed at its extreme. The cause of this fatigue are those toxic humours and putrid substances that, if they enter the vessels and mix with the blood, then their corrosiveness and toxicity is mitigated, but since the medicatrix naturae diverts them towards the skin, they reach the skin in their pure form, and their corrosiveness remains intact. Thus, the minimum harmful effect caused by these putrid substances is fatigue. However, if this substance is stimulated and undergoes a crisis, it may cause shivering; if it increases, it can also result in trembles. The concoction and stability of the putrid substance require time, and until this substance is concocted, it cannot be expelled; such substances are called raw humours. This substance sometimes enters the vessels and can be found in raw states in the muscles.

Distension (Tamaddudi) Fatigue: The person feels like his body has been crushed and feels movements and pressure. In this condition, even small movements such as stretching are unpleasant for the person, especially when the fatigue is due to excessive work.

The cause of this distension is those waste materials of the body (Fudlat) present in the organs' structures, but these waste materials of the body, in terms of their essence, are not toxic nor burning, and their cause may be Rih (Air/gas).

---

[214] اعیاء

Fatigue maddi (substance-related) and fatigue rih (Air/gas) are differentiated in lightness and heaviness. Fatigue maddi is heavy, and fatigue rih is light.

This type of fatigue is often due to lack of sleep, and so it is cured after proper sleep.

Inflammatory (Waram) fatigue: It is fatigue in which the body is hotter than its normal condition, as the organs are swollen in size and colour, are irritable on touch and movement and are also tensed.

The swelled organs are red and shiny because the skin is stretched due to the tension, which increases the skin's brightness. It results from standing for a long duration or taking long walks.

Another type of fatigue is when the person feels as if his body is suffering from excessive dryness. Its cause is excessive exercise and rough massage as a restoratory massage after the exercise, and sometimes its cause may also be fewer nutrients, fasting and sometimes excessive intercourse and evacuation.

Causes Related To The Four Qualities

Causes that produce heat (Asbab Musakhkhin)

The factors or causes that produce or induce heat in the body are as follows:

- Excessive activities (such as running or weight).
- Exposure of the body to moderate heat-producing substances (such as drugs).
- Hot Mizaj food and drinks (e.g., certain spices).
- Exposure to any condensation (e.g., sauna).
- Diseases that cause inflammation or fever.
- Emotional states like anger or extreme excitement.
- Extensive exposure to hot climates.

Causes that produce coldness (Asbab Mubarrid)

The causes that produce coldness in the body are as follows:

- Excessive rest.
- Interaction of refrigerants with the body.
- Cold Mizaj food and drinks (e.g., cucumbers).
- Low food or excessive food intake.

Causes that produce moisture (Asbab Murattib)

- Rest and peace.
- Excessive sleeping.
- Retention of abnormal fluids in the body.
- Improper or excessive bodily excretion, such as sufra (yellow bile).
- Excessive consumption of food.
- External application of moisture-producing products.
- Use of emollients (Murattibat).
- Use of light soothing agents (Musakkinat[215]).
- Use of refrigerants (Mubarridat)
- Moderate joy.

Causes that produce dryness (Asbab Mujaffif)

The causes that produce dryness in the body.

- Movements.
- Wakefulness.
- Excessive evacuation.
- Low food intake.
- Use of dry (Yabis) food and drugs.
- Excessive emotional stress or activities such as intercourse.
- External application of dryness-producing products.
- High intake of hot food and drinks, which produce dryness by causing excessive dehydration.

Causes of Deformities (Asbab Fasad Shakl[216])

Some causes are related to foetal life and alter the formative faculty.

1. The causes are due to the abnormal position of the foetus during childbirth, for example, breech delivery.
2. The causes are related to the abnormal grip of the baby during childbirth, which deforms the baby's shape.
3. External causes, for example, stroke or apoplexy.
4. Causes produced by the early movement and positioning of the foetus during childbirth.
5. Some causes are nervine-related—for example, facial palsy, hemiplegia, oedema, tremors, convulsions, and spastic conditions.

---

[215] Agent which calms a patient, eases agitation and induces sleep; also used to neutralize the hotness of humours.
216 اسباب فساد شكل

6. Sometimes, the shape deforms after the resolution, healing of the wound or inflammatory tumours.
7. Other diseases that deform the shape include leprosy, syphilis, smallpox, etc.
8. Sometimes, after a swelling or healing of a wound, there is a deformity in shape.
9. Old age and extreme weakness.

Causes of obstruction[217] and constriction of ducts (asbab sudad wa diq majari[218])

1. Obstruction can sometimes result when an abnormal object becomes trapped in a duct. It has two forms.
   a. Due to objects of unusual structure, such as stones or an excessive accumulation of certain substances, such as large deposits of sediments in the intestines.
   b. The object may have distinct properties, such as being overly thick and adhesive.
2. After an ulcer heals, it can result in the narrowing of a duct. For instance, an intestinal wound can lead to a narrower intestine.
3. Cysts or similar structures can develop inside a duct, causing blockage.
4. Inflammation or a cyst in the canal of a duct can exert pressure, narrowing the duct.
5. Cold conditions can cause ducts to constrict.
6. Using powerful astringents can lead to obstructions.
7. Applying tight bandages can also constrict ducts.

Causes of duct dilatation (asbab ittisa majari[219])

1. Retentive faculty (Quwwat Masika) weakness.
2. Expulsive faculty (Quwwat Dafi'a) strength.
3. Use of purgative (Mushila) drugs.
4. Use of drugs that temporarily dilate (Murkhi) the tract.

Causes of roughness (asbab khushunat[220])

1. Penetrating resolvent drugs (Miqatat[221]) or detergent (Jali[222]) drugs.
2. Mild astringent drugs that are dry.
3. Medications that have a cold effect.

---

[217] embolus
[218] اسباب سدد و ضیق مجاری
[219] اسباب اتساع مجری
[220] اسباب خشونت
[221] مقطعات
[222] جالی

Causes of smoothness in skin or mucous membranes (asbab malasat)

1. Application demulcents.
2. Use of mild resolvents that increase the flow of fluids.
3. Use of cold and viscous medications.

Causes of dislocation and separation of structures (asbab khila mufariqat-i-wada')

1. Factors that induce tension, causing a joint to dislocate and a cavity to form in the structures.
2. Interruptions in an organ's support during movement, resulting in a structural separation, as seen in sprains.
3. Conditions or factors that relax or moisten, weakening the fibrous structures, such as in hernias.
4. Factors leading to the decomposition or decay of the structure.

Causes of abnormal connections between organs (asbab su mujawirat[223])

1. Stiffness of adjacent organs.
2. Spasms.
3. Flaccidity or weakness of neighbouring organs.
4. Inflammation.
5. Healing from ulcers.
6. Fractures or dislocations.
7. Calcification of joints.
8. Congenital malformations.

Causes of abnormal movements (asbab ghayr tab'i)

These causes lead to abnormal organ movements such as tremors, convulsions, hiccoughs, shivering, burping, sneezing, pandiculation, and yawning. The causes include:

1. Dryness increases to such an extent that it causes weakness, resulting in tremors.
2. The dryness that induces convulsions can lead to hiccoughs, while dryness affecting the nerves can result in convulsions.
3. Waste materials in the body (Fudlat) that cause convulsions.

---

[223] اسباب سوء مجاورت

4. Waste materials in the body that support nerve function can lead to conditions like tremors, often resulting from congestion. In cases of complete obstruction, it can result in hemiplegia or apoplexy.
5. Due to their cold nature or specific physical properties (Kayfiyat), certain waste materials in the body can induce symptoms like trembling and shivering.
6. Retention of innate heat in the body, due to which the body becomes cold externally and hot internally.
7. Gas or air (Reeh) trapped in the muscles may cause fasciculations (Ikhtilaj) in organs.
8. The collection of gas (Reeh) and vapour (Bukhari) substances causes pandiculation and yawning.

Causes of increased size and number of organs (asbab ziyadati miqdar wa adad a'da')

The causes for an increase in the size and number of organs include:

1. A large amount of madda (matter).
2. Abnormal enhancement of the absorptive faculty (quwwat jadhiba), such as through massage.
3. Abnormality in the function of formative faculty[224] (Quwwat Musawwira[225]). This form is usually congenital, but it can sometimes be due to diseases like facial and skin moles.

Causes of discontinuity/separation (asbab tafarruq ittisal) Internal causes

Internal causes of discontinuity (Tafarruq Ittisal), relate to the interruption or loss of connection between bodily elements. A number of factors can produce this state, including:

- **Corrosive humour (Khilt Akkal):** As in caseation and loss of tissue in leprosy.
- **Escharotic (Muharriq):** Substances that can cause tissue to die and peel away.
- **Laxity (Murkhi):** Weakened or slackened tissues that may not maintain their structural integrity.
- **Excessive moisture (Murattib):** Overhydration or over-moistening of tissues that can lead to breakdown.
- **Drying (Mujaffif):** Excessive dryness that causes tissues to become brittle or separate.

---

[224] One of the reproductive faculties that shapes each organ of the body according to the species or race.
[225] قوت مصوّره

- **Accumulation of gas (Reeh):** Gaseous build-ups that might pressure and potentially rupture connections.

These factors, whether from excessive heat or an abundance of specific substances/matter (madda), lead to Tafarruq Ittisal. This occurs as the intense heat or surplus of matter amplifies the expulsive faculty (Quwwat Dafi'a), triggering a rupture in vessels or inducing inflammation, which can provoke tearing and a loss of continuity in bodily structures.

External causes

1. **Tension-producing causes:** Factors that place an unusual amount of strain or stress on a part of the body, causing it to lose its normal connectedness.
2. **Dissecting causes:** Factors that involve separating or tearing tissues, causing a breakdown in their physical integrity.
3. **Inflammatory causes:** Factors that induce inflammation can lead to swelling and possible rupturing of tissues.
4. **Compressive causes:** Factors involving compressive forces could damage and create disunity in tissue or organ structures.
5. **Scratching/Peeling causes:** Factors that involve abrasive or peeling forces, leading to a disintegration of the tissues.
6. **Biting/Pinching causes:** Factors that involve concentrated, often sharp pressure, which could potentially puncture or tear tissue.

Causes of ulcers (asbab qarha)

Ulcers can form for various reasons, such as ruptured inflamed masses, pustules, abscesses, or pus accumulation in wounds.

Causes of swelling (asbab waram)

Swelling originates from two primary sources: either related to 'Madda' (substances, i.e., humours) or specific to organs. While the causes related to Madda have been described in a previous section on diseases, we discuss organ-related causative factors of swelling here.

The following are the causes of swelling produced in the organs:

1. If an organ's expulsive faculty (Quwwat Dafi'a) is insufficient, the Madda expelled from a stronger organ causes swelling.
2. If the recipient organ becomes weak, it cannot expel the Madda (substances), and this causes swelling.
3. Organs are ready to accept waste materials from the body (Fudlat) in the following few cases:

a) The substance (madda) or its essence is of such type that it is made to be accepted by the body and absorbed by the body. However, some bodily wastes can remain on the body and need to be washed off and removed, and in some cases, these wastes can become even toxic or putrid and may provoke eruptions and swelling.
b) The structure of the organ is weak, for example, postauricular glands or nodes of axilla thighs for buttocks.
c) The route for the Madda (substances) to enter the organ is wide, but the route of the Madda (substances) expulsion from the organ is narrow.
d) Lower-located organs might accumulate Madda above, contributing to swelling.
e) The organ is smaller in size than the quantity of Madda (substances), and the organ cannot expel the substance.
f) When an organ cannot digest, absorb and transform the food due to some weakness, it becomes swollen.
g) Cessation of exercise could hinder Madda's dissolution (Tahlil). For instance, athletes stopping their training might encounter polyarthritis, digestive issues, and related swellings.
h) Whether normal or abnormal, an organ undergoing undue irritation or heat may result in swelling.

Pain

Pain and pleasure are subjective experiences that can positively or negatively affect a person's physical or mental state.

There are two types of causes of pain. The first is Su-e-Mizaj Mukhtalif (unstable morbid temperament), which occurs when an organ's temperament changes to an opposing one, causing unwanted effects on the organ. For example, if an organ with a natural hot temperament suddenly changes to a cold one, it can lead to disturbances or dysfunctions.

The second type is Tafarruq Ittisal (loss of continuity). According to Galen, this is the real cause of pain. When organs lose their connectivity, they can cause pain. This is why Su-e-Mizaj Harr Yabis (morbid hot and dry temperament) and Su-e-Mizaj Barid Yabis (morbid cold and dry temperament) can cause pain.

Su-e-Mizaj Mustawi (stable morbid temperament) does not cause pain because it gradually increases, allowing the body to adapt to the changes. This is why patients with hectic fever (humma Diqqiyya), which progresses slowly, may not feel as sick as those with ephemeral fever (humma yawm), which has a sudden onset and is more painful.

Causes of pain (asbab waja')

According to Galen and Ibn Sina, pain has been classified into 15 types. These types are as follows:

1. **Itching (Hakkak):** This is a skin-related pain that causes an itchy sensation due to the presence of a bitter Khilt (yellow bile humour or black bile humour) or due to a salty humour (abnormal phlegm humour).

2. **Rough (Khashin):** This type of pain occurs when a thick or sticky humour causes stretching between muscle fibres and their protective sheaths. For example, psoriasis can cause this type of skin pain.

3. **Stabbing (Nakhis):** This kind of pain produces a pricking sensation and is caused by the presence of Ikhlat (humours) that create distension and hardness in the organs. This is a lung-related pain, for example, pleurisy, produced from stretching and inflammation of membranes.

4. **Distension (Moumadid):** This pain is related to the stomach and is caused by an accumulation of gas or Ikhlat (humours) that leads to expansion within an organ's cavity or its membranes. The pain produces a distended sensation and can be due to gas or flatus, always associated with a feeling of lightness. Alternatively, it can be due to the build-up of corrupted Ikhlat, which tends to be associated with a sensation of heaviness.

5. **Pressure/squeezing (Dhaghaz):** This pain is produced by the accumulation of Madda (matter) or Reeh (air) that causes constriction as it surrounds an organ.

6. **Incisive pain (Mufasikh):** This is a type of muscular pain that arises when Ikhlat accumulate within the muscle fibres, causing them to become distended and generate a sharp, cutting, or incisive pain sensation.

7. **Breaking/Bony (Mukassir):** This type of pain originates in the bones and is triggered by the accumulation of Reeh or Ikhlat between the bone and its surrounding membrane, the periosteum. Specifically, the pain arises due to coldness, which induces constriction within the periosteum.

8. **Softening/Dull (Rakhou):** This is a type of low-intensity pain in the muscles' soft tissue produced from madda (substance), which creates pressure in the muscles but not in their tendons. It is called softening because the muscle is more extended than its nerve, tendon, or membrane.

9. **Boring/perforating (Thaqib):** This type of pain feels as if tissues are being drilled into. It is commonly experienced in the site where visceral/colicky pain occurs, such as in the abdomen. The cause of this pain is the retention of gross matter or off gas between the layers of a hard and thick organ, like the colon, which continually goads it and tears its parts asunder, boring into the interstices like a drill. An example of this type of pain can

be seen in conditions like diverticulitis, where inflamed pouches in the colon wall cause intense, boring pain.

10. **Stabbing/Piercing (Masalli):** This is a similar kind of pain to the above 'Boring/perforating' pain and arises when a substance, such as flatus or a humour (Khilt), accumulates in the compartment of the large intestine. This accumulation causes a sideways stretching of the intestine's layers, producing a pain that feels like a spindle is being pushed into the area.

11. **Neuropathic/Dull (Khader):** This is a neuropathic type of pain characterised by pain with paraesthesia caused by the blockage of sensory nerve endings due to extreme cold or cold temperament (mizaj), congestion, or other reasons.

12. **Throbbing (Dharabani):** This type of pain is pulsating in nature and is caused by hot swelling or the accumulation of irritating and sour matter, such as in a migraine.

13. **Heavy (Thaqeel):** This is a sensation of heaviness experienced in less sensitive organs or viscera, such as the lungs, kidneys, or spleen. It can also occur in typically sensitive areas, like the cardiac end of the stomach, particularly when their sensory capabilities are compromised, as might happen when carcinoma affects it, resulting in a pronounced heavy pain.

14. **Fatigue (Ayai):** This type of pain is caused by fatigue due to overwork, which produces discomfort in the body. It is also caused by tension from a humour or distension from reeh. It may also result from an irritating humour, which hurts like an ulcer. Combinations of these factors lead to several compound varieties of fatigue pain.

15. **Irritant (Ladhi'):** This is also a type of fatigue pain. It is produced from a sour humour that causes irritation.

Factors Leading to Cessation of Pain

When the source of pain is addressed or removed, relief follows. Some strategies to alleviate pain involve increasing moisture since wetness is not inherently painful, such as applying wet sedatives. Additional methods include:

- **Using of hypnotics for pain:** Sleep-inducing agents like opium can be employed to manage pain.
- **Utilising Anaesthetics:** These substances can cause a loss of sensation and reduce pain.
- **Spiritual Diversion:** Engaging the mind and soul in spiritual activities or practices can also divert attention away from the pain.

Fundamental approach to pain management

The paramount step in treating pain is to address its root cause. Some approaches to managing distinct pain types, such as Su-e-Mizaj (impaired temperament) or Su-e-Mizaj Madda (impaired temperament with matter), and Tafarruq Ittisal (discontinuity) include:

a. If the pain is due to Su-e-Mizaj, opposing (heteropathic) treatments can be beneficial.
b. In cases of pain caused by morbid matter or Su-e-Mizaj Madda, strategies to divert or evacuate this matter should be implemented, such as purgation, emesis, wet cupping massage, and hammam (bathing).

Effects of Pain

1. Pain can hinder an organ's functionality, potentially leading to weakness or even syncope. Examples include the discomfort experienced during colicky pain, angina pectoris, or renal pain.
2. The specific functions of an organ can be inhibited by pain.
3. Initially, pain tends to generate heat within the affected organ, but eventually, it produces coldness.

Why movement can cause pain

Movement causes a stretch in muscles and nerves, which produces discontinuity in the structures and thus causes pain.

Why Ikhlat Radi[226] (abnormal humours[227]) cause pain

1. Certain abnormal humours, like irritants (e.g., Safra Zanjari - verdigris green yellow bile) or hot humours (e.g., Safra-e-Har - hot bile), can induce pain because of their inherent characteristics.
2. Excessive abnormal humours can generate pain by creating stretching or discontinuity in bodily structures.
3. In some instances, the pain arises due to the amount and the properties of the humours.

Why Reeh (air) causes pain

Dense air, or Reeh, can gather in the cavities of organs, causing pressure and pain, as can be observed in flatulence. In some cases, Reeh can spread between structures, such as the

---

[226] Or known as Ikhlat Fasid/ Ikhlat Ghayr Mahmud.
[227] The kind of corrupted humours which are incapable of becoming part of an organ.

intestines, resulting in pain in different body areas, including the bladder. The dispersion or dissolution of Reeh and Bukharat (vapours) can depend on their density, consistency, and organ characteristics.

Causes of congestion

External Causes:

- Engaging in activities that increase bodily moisture, like bathing after eating.
- Excessive sleeping and resting or stopping exercise.
- Overeating and not properly evacuating waste.

Internal Causes:

- Weakness in the digestive faculty (Quwwat Hadima).
- A strong retentive faculty (Quwwat Masika) and narrow ducts that impede flow.

Causes of infection

According to ancient physicians like Ibn Sina and others, the causes of infection are:

- Consumption of spoiled or decayed food.
- Obstruction in a vessel or duct retains madda (substance). This retention leads to Su-e-Mizaj (impaired temperament). Consequently, respiration through pores is affected, and digestion is incomplete, culminating in infection.
- Malodorous winds, especially those passing over stagnant water, can reach and affect the body's humours through respiration and pores and infect the madda (substance).

From the above points, we can see that there are two main causes of infections that are produced in the humours: toxic food and air and abnormal digestion due to Su-e-Mizaj (impaired temperament).

Causes of retention and evacuation (Asbab ihtibas wa istifragh)

Causes of abnormal retention

1. Weak, expulsive faculty (Quwwat Dafi'a).
2. Strong, retentive faculty (Quwwat Masika).
3. Weak digestive faculty (Quwwat Hadima).
4. Constricted or obstructed ducts.
5. Thick, adhesive or large amount of madda (substance) that the expulsive faculty (Quwwat Dafi'a) cannot expel.

6. There is a loss of or decrease in the sense of the need for expulsion, like the loss of sense for defecation when the sufra (yellow bile) does not reach the intestines.
7. During crises, natural healing mechanisms (medicatrix naturae) might prioritise other processes like sweating or nosebleeds (epistaxis), neglecting regular expulsion actions.

Causes of abnormal evacuation

The following are the causes of the expulsion of the substance that should stay in the body:

1. Strong expulsive faculty (Quwwat Dafi'a).
2. Weak, retentive faculty (Quwwat Masika).
3. Substance (Madda) that becomes harmful through its volume, pressure effects of air (Reeh), or by acquiring qualities like roughness and heat, generating irritation swellings.
4. The thinness of madda (substance).
5. Dilated duct as during haemorrhage and frequent discharge of thin semen.
6. A tear through the length and width of the duct or its opening, as in epistaxis.

Causes of weakness of organs (Asbab du'f a'da[228])

Weakness of organs occurs in three forms. The target organ is affected, Ruh (pneuma), which is the source of the Quwwat Tabi'iyya (physical or natural faculties), is affected, or the Quwwat Tabi'iyya (physical or natural faculties) is affected.

1. **Target organ is affected:** The causes that directly affect the organ and produce weakness have two types: a. Su-e-Mizaj (impaired temperament) b. Amrad Su-e-Tarkib (Structural Diseases)

    a. Su-e-Mizaj, especially Su-e-Mizaj Barid (morbid cold temperament), is more harmful than Su-e-Mizaj Harr (morbid hot temperament), which also causes weakness. For example, the effect of extreme heat on the body or a long stay in a bath can cause syncope. Similarly, due to thickened and blocked pores, Su-e-Mizaj Yabis (morbid dry temperament) causes weakness. Whereas Su-e-Mizaj Ratb (morbid moist temperament) loosens the pores of the organ such that no faculty affects them.

---

228 اسباب ضعف اعضاء

b. In Amrad Su-e-Tarkib (Structural Diseases), the most important thing is that the structures become loose. The patient does not feel any pain, but weakness increases.

1. **The Ruh (pneuma) is affected:** The causes that directly affect the Ruh (pneuma) and cause weakness are first the Su-e-Mizaj of the Ruh, and second is the dissolving of the pneuma. This could be due to the resolution of psychic reactions [229](Infi'alat Nafsaniyya[230]) factors or evacuation through venesection.
2. **The Quwwat Tabi'iyya (physical or natural faculties) is affected:** When natural faculties are overused or exposed to repetitive and severe stressors, they can weaken. This can cause an imbalance in the body's pneuma/ vital force (Ruh) and organs, leading to exhaustion and potential harm if not given proper rest.

Other causes of weakness

Several causes of weakness can affect the body. One of them is an abnormality in air, water, and food, which can lead to putrefaction in the temperament of blood, Ruh (pneuma), and organs, eventually causing weakness.

Another cause of weakness is related to evacuation and includes conditions like haemorrhage, diarrhoea, oedema, and swelling with pus accumulation.

All types of pain, such as stomach ache, colic pain, angina pectoris, and renal pain, can also cause weakness.

Fevers can also lead to weakness as they cause the pneuma to have a morbid hot temperament, ultimately resulting in vitality dissolving.

Dilation of skin pores can also cause weakness by aiding the dissolving of vitality.

Hunger is yet another cause of weakness.

Lastly, some organs are inherently weak, such as the brain, eyes, heart, etc., and nature has protected these organs from injuries and trauma.

---

[229] Reactions produced from factors affecting the psychic faculty, e.g., happiness, sorrow, anger, fear, etc.
[230] انفعالات نفسانیہ

SIGNS AND SYMPTOMS ('ILM AL-DALA'IL WA'L 'ALAMAT)

Clinical Manifestation Of Diseases (A'rad Amrad[231])

'Ard[232] is the singular form of A'rad[233], meaning both diseases and signs. Signs that indicate health are known as signs of health, while signs that indicate disease are known as signs of the disease.

Ibn Sina says that, 'the symptoms and signs that indicate the state of a patient's health can point to one of three situations. Firstly, a present condition that requires the patient to take certain actions to benefit their own health. Secondly, a past condition that highlights the physician's progress in their profession and builds trust in their judgement. And thirdly, a future condition that benefits both the physician, as it enhances their knowledge, and the patient, as it provides insight into how to manage their illness.' Galen believed that these situations were key indicators of a patient's health status and could guide physicians in their treatment plan.

Signs of health

There are three types of signs that indicate a person's health status:

1. Signs that relate to an organ's structure, position, quantity, and numbers, whether in a healthy or diseased state (Alamat Jawhariyya).

2. Signs of temperament are signs that show a balanced or moderate temperament and are related to the shape and appearance of organs, as well as their aesthetic appearance (Alamat Imzijah).

3. Signs that are related to the structure of the organ pertaining to its functional ability (Alamat Tamamiyya).

Signs of disease

The presence of a disease can be indicated by various signs. Some of these signs can inform us about the nature of the disease, such as a rapid pulse rate during fever, which indicates the severity of the fever. Others can indicate the site of the disease, such as pulse fluctuations indicating pain or swelling in the chest area or pleurisy. Certain signs are specific to a particular disease, for instance, signs of congestion. Additionally, there are specific signs that are time-limited, such as the onset of high fever in pleurisy, dry cough,

---

231 اعراض امراض
232 عرض
233 اعراض

shortness of breath, impaired or stinging pain, and Nabd Minshari (serrate pulse[234]). These signs begin with the disease and end with it.

Conversely, some symptoms can be chronic, such as a headache that persists even after the fever subsides, while others occur only during the extreme stages of the disease. Furthermore, certain signs indicate diseases of the external organs, such as discoloration, softening or hardening, and coldness or hotness of the organs.

Movements can also be indicative of internal diseases, with puffiness of the lips indicating facial palsy or hemiplegia. Rest-related signs, including epilepsy, seizures, syncope, and hemiplegia, can also occur. Signs related to movement, such as tremors, shivers, sneezing, hiccups, coughing, or convulsions, indicate increased movements. Among these movements, some are relevant to the medicatrix naturae's functions, such as sneezing and hiccups, which occur in a healthy state, while others are related to a temporary function of the medicatrix naturae, such as shivers, tremors, and convulsions.

Signs of external diseases

According to Ibn Sina, external diseases are characterised by observable and objective signs that can be perceived through the senses. For instance, the colour of the affected area can be visually identified, while temperature and consistency can be determined through touch. On the other hand, the assessment of complex perceptions such as form, position, activity, or inactivity of organs may require the use of multiple senses. Signs that indicate the internal condition of the body are primarily related to movement. For example, twitching of the lower lip is indicative of vomiting, while changes in organ size or number can signify an underlying disease. Abnormal stool colour, rumbling noises in the abdomen, and tastes and odours can also indicate abnormal conditions of the body.

Loss of activity is observed in conditions such as apoplexy, epilepsy, syncope, and paralysis. Abnormal motor activity, on the other hand, is characterized by shivering, rigors, hiccups, sneezing, yawning, stretching, coughing, jactitation, and convulsions. Some of these movements are physiological, such as sneezing and hiccups, while others are symptomatic, such as tremors and convulsions.

Movements can either be voluntary or partly voluntary and involuntary. For instance, coughing and micturition are partly voluntary and involuntary, while restlessness and tossing about in bed are voluntary movements. In some composite movements, such as coughing, the movement may be initiated by volition but later becomes involuntary. The strength, extent, severity, support, location, faculty concerned, and humours of movements differ from one another.

The various signs and symptoms discussed above are mainly associated with external organ diseases. However, some of these signs may also indicate the condition of internal

---

[234] Compound pulse resembling wavy pulse but firm and hard

organs. For example, flushing of the cheeks in pneumonia is an external sign that can indicate internal organ disease.

Signs of internal diseases

The diagnosis of internal diseases necessitates an understanding of anatomy, which provides insights into the substance, form, product, site, relationship, nature of excretion, and nature of functions of organs. This knowledge aids in distinguishing between organs and their swellings, locating pain or swelling within or outside organs, determining the origin of morbid matter, and establishing whether the excreted material corresponds to the involved organ.

The diagnosis of internal disease is founded upon six laws: Functional disturbances, which offer direct and dependable evidence of internal disease; excretions, which offer indirect clues to the presence or absence of normal digestion and maturation; pain; swelling; form and relationship; and special symptoms, which do not necessarily furnish direct and dependable evidence of disease.

Functions of the organs as an indicator

Functional disturbances are an indication of disease, resulting from weakness or other causative factors. These disturbances manifest in various forms, including impairments such as defective vision or a weak stomach resulting in difficulties and delays during digestion, dysfunction such as visual hallucinations or food derangement, and loss of function, such as complete absence of digestion or loss of vision.

Retention and depletion as indicators

Retention and depletion are two important bodily processes that play a vital role in keeping the body healthy. Retention refers to the natural process by which the body retains certain materials such as urine and faeces. This process is essential for maintaining the balance of fluids in the body and ensuring that the body's waste products are eliminated properly.

Depletion, on the other hand, is an abnormal loss or evacuation of materials that are typically retained in the body. Such depletion may be derived from a specific organ, and can help in the diagnosis by way of its nature, quality, or colour.

For example, the expectoration of cartilaginous pieces from bronchial rings may indicate ulceration of the bronchi. The quality of the depleted material can also be used for diagnosis, such as thick mucus indicating ulceration of the colon and thin mucus indicating ulceration of the small intestine. The colour of the depleted material can also provide important diagnostic information, such as red flaky deposits in urine indicating a disease of some fleshy organ such as the kidneys and white deposits indicating a disease of some nervous organ, such as the bladder.

Pain as an indicator

Pain is an indicator of disease, and it can reveal the affected area and the cause of the disease. The location of pain can help identify the organ involved, for example, pain in the right chest can indicate liver involvement while pain on the left side can indicate spleen involvement. The nature of pain can also help indicate the cause of the disease. For instance, a dull ache can sometimes indicate involvement of an insensitive organ or of an organ that has been made insensitive by disease. Bursting pain, on the other hand, indicates an excess of morbid material, while irritant pain (waja' ladhi') is a sign of active substance and crisis.

Swelling as an indicator

Swelling is an indication of a disease and can provide valuable information about the type, site, and shape of the disease. The type of swelling, such as erysipelas, can indicate the presence of dense sufra (yellow bile humour), while a hard swelling can indicate Suda (black bile). The location of the swelling is also important. For example, a swelling in the lower right chest can be a sign of liver inflammation, while swelling in the lower left chest can indicate spleen inflammation. The shape of the swelling is also significant. A swelling that is crescent-shaped on the right side of the abdomen is likely connected to the liver, while a longitudinal swelling may indicate the abdominal muscles in front of the liver.

Location and relationship as indicators

Diagnosis can be aided by considering the site of the symptoms and the relationship between organs. Sometimes, the connections and relationships of organs can also provide evidence of disease. For instance, pain in the fingers may be an early sign of disease or injury to the sixth cervical nerve.

Primary and Secondary diseases

It is important to identify the order of occurrence of diseases, i.e., the primary and secondary diseases. The disease that occurs first is considered as the primary disease and the one that occurs later is the secondary disease. Also, it needs to be determined which disease persists after the resolution of other diseases. The disease that remains is the primary disease, whereas the one that disappears is considered as the secondary disease. Furthermore, the disease that would be eradicated due to the causes of another disease is considered as the secondary disease, and the other is the primary disease. In cases where one disease is imperceptible, and another occurs simultaneously, the primary disease intensifies. Therefore, a physician must understand the association of organs, the related diseases, and their early and late signs to avoid errors in diagnosis.

Signs indicating temperament

The signs which indicate the quality of temperaments are of ten types:

(1) Touch or feel of the body: This can be determined by comparing the feel of their body to that of a person with a balanced temperament. If the feel is the same in both cases, the temperament is balanced, however, it can still be relatively hot or cold. If a person with a balanced temperament finds that the feel of another's body is hot or cold, hard or soft, smooth or rough, the other person's temperament is likely to be abnormal, provided there is nothing external such as atmospheric changes or baths that could affect the body's feel.

The conclusions drawn from a soft or hard feel depend on the body's proper balance of heat and cold. Excess heat after dispersing the moisture makes the body soft and moist even if it was originally hard, while cold makes the normal or even soft body hard, like ice or solid fats.

However, it is important to note that people with cold temperaments may feel soft even if they are thin and weak because of an excess of immature humours.

(2) The quantity of flesh and fats: A well-developed muscular structure suggests increased heat and moisture, while underdeveloped muscles and deficiency of adipose tissue indicate dryness. Excess adipose tissue and oily skin can indicate a colder temperament.

Narrow veins suggest a lack of pure blood, leading to anaemia and hunger, indicating a cold temperament. The absence of both liquid and solid adipose tissue indicates a hot temperament.

The heart's affinity towards fat and excessive adipose tissue in the body cause a higher concentration of fat accumulation. Concentration of adipose tissue in the body depends on the excess or deficiency of heat.

Leanness of the body is most notable in cases of excessive coldness and dryness.

(3) The nature of the hair: When it comes to hair, there are several things to consider. These include how fast or slow the hair grows, whether there is a lot or a little of it, whether it is thin or thick, and whether it is straight or curly. The colour of the hair is also an important factor to take into account.

If hair growth is slow or non-existent, this can indicate a wet temperament, while fast growth can indicate a dry temperament. Thick, fast-growing hair is a sign of heat and dryness, while thin hair can indicate both wetness and dryness. Curly hair is a sign of heat and dryness as well and can also indicate complications with skin pores.

In terms of hair colour, black hair suggests a hot temperament, while brown or white hair reflects a cold temperament. Red and blonde hair indicate a moderate temperament. It's important to note that these generalizations can vary depending on race, with northern Europeans and Slavic races having different characteristics than those from the African continent, for example.

In children, having excess hair may indicate an excess of black bile. However, in elderly individuals, excess hair may be a sign that their black bile is already excessive.

(4) The skin colour: Pallor denotes loss or deficiency of blood and, therefore, a cold temperament. Yellow complexion may indicate an excess of sufra (yellow bile). A rosy complexion is a sign of excess heat and more blood. A bluish tinge points to an excess of cold, meaning that blood formation is less, and whatever little blood is formed is being congealed, thus becoming dark.

A wheaty complexion suggests heat, while purple denotes cold and dryness. A chalky colour indicates cold and phlegm, while a leaden hue indicates a cold and moist temperament tinged with black bile. This colour results from a trace of green colour in the white complexion. Ivory complexion points to a small quantity of yellow bile mixed in the cold phlegm and is often found in liver disorders. A dark yellow colour is generally seen in spleen disorders, while piles temporarily produce a greenish-yellow complexion.

The colour of the tongue can also indicate the condition of our blood vessels. Sometimes, in the same disease, the colour of one organ may differ from that of the other. For example, in the case of excessive combustion of bile, the tongue may be white, but the face may be dark.

(5) Physique or shapes of organs: A person with a hot temperament due to heat in their body will have a broad chest, long limbs, high and strong pulse and thick muscles, whereas the appearance of a person of cold temperament will have the opposite characteristics because cold hinders the growth and functional maturity of organs. The dry temperament is characterized by dry and rough skin, prominent joints, thin and prominent nasal and tracheal cartilages, and an erect nose.

(6) Reactivity of organs: If a person's organs become hot rapidly due to any cause, then they have a hot temperament, and if they become cold then the person has a cold temperament but if the skin is not affected then this is a sign of moderate temperament.

(7) Sleep and wakefulness: Moderation in sleep and wakefulness is a sign of moderate temperament, excessive sleep is a sign of moisture and coldness whereas excessive wakefulness is a sign of heat and dryness.

(8) The functions of the organs: When the organs function at a normal pace, it is an indication of a moderate temperament. On the other hand, if the rate of these functions increases, it may indicate heat, such as rapid growth of nails or hair. Extreme heat may impair several physical functions, including decreased sleep or no sleep due to Su-e-Mizaj (impaired temperament). Conversely, if there is a decrease in function, such as sluggishness and weakness, it is a sign of a cold temperament.

(9) The waste materials of the body (Fudlat): The condition of excretions such as stools, urine, and sweat can reveal whether the body is hot or cold. If the excretions have strong odours, bright colours, full maturity, and proper consistency, it is a sign of heat. On the other hand, if the excretions lack these features and have opposite characteristics, it indicates the coldness of temperament.

(10) Psychological reactions: The signs of heat-induced psychological activity are high levels of anger, deep sadness, heightened perception and memory, excessive initiative, lack of scruples, over trust, optimism, callousness, vigilance, courage, active habits, and insensitivity. Conversely, a cold temperament is characterized by opposite traits. Dryness is indicated by the persistence of joy or anger and good memory, whereas forgetfulness is a sign of excessive moisture.

The aforementioned signs are used to diagnose both innate and congenital temperaments. Below are signs that are indicative of temporarily acquired temperaments:

Signs indicating a temporarily acquired temperament

1. **Abnormal heat**: A temporary hot temperament may present with symptoms such as discomforting heat, undue distress during fevers, quick exhaustion of energy due to increased body heat, excessive thirst, inflammation of the stomach mouth (gastritis), a bitter taste in the mouth, a weak, quick, and rapid pulse, intolerance of hot foods, comfort from cold things, and distress in hot weather.

2. **Abnormal cold**: A temporary cold temperament may manifest as weak digestion, reduced desire for drinks, lax joints, a tendency for catarrhal conditions and phlegmatic fevers, improvement with hot food, and adverse conditions in the winter.

3. **Abnormal moisture**: This temperament is comparable to a cold temperament, with additional symptoms such as flabbiness, excessive salivation and nasal discharge, the tendency toward diarrhoea and indigestion, adversity from moist food, excessive sleep, and puffiness of eyelids.

4. **Abnormal dryness**: Signs of abnormal dry temperament include dry skin, insomnia, abnormal weight loss, intolerance of dry foods but comfort from eating moistening things, making the condition worse in autumn, and the body's quick absorption of hot water and light oils.

Signs of a balanced temperament

A balanced temperament is characterized by moderation in various aspects. Such aspects include heat, cold, dryness, moisture, softness, and hardness on touch. The skin colour should be intermediate between white and red, though this may vary depending on race.

The individual's physical constitution should not be excessively weak or overweight, nor should the body's vessels be too prominent or compressed. The thickness, quality, and curl of hair should be moderate. Balanced sleep and wake cycles and other bodily functions are crucial indicators of a balanced temperament. Imagination and thoughts should also be moderate, and morals, habits, and manners should be balanced and moderate as well.

Signs and symptoms of plethora/fullness ('alamat-i-imtila)

There are two types of fullness:

1. Quantitative fullness[235] of blood vessels
2. Qualitative fullness of blood vessels

a) Blood vessels can become filled and tense if the quantity of Ikhlat (humours) is increased, even if their quality is correct. This is known as quantitative fullness of blood vessels. Individuals with this condition are at risk of dangerous movements, as they may cause the vessels to rupture, potentially resulting in serious ailments like palpitation, epilepsy or hemiplegia.

There are various signs that indicate the body is full due to excessive food intake. These signs include feelings of heaviness in the organs and general weakness, the reddish colouration of the body, swelling and tension in the vessels, voluminous pulse, thickening and discolouration of the urine, impaired vision, and dizziness. Some other symptoms may include dark circles under the eyes and a general feeling of giddiness.

b) The term 'qualitative fullness of blood vessels' refers to the type of pain experienced, which is not solely caused by an excess of humours but also due to their quality. This decrease in the body's faculties can impair digestion function. If the quantity of humour is also increased, it can lead to infectious diseases such as pyaemia, toxaemia, and septicaemia.

When there is a qualitative fullness, the signs of fullness are normal as long as the amount of humour is not excessive and only the quality is compromised. However, if the humoral quantity is high and the quality is also affected, it leads to infectious diseases.

---

[235] Or repletion

Signs that indicate a dominant humour

Khilt Dam (blood humour)

Blood humour predominance and quantitative fullness share similar symptoms, including body heaviness, drowsiness, poor perception, and a dull mind. Excessive fatigue, sweet taste in the mouth, red tongue, bleeding from gums, bleeding from the nose or anus (epistaxis or haemorrhoids) are common. Boils on the body and ulcers on the tongue may also occur. The characteristic dreams include seeing red things, flowing blood, and being immersed in blood.

Khilt Balgham (phlegm humour)

Phlegm humour predominance is identified by signs like excessive pallor, flabbiness, cold and moist skin, excessive salivation, and viscid saliva. Thirst is diminished, except when acid phlegm predominates. It's typical of weak digestion, with sour belching, pale urine, sleepiness, flabby muscles, mental dullness, and a soft and slow pulse. Dreams about water, canals, cold, ice, rain, and hailstorms may denote an excess of phlegm.

Khilt Sufra (yellow bile)

Yellow bile humour predominance is identified by signs like yellowish discolouration of the eyes and skin, bitter taste in mouth, dryness and roughness on the tongue and skin, and dry nostrils that are relieved by cold air and cold water. Increased thirst and rapid and voluminous pulse. Bilious vomiting and stools, irritation in throat and stomach, tremors in the body or needle-like stinging sensation. Characteristic dreams include fire and yellow flags.

Khilt Sauda (black bile)

Black bile predominance is identified by signs like blackish discoloration of the body, dry skin, impaired senses, irritation and burning, concentrated and dark urine, excessive hair growth, black spots on the skin, and repeated spleen diseases. People with this condition often have anxiety-filled dreams that involve dark places, trenches, and frightening objects.

Signs of obstruction ('alamat-i-sudad)

When a substance is stuck in the body and causes dilation, congestion is found in the body. Such situations indicate the presence of obstruction. Obstruction can be distinguished from inflammation by the absence of fever in obstruction. The feeling of heaviness will be absent if the obstruction is formed in the narrow structures. However, there will be some disturbances in the function of the organs and some signs of anaemia.

Signs of swelling/inflammation ('alamat -i-awram)

External swellings/inflammation

Is diagnosed on inspection and palpation. But internal swelling is diagnosed by the following signs:

Signs of hot/acute swellings/inflammation (Awram harra)

The signs of acute or hot swelling can be diagnosed through visual examination and palpation. Fever is usually present in the case of hot swellings of internal organs. Sensitivity of the affected organ can result in pain, while insensitivity can cause a feeling of heaviness. Any accompanying functional disturbances can also provide important clues as to the severity of the condition. If the affected organ is accessible, it will feel swollen to the touch.

Signs of cold/chronic swellings (Awram barid)

Cold or chronic swellings do not usually present with pain and fever, but heaviness without pain is a sign of chronic swelling. Softness in swelling is a sign of phlegmatic inflammation, and hardness is a sign of melancholic inflammation.

All kinds of inflammation, i.e., inflammation that weakens the gut, hypochondria, peritoneum and abdominal wall, hurt like boils, with severe pain and fever, which causes weakness and sluggishness in the body with a tingling sensation. They also darken the eye circles. When pus is formed inside the inflammation, it reduces fever, pain and tingling sensation but causes itching instead of pain and increases heaviness.

When the swelling erupts, the burning substance produces tremors through pus, increasing the fever (toxaemia). The body becomes weak due to the evacuation of the substance, the pulse becomes parvus, slow and uneven, and the appetite is decreased. Sometimes, the hands and feet become cold after the eruption of swelling, and sometimes, the pus is excreted with faeces, urine or through the mouth.

The eruption of the swelling is sometimes beneficial and sometimes harmful. Thus, the signs of eruptions are:

- the complete cure of fever.
- the easiness in the shortness of breath.
- restoration of body faculties and substance excretion through its natural route (through faeces).

Sometimes, inflammation in the gut can spread to other organs, which can be either beneficial or harmful. It is helpful when the substance travels from the donor organ to a low organ. For instance, the inflammation in the brain can move towards the postauricular gland. However, it can be harmful when the substance moves from the lower organ towards a donor organ. For example, pleurisy can cause inflammation to travel towards the lungs or the heart.

Inflammation within the internal organs tends to spread either upwards or downwards in a characteristic manner.

When the substance inclines downwards, an individual may experience tension and heaviness in the epigastrium. Conversely, if madda (substance) inclines upwards, breathing difficulties and headaches may arise. If the substance reaches the brain, it can pose a significant threat. However, if a person experiences nosebleeds or the postauricular glands become inflamed, these are positive signs.

Signs of reeh

The presence of Reeh (Flatus or matter in a gas form) in the body can sometimes cause pain in various sensory organs. This pain can be caused by the movement of the organs or by a discontinuity in the flow of gas. The sounds of gas moving, also known as Reeh, can also indicate its presence. For instance, gurgling or palpation can be signs of Reeh. The pain associated with Reeh is usually a sensation of tension rather than heaviness.

Fasciculation, or muscle twitching, can indicate the movement of gas in the organs. This can mean that the gas is being expelled or is dissolving. Sometimes, the Reeh produces a sound, such as gurgling in the stomach. The presence of gas can also be detected through palpation of the abdomen. If there is an inflation, tumor, or swelling, it will not compress under the fingertips like Reeh does. By assessing the response of the abdomen to palpation, it is possible to determine the presence of Reeh or other conditions.

Signs of loss of continuity (alamat-i-tafarruqi-ittisa)

The loss of continuity in external organs is easily identifiable through inspection and palpation. In internal organs, the signs and symptoms of loss of continuity include:

(i) Pain which is boring, pricking, or of a corroding nature, especially without associated fever.

(ii) Discharge of some fluid, such as expectoration of blood or discharge of blood-stained pus from an existing inflammation or mature abscess. This discharge may or may not relieve the heaviness and fever, depending on whether it is from a mature inflammation.

(iii) Complete or partial displacement of an organ, as in the case of a hernia or fracture.

(iv) Stoppage of normal excretions of the body (Fudlat) expelled from ducts can cause abnormal discontinuity, for example, urine retention due to rupture of the urethra.

Sometimes, an injury may not be detected due to a lack of the signs above. In such cases, the knowledge of the specific characteristics of the damaged organ is used for diagnosis.

This can occur when an organ is insensitive, has no excretion, is too firmly attached for any displacement, or is prevented from being displaced by another organ. Inflammation and injuries of the extremely sensitive nervous tissues can be severe and may lead to fainting or convulsions. Inflammation and injuries of joints are also challenging to resolve due to movements and the predisposition of joint cavities to inflammation.

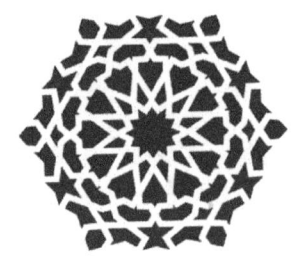

SECTION 3

PULSE, URINE & STOOL

'It's far more important to know what person the disease has than what disease the person has'.

– Hippocrates

Examining pulse, urine and stool in Unani medicine is very important in helping to diagnose a disease.

Here, the general principles of pulse, urine and stool and all their types have been explained.

Diagnosis through pulse, urine and stool is an art that can only be learned with the guidance of a good teacher. Therefore, if a student wishes to master this art, they should practice under the supervision of physicians in a clinical setting. However, the student will be able to master this art of assessment in the clinic only after learning and memorising the principles and rules related to pulse, urine and stool, which are explained in this section.

Examination of the condition and nature of the pulse is necessary to diagnose disease as abnormal changes in rhythm and regularity can indicate illness.

The Pulse (AL-NABD)

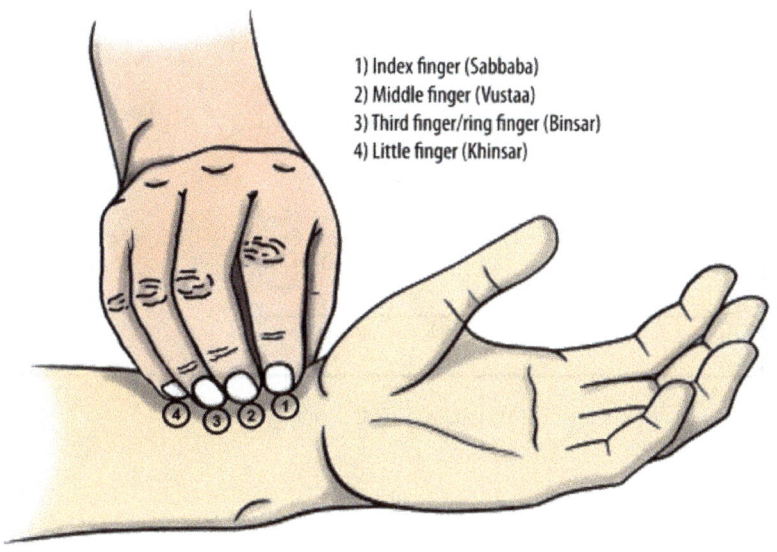

1) Index finger (Sabbaba)
2) Middle finger (Vustaa)
3) Third finger/ring finger (Binsar)
4) Little finger (Khinsar)

Definition of Pulse

The pulse refers to the rhythmic movement of the vasa of pneuma (Aw'iyah Ruh[236]) in the arteries, characterised by alternating dilatation/expansion (inbisat[237]) and contraction (inqibad[238]).

According to Ibn Sina, the main purpose of this rhythmic movement is to facilitate the modulation and management of the ruh through subtle air (Nasim[239]).

The vasa of pneuma are the vessels that contain the pneuma (life force or vital spirit). These include the heart, arteries, veins, and some vital pneuma (Ruh Haywaniyya). The pulse, however, specifically refers to the movement of the arteries and the heart.

In modern medicine, pulse is defined as the rhythmic expansion and contraction of an artery as blood is forced through it by the repeated contractions of the heart. The pulse wave results from the sudden ejection of blood into the aorta and its transmission throughout the arterial system. The pressure wave travels along the arteries much faster than the actual flow of the blood itself.

A pulse cycle

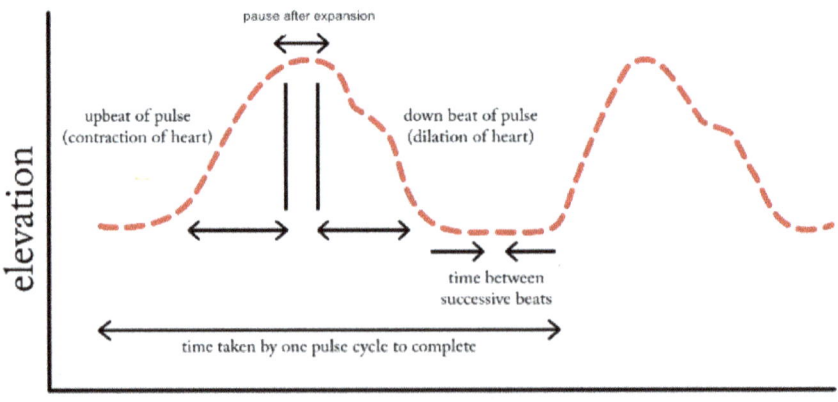

---

[236] اوعیہ روح
[237] انبساط
[238] انقباض
[239] نسیم Nasim is that part of air which is subtle or is subtle air, which through the lungs enters the blood and then to the heart to become Ruh Haywaniyya (Vital pneuma), giving life to the whole body, i.e., the process of oxygenation.

A pulse cycle consists of four components: two movements of contraction (systole) and two pauses of relaxation (diastole). These movements are: (1) contraction of pulse (Harakat-i-Inqibad), (2) pause, (3) dilatation or expansion of pulse (Harakat-i-Inbisat), (4) pause. The pause following contraction is called internal pause (Sukun Dakhili/Sukun Markazi), while the pause following dilatation is called external pause (Sukun Khariji/Sukun Muhiti).

Classical physicians have said that the reason for these pauses is that the medicatrix naturae, which is responsible for regulating the pulse, needs to rest after every contracting and dilating movement.

Movement of pulse

The movement of the heart, that is, the contraction of the heart, is related to the personal faculty of the heart, which is called the vital power (Quwwat Haywaniyya) by the physicians. This stimulating faculty is also affected by other factors. For example, when a frightening event occurs in front of someone, the heart is affected by the brain and nerves, and since the pulse is subject to the movement of the heart, in all these cases, the pulse's rate changes from the normal in proportional to the heart's response.

It's important to note that aside from the involuntary movement of blood through the arteries, there is also a natural ability for arteries to adjust their diameter as needed. This means that in the case of swelling, pain, or injury, the arteries at the affected site will dilate more than others, allowing for an influx of blood and Ruh (pneuma). Conversely, in other situations, the arteries will constrict, reducing blood flow and pneuma to the affected areas. At times, this personal movement of the arteries can even become systemic, with all the arteries in the body dilating or constricting at once for unknown reasons. It's worth noting that unlike breathing, the movement of the heart and pulse is involuntary.

What is the type of movement of the pulse?

Pulse movement have been categorised into four types:

1. Position/location change (Harakat Ayniyya[240]): This type of movement pertains to the changes in the position of the wall of an artery as it undergoes pulsations. Despite these changes, the artery remains in its fixed anatomical position within the body and does not physically shift or move. Instead, the pulsations result in dynamic changes in the artery's diameter or cross-sectional area, which gives the appearance of movement without actual displacement.
2. Change in shape or orientation (Harakat Wada'iyya[241]): This type of movement pertains to changes in the shape or size of the pulsating artery without causing significant displacement of its central position in the body. In simpler terms, the

---

[240] حرکت اینیہ
[241] حرکت وضعیہ

artery may alter its shape or size during pulsations while still maintaining its overall location within the body.
3. Quantitative movement (Harakat Kammiyya[242]): This type of movement refers to changes in the amount of certain substances that directly affect the pulse. These substances may include blood volume, hormone levels, or blood composition. Changes in the quantity of these substances can influence the characteristics of the pulse. These changes can either increase or decrease the amount of the substance, which may impact physiological processes, including the characteristics of the pulse.
4. Qualitative movement (Harakat Kayfiyya[243]): This type of movement refers to qualitative alterations within the pulsating artery. An example of such qualitative change includes variations in the temperature of the blood flowing through the artery. Changes in blood temperature can influence pulse characteristics, potentially leading to pulse rate, rhythm, or amplitude alterations. For instance, an increase or decrease in blood temperature can result in corresponding changes in pulse behaviour, reflecting the body's physiological response to temperature fluctuations.

There has been a significant debate about the nature of pulse movement. While most physicians believed that the movement of the pulse falls under the category of position change, Ibn Sina and others argue that the movement of the pulse is simply the movement of the dimensions of the artery (Harakat Wada'iyya), and the position of the artery does not change during pulsations.

Conditions for examination of pulse

1. During the pulse examination, the patient's hand should be extended towards the physician in such a way that the thumb is raised upwards. If the patient's hand is upward or downward facing, then the physician will not be able to feel the pulse properly. There will also be a difference in the normal position and length of the pulse.
2. The pulse should be observed at a time when the patient is not affected by the psychic emotions, the stomach is not full, the patient should not be experiencing severe hunger and the patient has not given up any of his habits/experiencing withdrawal.
3. The pulse of a patient should be studied in comparison with the normal pulse of a healthy and moderate person, i.e., moderate pulse should be considered as a standard[244].
4. In order to assess a patient's pulse, a physician should position their hand on the patient's wrist, specifically over the radial artery. They should then place the pulp

---

[242] حرکت کمّیہ

[243] حرکت کیفیہ

[244] Every time you take a patient's pulse, you should have a standard pulse in mind. This benchmark helps identify pulse deviations or abnormalities that can be crucial for diagnosis.

of their four fingertips: the index finger (Sabbaba[245]), middle finger (Vustaa[246]), third finger/ring finger (Binsar[247]), and little finger (Khinsar[248]), together at the end of the patient's wrist. The index finger should be oriented towards the patient's thumb, while the little finger should be directed towards the patient's elbow. This technique will enable the physician to detect the pulse and ascertain its characteristics.

5. The pulse in the patient's left hand should be checked using the right hand, while the pulse in the patient's right hand should be examined with the left hand. The physician's other free hand should support the patient's arm during the examination.
6. The fingers of the physician and especially the phalanges should not be hard and rough but they should be soft and smooth.
7. While examining the pulse, the physician should be free from all the physical and mental illnesses which can be distracting for him and disturbing his mind.
8. When examining a pulse, it is important to apply the appropriate amount of pressure based on the strength of the pulse. If the pulse is weak, apply less pressure; if it is strong, apply more pressure. This helps in estimating the strength and weakness of the pulse.
9. It is important to keep the patient's hand still when examining their pulse. Removing any bandages or other items that may apply pressure to the vessels is necessary to ensure an accurate assessment of the pulse and make a proper diagnosis.
10. The physician should not check the pulse immediately upon the patient's arrival, but it is recommended that the patient remains seated calmly in the clinic for a few minutes before the physician examines their pulse. This will help ensure an accurate reading.
11. The physician should examine the patient's pulse until they can understand the exact condition of the pulse. Some physicians have said examining the pulse for at least thirty cycles (expansion, pause, contraction, and pause) is necessary.
12. The physician and patient must be comfortable and calm during a pulse examination. They should avoid any distractions and focus solely on the examination. The physician should carefully observe the patient's face, eyes, and pulse condition with their expertise and understanding. Examining the pulse in a quiet environment is essential to accurately assess its condition and state. The physician should be satisfied with their observations before drawing any conclusions.

---

[245] سَبّابَه
[246] وُسْطىٰ
[247] بِنْصَر
[248] خِنْصَر

Methods of examining the pulse

Physicians have described different methods of examining the pulse.

1. Examining the pulse with one finger, place the index finger on the pulse in such a way that the third knuckle of the finger is towards the wrist. In this way, the different components of the pulse are felt with the same finger which is more reliable because, in the examination of the pulse with three or four fingers, all four fingers are different according to the sensory power, therefore, this difference leads to a difference in sensory input, which makes it difficult to make a definite and correct decision about the pulse.
2. Examining the pulse with three fingers. The method is common in India. Many physicians use this method to examine the pulse. In this method, the index finger is placed on the wrist together with the rest of the fingers that are positioned over the pulse of the artery. Some physicians place the index finger towards the elbow and the rest of the fingers joined together towards the thumb.
3. Examining the pulse with four fingers. It is more commonly practised in people whose pulse artery is long.
4. Some physicians usually examine the patient's hands with one hand, i.e., the right hand, and some physicians examine the pulse of the right hand of the patient with their right hand and the pulse of the left hand with their left hand.

However, assessing the symmetry of the pulse on both sides is crucial. The pulse can differ between the two sides for various reasons, including an anomalous radial artery, compression of the artery vessel, an atheromatous plaque from atherosclerosis, or embolization leading to blockage. Recognizing any discrepancies in the pulse is essential to diagnose these potential underlying issues.

Reason for examining the pulse at the wrist

1. The radial artery (Shiryan Zandi 'Ala[249]) is easily accessible and palpable.
2. This artery is more directly connected to the heart than other arteries, giving a clearer indication of heart activity.
3. For female patients, examining the radial artery avoids modesty concerns associated with exposing other body parts.
4. Its superficial location, not obscured by muscles, simplifies the examination process.
5. The radial artery carries a greater volume of blood and ruh (pneuma/oxygen) than narrower arteries, providing a more detailed assessment.

---

[249] شریان زندی اعلی

Parameters which describe the pulse (adilla nabd[250]):

The pulse's parameters, indicators, or clues are essential aspects related to the pulse that elucidate the body's conditions. There are ten primary parameters:

1. **Amount of Expansion of Pulse (Miqdar Inbisat[251])**: Reflects how much the artery expands during each pulse.
2. **Strength of Pulse (Kayfiy'e Qar'[252])**: This pertains to the force exerted by the pulse against the arterial wall.
3. **Duration of the movement of Pulse (Zamana-i-Harakat[253])**: Represents the active phase's length during each pulse cycle.
4. **Period of Pause (Zamana-i- Sukun[254])**: Indicates the length of rest between each pulse beat.
5. **Texture of the Arterial Wall (Qiwam-i-Ala[255])**: Describes the elasticity felt in the arterial wall during palpation.
6. **Emptiness and Fullness (Khala wa Imtila[256])**: Refers to the pulse's volume or fullness.
7. **The Feel of Touch/ Temperature Sensation (Malmas[257])**: Relates to the temperature or tactile feel of the pulse upon touch.
8. **Uniformity and Variability (Istiwa wa Ikhtilaf[258])**: Indicates whether the pulse is consistent (regular) or varies in its rhythm, possibly at different beats or within a single beat.
9. **Regularity and Irregularity (Nizam wa' Adm-i- Nizam[259])**: Defines the pulse's overall rhythm, discerning between rhythmic and arrhythmic patterns.
10. **Measurement (Wazn[260])**: Compares the durations of both the movement and the pause phases of the pulse.

---

[250] ادلّه نبض
[251] مقدار انبساط
[252] کیفیت قرع
[253] زمانه حرکت
[254] زمانی سکون
[255] قوام آله
[256] خلاء و امتلاء
[257] ملمس
[258] استواء و اختلاف
[259] نظام و عدم نظام
[260] وزن

Amount of Expansion of Pulse

(Miqdar Inbisat)

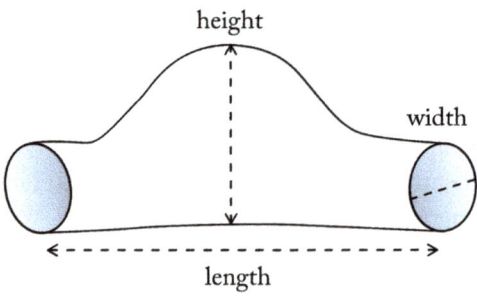

Three diameters of pulse

There are nine simple types of pulse in terms of Miqdar Inbisat of pulse:

Nabd Tawil[261] **(Long pulse - Pulsus longus):** This type of pulse exhibits an expansion that extends beyond the fourth fingertip when measured against the examining hand, indicating a longer duration of arterial expansion during the cardiac cycle.

Nabd Qasir[262] **(Short pulse - Pulsus curtus):** This pulse feels shorter in expansion compared to a moderate pulse, typically not reaching the length of four fingers when palpated, suggesting a quicker arterial contraction.

Nabd Mu'tadil[263] **(Moderate pulse in terms of length):** It represents a pulse that achieves a balanced state in terms of expansion, neither too long nor too short, extending approximately the breadth of four fingers.

Tawil pulse is the length of the pulsating artery felt under the fingers, not the actual resting length. The segment's length depends on the blood volume and pressure within the artery.

A weak pulse cannot resist the pressure of the physician's fingertips and disappears under two or three fingers. A strong pulse resists the pressure of the fingers and travels beyond all four fingers. A pulse felt under less than four fingers is Nabd Qasir or short pulse, and one felt beyond the four fingers is Nabd Tawil or long pulse.

A longer pulse often indicates normal or hyperdynamic cardiac output, but factors like vessel texture can also affect its length. Soft vessels compress easily, while harder ones require more pressure to obstruct blood flow.

---

261 نبض طویل
262 نبض قصیر
263 نبض معتدل

Nabd 'Arid[264] **(Broad pulse - Pulsus latus):** It is the pulse that pulse feels wider than the moderate state of width of the pulsating artery. The artery expands more in its transverse diameter. It also means that the area of contact between the artery and finger is more.

Nabd Dayyiq[265] **(Narrow pulse - Pulsus strictus):** Opposite of Broad pulse. Here the pulsating artery feels narrower or thinner than normal

Nabd Mu'tadil (Moderate pulse in terms of breadth): It is the pulse that is between the broad and narrow.

The 'Tawil pulse' is the length of the artery's expansion that can be felt under the examining fingers. The blood volume and the intravascular pressure at the time of examination determine this.

A weak pulse may disappear easily, notwithstanding the gentle pressure of two or three fingers, while a strong pulse can be felt even under pressure applied by all four fingers. A pulse felt under the breadth of less than four fingers is known as a 'Nabd Qasir' or short pulse, and one that travels beyond is recognized as a 'Nabd Tawil' or long pulse.

A longer pulse may indicate a higher volume of blood being pumped with each heartbeat or a dynamic state of the circulatory system. The texture of the vessels can also influence the perceived expansion; more compliant vessels may present a different palpation experience compared to those with less compliance.

Nabd Mushrif[266] **(Elevated pulse):** The expansion of this pulse is significant in terms of height, presenting an outward-extending appearance. Classically compared to the 'water hammer pulse,' due to the similar sensation of a forceful and rapid pulsation. In modern terminology, it closely resembles the 'bounding pulse'. With this type, the upbeat notably rises above its customary level.

Nabd Munkhafid[267] **(Low pulse/depressed pulse):** This pulse contrasts the elevated pulse with its diminished expansion, resulting in a pulse height below the standard norm. This suggests the artery might be refraining from its usual expansion, giving off a feeling of a subdued or weakened pulse.

Nabd Mu'tadil (Moderate pulse in terms of height): A pulse that is neither too high nor too low is considered 'Mu'tadil' or moderate. This type of pulse indicates a balanced state where the qualities of the pulse are neither excessive nor deficient, implying a state of equilibrium within the body.

---

[264] نبض عريض
[265] نبض ضيق
[266] نبض مشرف
[267] نبض منخفض

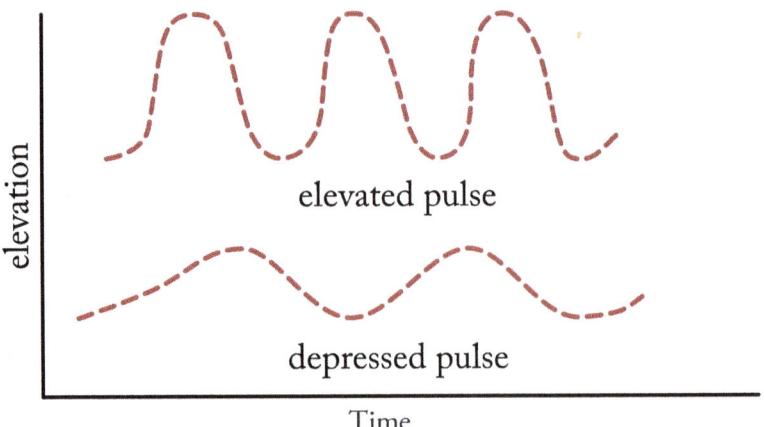

Comparison of Elevated and Depressed Pulse Patterns

There are three types of pulse in terms of length, breadth and height: (1) long, broad and elevated pulse, (2) short, broad and elevated pulse (3) moderate, broad and elevated pulse, then each of them has nine types (9). Thus, according to the quantity (3 x 9 = 27) types are formed as mentioned in the table below.

No.	Length	Width	Height
1	Long (Tawil)	Broad (A'rid)	Elevated (Mushrif)
2	Long (Tawil)	Broad (A'rid)	Moderate (Mu'tadil) in Height
3	Long (Tawil)	Broad (A'rid)	Low (Munkhafid)
4	Long (Tawil)	Moderate (Mu'tadil) in Width	Elevated (Mushrif)
5	Long (Tawil)	Moderate (Mu'tadil) in Width	Moderate (Mu'tadil) in Height
6	Long (Tawil)	Moderate (Mu'tadil) in Width	Low (Munkhafid)
7	Long (Tawil)	Narrow (Dayyiq)	Elevated (Mushrif)
8	Long (Tawil)	Narrow (Dayyiq)	Moderate (Mu'tadil) in Height
9	Long (Tawil)	Narrow (Dayyiq)	Low (Munkhafid)
10	Moderate (Mu'tadil) in Length	Broad (A'rid)	Elevated (Mushrif)
11	Moderate (Mu'tadil) in Length	Broad (A'rid)	Moderate (Mu'tadil) in Height
12	Moderate (Mu'tadil) in Length	Broad (A'rid)	Low (Munkhafid)
13	Moderate (Mu'tadil) in Length	Moderate (Mu'tadil) in Width	Elevated (Mushrif)
14	Moderate (Mu'tadil) in Length	Moderate (Mu'tadil) in Width	Moderate (Mu'tadil) in Height
15	Moderate (Mu'tadil) in Length	Moderate (Mu'tadil) in Width	Low (Munkhafid)
16	Moderate (Mu'tadil) in Length	Narrow (Dayyiq)	Elevated (Mushrif)

17	Moderate (Mu'tadil) in Length	Narrow (Dayyiq)	Moderate (Mu'tadil) in Height
18	Moderate (Mu'tadil) in Length	Narrow (Dayyiq)	Low (Munkhafid)
19	Short (Qasir)	Broad (A'rid)	Elevated (Mushrif)
20	Short (Qasir)	Broad (A'rid)	Moderate (Mu'tadil) in Height
21	Short (Qasir)	Broad (A'rid)	Low (Munkhafid)
22	Short (Qasir)	Moderate (Mu'tadil) in Width	Elevated (Mushrif)
23	Short (Qasir)	Moderate (Mu'tadil) in Width	Moderate (Mu'tadil) in Height
24	Short (Qasir)	Moderate (Mu'tadil) in Width	Low (Munkhafid)
25	Short (Qasir)	Narrow (Dayyiq)	Elevated (Mushrif)
26	Short (Qasir)	Narrow (Dayyiq)	Moderate (Mu'tadil) in Height
27	Short (Qasir)	Narrow (Dayyiq)	Low (Munkhafid)

Unani medicine recognizes six of the twenty-seven types of pulse shown in the table above as particularly important, and these are described below:

1. **Nabd 'Azim (Great/Large Pulse - Pulsus Magnus):**
   The pulse is described as being long (Tawil), broad (A'rid), and elevated (Mushrif), which often indicates a condition of excess or strong vitality in the body. Such a pulse might be associated with inflammation or an abundance of certain humours.
   Significance: This pulse type is critical as it may point to the acute phase of an illness or an inflammatory condition requiring immediate attention.

2. **Nabd Saghir (Small/Shrunken Pulse - Pulsus Parvus):**
   This pulse is described as being short (Qasir), narrow (Dayyiq), and low (Munkhafid), reflecting a weakened state or deficiency of humours.
   Significance: Its presence usually indicates a lack of strength, possible undernourishment, or a chronic condition, informing the practitioner about the body's lack of robustness.

3. **Nabd Mu'tadil (Moderate Pulse):**
   This pulse is of moderate length, breadth, and height, indicating a balanced state between the large and small pulses.
   Significance: As the ideal and balanced pulse, it suggests good health and is what practitioners aim to achieve with their treatments.

4. **Nabd Ghaliz (Thick Pulse - Pulsus Grossus):**
   This pulse is broad (A'rid) and elevated (Mushrif) regardless of its length, suggesting a concentration of certain humours, like phlegm.
   Significance: This type of pulse is important for indicating sluggish bodily functions or an excess state, which might require therapeutic measures to balance or invigorate the system.

5. **Nabd Raqiq (Slender Pulse - Pulsus Subtilis):**
   This pulse's breadth and elevation are less pronounced than in a normal pulse, regardless of the length of the pulse.
   Significance: It points towards a state of dryness or a decrease in the body's fluids, which can be important in diagnosing conditions related to dehydration or humoral deficiency.
6. **Nabd Mu'tadil (Balanced Pulse in Terms of Breadth and Height):**
   The pulse's breadth and height lie between the thick (Nabd Ghaliz) and thin (Nabd Raqiq) pulses.
   Significance: This pulse indicates a state of relative equilibrium, with slight tendencies toward excess or deficiency, and it helps practitioners fine-tune their diagnosis and treatment plans.

Strength of Pulse (Kayfiy'e Qar')

The second parameter of the pulse (adilla nabd) is the strength of the pulse (Kayfiy'e Qar'), and it refers to the impact or pressure of the pulse against the fingertips. It has three types:

1. **Nabd Qawi[268] (Strong Pulse - Pulsus Fortis):** Strong pulse, is a pulse that feels forceful against the fingertips during artery expansion. This type of pulse remains pronounced even under applied pressure, indicating that it cannot be easily suppressed. It is associated with high lateral blood pressure within the arteries and corresponds to what is commonly referred to as a bounding pulse in western medical terminology. It is often observed in individuals with high blood pressure.
2. **Nabd Da'if[269] (Weak Pulse - Pulsus Debilis):** Less forceful at expansion and can be suppressed with slight pressure. Typically seen in conditions with reduced cardiac output, like shock. Analogous to the thready pulse described in western medicine.
3. **Nabd Mu'tadil (Balanced Pulse in Strength):** It is a balanced pulse in strength and is characterized by a moderate impact that is neither too strong nor too weak. Although a moderate pulse is generally considered ideal, a stronger pulse is preferred as it indicates robust health and vitality (Quwat).

Note on Pulse Strength Evaluation:

A stronger pulse is considered favourable for individuals with normal blood pressure, reflecting better overall health and vitality. However, it is important to note that this assessment does not imply that high blood pressure is also advantageous. Instead, a more pronounced pulse is seen as a positive sign within a normal range.

---

[268] نبض قوى
[269] نبض ضعیف

It is crucial to differentiate these evaluations from those made under pathological conditions such as hypertension, where the criteria for assessment would differ.

Duration of the movement of Pulse (Zamana-i-Harakat):

Understanding the time-related aspects of arterial wall movements, or pulsations, is a key element of pulse assessment. Classical texts describe each pulse cycle as having four stages: two active motions and two pauses. Under the parameter of Zamana-i-Harakat, we analyse these active stages. Pulses are categorized into three types based on their movement duration:

Nabd Sari'[270] **(Rapid pulse - Pulsus Velox):** is characterized by a faster completion of one pulse cycle with shorter expansion and contraction phases compared to normal. This is different from a fast pulse rate, which refers to the number of cycles per minute. Often observed in systolic hypertension.

Nabd Bati'[271] **(Slow pulse - Pulsus tardus):** Opposite to Nabd Sari', the pulse cycle, including the upbeat and downbeat, takes longer to complete.

Nabd Mu'tadil (Moderate in Duration of movement): The duration of the pulse cycle is neither too rapid nor too slow, representing a balanced or intermediate rate of expansion and contraction.

Note:
The term 'Sari' refers to the rapidity of a single pulse cycle rather than the overall pulse rate. To assess these durations, we focus on the time it takes for one complete cycle and not the number of pulse cycles. A 'Sari' pulse may indicate a heightened vital force (Quwat) in the body.

Period of Pause (Zamana-i- Sukun)

The pulse cycle is observed through four distinct phases: two active movements and two resting stages. The resting stage (Zamana-i-Sukun) helps assess the vitality and rhythmic quality of the heartbeat, providing insights into the individual's overall health. The evaluation of the pause between pulses leads to the identification of three pulse types:

1. **Nabd Mutawatir**[272,273] **(uninterrupted pulse - Pulsus frequens):** Characterised by a brief resting stage between beats, resulting in a sensation of almost continuous pulses. The short pauses give the impression of a rapid succession of pulses.

---

[270] نبض سریع

[271] نبض بطی

[272] نبض متواتر

[273] Also known as Nabd Mutadarik (نبض متدارک) and Nabd Mutakathif (نبض متکاثف).

2. **Nabd Mutafawit**[274] **(interrupted pulse - Pulsus rarus):** When the heart takes a longer pause than usual between consecutive beats, it is known as a prolonged resting phase. A slower pulse rate characterizes this pattern and can be normal in athletes or could indicate an abnormally slow resting heart rate (bradyarrhythmias) and heart blocks. The intervals between pulses may be consistent (regularly interrupted) or irregular (irregularly interrupted).
3. **Nabd Mu'tadil (Moderate in period of pause):** The pulse type that represents a balance between the uninterrupted and interrupted pulses, with pauses that are neither too short nor too long, is considered moderate in rhythm. It is typically viewed as a sign of a balanced physiological state.

Distinguishing Rapid Pulse (Pulsus Velox) from Uninterrupted Pulse (Pulsus Frequens):

- **Pulsus Frequens** is characterized by a shortened period of pause between beats. The focus here is on the frequency of the pulse—the beats are frequent, and the pauses are minimal, making the pulse feel almost continuous.
- **Pulsus Velox**, on the other hand, is recognized by a shortened period of movement during each beat. This means that the expansion and contraction of the artery occur more quickly, but this does not necessarily affect the frequency of the pulse.

The key difference lies in the aspect of the pulse cycle being shortened: **Pulsus Frequens** affects the pause, and **Pulsus Velox** affects the movement. Clinically, this distinction is important because it may point to different underlying conditions or states of the body.

Texture of the Arterial Wall (Qiwam-i-Ala)

The texture, which includes the hardness or softness of the arterial wall, can be categorized into three types

1. **Nabd Layyin**[275] **(Soft pulse - Pulsus Mollis):** This type of pulse is characterized by its ease of compression when pressure is applied. It indicates a soft arterial wall, which can be compressed without much resistance.
2. **Nabd Sulb**[276] **(Hard pulse - Pulsus Durus):** In contrast, this pulse signifies an arterial wall that feels hard and is difficult to compress. This is often due to arteriosclerosis, where vessels become stiff. This rigidity can lead to a decrease in the internal diameter of the artery, giving it a hard feeling upon examination.
3. **Nabd Mu'tadil (Moderate in terms of softness and hardness):** The texture of an arterial wall can be classified as moderate when it does not feel too hard or

---

274 نبض متفاوت
275 نبض ليّن
276 نبض صلب

too soft. This indicates that the wall tension is balanced, which is an ideal state for arteries. It implies a healthy balance, enabling blood to flow smoothly through the arteries.

Emptiness and Fullness (Khala wa Imtila)

The feeling of emptiness or fullness of a pulse is related to the volume of blood in the circulatory system. Changes in blood volume can result from various clinical conditions:

1. **Nabd mumtali**[277] **(Full Pulse - Pulsus Plenus):** This is a strong, full pulse that resists compression, indicating a higher volume of blood within the artery. This type of pulse might be observed in conditions where the heart is forcefully pumping a large volume of blood, such as in hypertensive states or during fever.
2. **Nabd khali**[278] **(Empty pulse - Pulsus Vacuus):** This pulse feels weak and is easily compressed, suggesting a lower volume of blood in the artery. It can be felt in conditions such as dehydration, after significant blood loss, or in cases of shock where peripheral vasoconstriction leads to a diminished pulse.
3. **Nabd Mu'tadil (Moderate fullness):** A pulse with a moderate feeling of fullness; it represents a balanced state between emptiness and fullness. This is the normal pulse one might expect to find in a healthy individual, with neither an excess nor a deficit in blood volume.

The Feel of Touch/ Temperature Sensation (Malmas)

When examining a patient, a physician may touch the artery to evaluate the temperature of that particular location. The pulse temperature may be cooler or warmer than the surrounding body area. In Unani medicine, it is understood that the temperature of a pulsating artery can be distinct from the rest of the body's surface based on the concept that arteries, which transport oxygen-rich blood and the vital spirit (Ruh), directly connect with the heart's activity. Therefore, a temperature variation may be felt where the artery is palpated. Based on the temperature felt at the pulsating artery, the pulse is classified into three categories:

1. **Nabd Harr**[279] **(Hot Pulse):** The artery feels warmer than the patient's general body temperature. This could be indicative of inflammatory processes or feverish conditions.
2. **Nabd Barid**[280] **(Cold Pulse):** The artery feels cooler than the surrounding body temperature upon palpation, which may suggest poor circulation or systemic conditions affecting blood flow (e.g., due to blockages).

---

277 نبض ممتلى
278 نبض خالی
279 نبض حار
280 نبض بارد

3. **Nabd Mu'tadil (Moderate temperament):** The temperature of the artery is typically in balance with the patient's body temperature, indicating a healthy state.

Uniformity and Variability (Istiwa wa Ikhtilaf)

In the study of Uniformity and Variability (Istiwa wa Ikhtilaf), we examine the pulse for consistency across:

1. Different pulse cycles.
2. Various stages within the same pulse cycle.
3. A particular stage of a pulse cycle, in terms of five variables: largeness and smallness, strength and weakness, swiftness and sluggishness, rapidity and slowness, and hardness and softness.

Pulses are classified based on their uniformity into two main types:

1. Nabd Mustawi[281] (equal/uniform pulse - Pulsus aequalis)
2. Nabd Mukhtalif[282] (unequal/Variable pulse - Pulse Pulsus inequalis)

Nabd Mustawi (Uniform/Equal Pulse - Pulsus aequalis): Has two types:

- **Nabd Mustawi Mutlaq[283] (Absolutely Uniform Pulse):** This pulse is uniform across all five mentioned properties
- **Nabd Mustawi Muqayyad[284] (Specifically Uniform Pulse):** The pulse is uniform in one of the five properties but varies in the others. For example, a pulse uniform in strength alone would be termed 'Uniform in strength'.

Nabd Mukhtalif (Variable/Unequal Pulse - Pulsus inaequalis): Has two types:

- **Nabd Mukhtalif Mutlaq[285] (Absolutely Variable Pulse):** This pulse varies in all five properties.
- **Nabd Mukhtalif Muqayyad[286] (Specifically Variable Pulse):** The pulse varies specifically in one property. For example, if it varies in rapidity, it would be termed 'Variable in rapidity'.

---

[281] نبض مستوی
[282] نبض مختلف
[283] نبض مستوی مطلق
[284] نبض مستوی مقید
[285] نبض مختلف مطلق
[286] نبض مختلف مقید

Pulse Segmentation Based on Examining Fingers:

The pulse is also analyzed based on the segments under the examining fingers — index, middle, ring, and little finger — with each segment potentially exhibiting different characteristics.

Variability in Pulse Segmentation:

- **Ikhtilaf Sanai** [287] **(Two-Segment Variability):** Variability is present in two properties, with no variability in the other two.
- **Ikhtilaf Salasi** [288] **(Three-Segment Variability):** Variability is present in three properties, with no variability in one.
- **Ikhtilaf Rubai'** [289] **(Four-Segment Variability):** Variability is present in all four properties.

Variability in Movement and Position:

Variability can occur in terms of position (directions: up, down, front, back, right, and left) or in the nature of the pulse's movement (fast and slow, early and late, strength and weakness, big and small).

Specific Forms of Irregular Pulse:

- **Nabd Munqati'** [290] **(Intermittent Pulse or Dropped Pulse):** Characterized by a perceivable gap in the pulse under one finger, indicating a temporary cessation of the pulse wave.
- **Nabd 'A'id** [291] **(Reverting pulse):** A pulse that changes in size (from large to small or vice versa) as it moves to a different segment.
- **Nabd Mutassil** [292] **(Continuously Irregular Pulse):** Characterized by a continuous, gradual variability without distinct separation between changes.
- **Nabd Mutadakhil** [293] **/Nabd Dhu'l Qar'atayn** [294] **(Pulsus duplex/Dicrotic Pulse):** A pulse where two beats are felt as one due to overlapping beats.

Examples of continuously irregular pulse include:

- A pulse that gradually transitions from small to large, or vice versa.

---

[287] اختلاف ثنائی
[288] اختلاف ثلاثی
[289] اختلاف رباعی
[290] نبض منقطع
[291] نبض عائد
[292] نبض متصل
[293] نبض متداخل
[294] نبض ذو القرعتین

- A pulse that changes from fast to slow, or vice versa.
- A pulse that varies from moderate to either fast or slow, or vice versa, without abrupt changes.

Regularity and Irregularity (Nizam wa' Adm-i-Nizam)

In the study of pulse, we observe variations that may occur within a single pulse cycle or across several cycles. The pattern of these variations leads to the classification of the pulse into two main categories:

1. **Nabd Mukhtalif Muntazim**[295] **(Regularly Irregular Pulse):** This type of pulse displays variations that follow a recognizable pattern. It is subdivided into:
   - **Nabd Mukhtalif Muntazim mutlaq**[296] (Generally Regularly Irregular Pulse): Here, one particular irregularity repeats consistently.
   - **Nabd Mukhtalif Muntazim Da'ir**[297] (Cyclically Regularly Irregular Pulse): This pulse exhibits a cycle where two or more irregularities recur in a predictable sequence.
2. **Nabd Mukhtalif Ghayr Muntazim**[298] **(Irregularly Irregular Pulse):** This pulse does not follow any discernible order in its variations and is frequently an indication of serious underlying health issues.

Modern western medicine employs similar classifications, particularly in diagnosing cardiac arrhythmias, and in Unani medicine, the patterns of arterial pulses can also indicate irregularities due to various cardiac conditions.

Measurement (Wazn/Comparison of Duration of Movements and Pauses)

In Unani medicine, the term 'Wazn' refers to the measurement or comparison of the durations of active pulse movements, which include both contraction and dilatation and the pauses or rest periods between them. This principle was described by Ibn Sina.

The main objective of Wazn is to compare the duration of the active phase (movement) with that of the passive phase (pause) and not to compare one active movement of the pulse with another. This is because the latter falls under the scope of uniformity and variability (Istiwa wa Ikhtilaf) and discussed there.

According to the principle of Wazn, pulses can be categorized based on their rhythmic quality, which should correspond to the individual's age:

---

[295] نبض مختلف منتظم
[296] نبض مختلف منتظم مطلق
[297] نبض مختلف منتظم دائر
[298] نبض مختلف غير منتظم

1. **Nabd Jayyid al-Wazn**[299] **(Eurhythmic Pulse):** This pulse has a rhythm that is considered normal or appropriate for the person's age group, indicating a balance between the active and passive phases.
   Clinical Implication: This rhythm is usually found in a state of health and does not require intervention.
2. **Nabd radi-al Wazn**[300] **(Dysrhythmic Pulse):** This pulse has a rhythm that deviates from what is expected for the individual's age. Dysrhythmic pulses can be further classified into:
   a. **Nabd Mutaghayyir al-Wazn**[301] **(Pararythmic Pulse):** The pulse rhythm resembles that of an adjacent age group, such as when the pulse of a child takes on characteristics typical of a young adult's pulse.
   Example: A teenager exhibiting a pulse characteristic of a child may be undergoing certain developmental changes or experiencing a humoral imbalance.
   Clinical Implication: The practitioner might consider lifestyle adjustments or interventions to support the transitional phase or address the imbalance.
   b. **Nabd Mubayan al-Wazn**[302] **(Disproportionate Rhythm Pulse):** Here, the pulse rhythm shifts to resemble that of a non-adjacent age group, such as a child's pulse mimicking the rhythm of an elderly person's pulse.
   Example: An elderly person whose pulse resembles that of a much younger individual could indicate excessive or depleted vital energy or an underlying pathological condition.
   Clinical Implication: Detailed assessment and possibly immediate therapeutic measures may be warranted to address the underlying issues.
   c. **Nabd Kharij al-Wazn**[303] **(Arrhythmic Pulse):** The pulse's rhythm is irregular and does not align with any standard age-related pattern.
   Example: A pulse that does not correspond with any age-related pattern could be observed in severe systemic conditions or complex humoral disturbances.
   Clinical Implication: Such a pulse often suggests a critical state requiring urgent and comprehensive medical attention.

By analysing the rhythm and comparing it with the individual's age, Unani practitioners gain insight into the humoral dynamics at play within the body. The pulse serves as a window into the patient's inner workings, and changes in Wazn may signal shifts in humoral balance, pointing to potential health issues that may require intervention.

---

[299] نبض جيد الوزن
[300] نبض ردّى الوزن
[301] نبض متغير الوزن
[302] نبض مباين الوزن
[303] خارج الوزن

Compound pulses

We have discussed how a pulse can vary in measurable parameters (Adilla Nabd). To assess the pulse correctly, we need to focus on all its parameters. An abnormal or compound pulse deviates in multiple ways, creating a unique pattern that Unani physicians can recognize and classify. For instance, a long pulse (Nabd Tawil) can also be broad (Nabd' Arid) and elevated (Mushrif) at the same time, which makes it a compound pulse. In theory, there can be an endless number of compound pulses if we combine different parameters. However, physicians have identified and named fourteen clinically significant compound pulses, which we will discuss now:

1. Nabd misalli[304] (Spindle-shaped / Tubercular pulse - Pulsus mesalius)
2. Nabd Dhu'l Fatra[305] (Intermittent pulse - Pulsus intercidens)
3. Nabd Waqi' fi'l Wasat[306],[307] (Supernumerary pulse)
4. Nabd Dhu'l Qar'atayn[308] (dicrotic pulse)
5. Nabd Dhanab al-Far[309] (Mouse-tail pulse- Pulsus myurus)
6. Nabd Ghazali[310] (Deer-leap/Jerking pulse)
7. Nabd Mawji[311] (wavy/ bounding pulse - Pulsus fructuous)
8. Nabd Dudi[312] (vermicular pulse - Pulsus vermicularis)
9. Nabd Namli[313] (Pulsus formicans)
10. Nabd Minshari (Pulsus serratus)
11. Nabd Mutashannij[314] (Spasmodic pulse)
12. Nabd Multawi[315] (Twisting/Wiry pulse - Pulsus retortus)
13. Nabd Murta'ish[316] (Pulsus tremulus)
14. Nabd Mutawattir[317] (Cord-like pulse - Pulsus Chordosus)

1. Nabd misalli (Spindle-shaped / Tubercular pulse - Pulsus mesalius)

Named after 'sil,' the word for tuberculosis, this pulse is rare in modern times and was historically linked to late-stage TB. This pulse appears weak and dry; it manifests in varying thicknesses along its length and may present in six distinct forms based on fluctuations in amplitude.

---

[304] نبض مسلى

[305] نبض ذو الفترة

[306] Also know as Nabd Mutadakhil or Nabd Mitraqi

[307] نبض واقع في الوسط

[308] نبض ذو القرعتين

[309] نبض ذنب الفار

[310] نبض غزالى

[311] نبض موجي

[312] نبض دودي

[313] نبض نملى

[314] نبض متشنج

[315] نبض ملتوى

[316] نبض مرتعش

[317] نبض متوتر

It has the following forms:

1. Fluctuate from low to high order and then ends at low from high order. This pulse is thick in the middle and thin on the ends. It is also called Nabd Ma'il al-Wast[318] and Nabd Munhadir[319].
2. It tends to fluctuate from high to low order and then returns to high from low, i.e., it is thin in the middle and thick on the ends. This type of pulse is also called Nabd 'Amiq Munhani[320] and Ma'il al Tarfayn.[321]
3. Fluctuates from low to high order and then moves from high to low but stops before the extremity.
4. Fluctuates from high to low order and then moves from low to high order but stop before extremity.
5. Fluctuates from low to high order and then moves from high to low but go beyond extremity.
6. Fluctuates from high to low order and then moves from low to high order but go beyond extremity.

2 & 3. Nabd Dhu'l Fatra (Intermittent pulse - Pulsus intercidens) and Nabd Waqi' fi'l Wasat (Supernumerary pulse)

A pulse cycle consists of four stages, with two pauses between opposite motions. At the peak of each relaxation or outward movement of the vessel, there is a brief pause before the contraction or inward movement occurs. If we feel a loss of motion or pause during the expanding stage of the arterial wall before reaching the highest peak, it is called Nabd Dhu'l Fatra (Intermittent pulse). This pulse refers to an abnormal, extra, and unexpected pause in the moving phase of the pulse. On the other hand, if we find movement in the arterial wall at a point when rest is expected, it is known as Nabd Waqi' fill Wasat (Supernumerary pulse). This pulse is the opposite of Nabd Dhu'l Fatra. In between the opposite motions of expansion and contraction movement, there is supposed to be a brief pause. However, in the Nabd Dhu'l Fatra pulse, we feel that the pause is masked by an abnormal movement at this stage. Therefore, an extra stroke appears between two movements, which is named as such. In the case of the Nabd Waqi' fi'l Wasat pulse, an abnormal pulse beat overlaps the normal pulse cycle during the phase of normal pause. According to Unani medicine, the cause of Nabd Waqi' fi'l Wasat pulse is believed to be due to extra heat. Various hot mizaj diseases may cause this extra heat. It is believed that this extra heat energy sets the pulse in motion at the pause stage. However, this extra energy is always abnormal.

---

318 نبض مائل الوسط
319 نبض منحدر
320 عميق منحنى
321 مائل الطرفين

4. Nabd Dhu'l Qar'atayn (Dicrotic pulse – Pulse with two beats)

The concept of a compound pulse can be interpreted differently by different physicians. Some consider it to be a single-beat pulse, while others consider it to be a coupled beat pulse. Essentially, a compound pulse occurs when two pulse cycles overlap to appear as one, or when one pulse cycle appears to be composed of two overlapped pulses.

5. Nabd Dhanab al-Far (Mouse-tail pulse- Pulsus myurus)

It is a type of pulse in which the inequality gradually increases from low to high or decreases from high to low. This inequality occurs regarding largeness and smallness, strength and weakness, or rapidness and slowness. However, the inequality, which is more characteristic of this pulse, is large and small.

There are three types of Nabd Dhanab al-Far (Mouse-tail pulse):

1. **Nabd Dhanab al-Far Munqadi**[322] **(elapsed mouse-tail pulse)** : Mouse-tail pulse which is irregular in the expansion of the beat and starts as a large pulse but does not end on a definite limit of smallness.
2. **Nabd Dhanab al- Far Thabit**[323] **(continuous mouse-tail pulse)** : Mouse-tail pulse which starts as a large pulse and ends as a small pulse.
3. **Nabd Dhanab al- Far 'A'id**[324] **(recurrent mouse-tail pulse)** : Mouse-tail pulse which starts as a large pulse and ends as a small pulse, after that rebounding to the state of a large pulse.

6. Nabd Ghazali (Deer-leap/Jerking pulse)

A compound pulse which has its beats sluggish in the initial phase but then increases its speed and becomes fast, similar to a deer's leap.

The difference between Nabd Ghazali (Deer-leap pulse) and Nabd Waqi' fi'l Wasat (Supernumerary pulse) is that in the jerking pulse, the second beat occurs before the first beat ends. On the other hand, in Nabd Waqi' fi'l Wasat pulse, the beat of the second movement occurs during the pause period after the first beat ends.

In a Deer-leap, the segments of the same expansion vary in terms of rapidness and slowness. This means that the first part of an expansion becomes slow and the second part becomes fast. In Nabd Waqi' fi'l Wasat pulse, the period of pause occurs after the second beat ends.

---

[322] نبض ذنب الفار منقضي
[323] نبض ذنب الفار ثابت
[324] نبض ذنب الفار عائد

7. Nabd Mawji (Wavy/ bounding pulse - Pulsus fructuous)

Is a type of pulse that can fluctuate in many ways. It can be large or small, elevated or depressed, broad or narrow, fast or slow, frequent or rare, and hard or soft. This type of pulse is compared to the waves of a river due to its similarity, hence the name wavy pulse.

8. Nabd Dudi (Millipede or vermicular pulse - Pulsus vermicularis)

Similar to the wavy pulse, yet distinguished by its small size and frequent beats, this pulse imitates the movement of a many-legged worm.

9. Nabd Namli (Ant-like pulse - Pulsus formicans)

Smaller and more frequent than the vermicular pulse, the ant-like pulse is faint and can resemble the sensation of an ant's motion under the fingers.

10. Nabd Minshari (Pulsus serratus)

Rapid, frequent, and varying in hardness, the segments of this pulse are reminiscent of saw teeth, giving it its name (Minshari).

The main difference between Nabd Mawji (wavy pulse/bounding pulse) and Nabd Minshari (Pulsus serratus) is that while both have segments that are unequal in terms of elevation, depression, breadth, narrowness, progression, and delay, but the Nabd Minshari (Pulsus serratus) pulse may feel harder, even though its segments may vary in hardness.

11. Nabd Mutashannij (Spasmodic pulse)

This pulse is marked by repetitive convulsive movements, similar to spasms.

12. Nabd Multawi (Twisting pulse/Wiry pulse - Pulsus retortus)

It can feel like a twisted thread or a tense wire, offering a tactile sensation that indicates its wiry quality.

13. Nabd Murta'ish (Pulsus tremulus)

Compound pulse, which is feeble and trembling.

14. Nabd Mutawattir (Cord-like pulse - Pulsus Chordosus)

This is a type of pulse that is similar to the Nabd Murta'ish (Pulsus tremulus). The difference between them is that the Nabd Mutawattir feels tense rather than vibrating. It is similar to a string that is pulled from one side and becomes tense. Moreover, the tension in Nabd Mutawattir may be inclined towards one side or both sides.

Normal pulse (Nabd tibbi[325])

A Normal Pulse, is a composite assessment of pulse characteristics within normal ranges. These characteristics serve as a baseline for understanding variations indicating specific health conditions.

1. **Expansion of the Pulse:** It expands moderately, suggesting a balanced blood flow without excessive force or weakness.
2. **Strength of Pulse:** The pulse feels firm, indicating healthy cardiac output and vital energy without being overly forceful or feeble.
3. **Period of Movement:** The duration of each pulse beat is consistent, reflecting a steady heart rate and regular circulation.
4. **Consistency of the Arterial Wall:** The arterial wall presents a normal tension, implying healthy vessel integrity and tone.
5. **Volume of the Pulse:** It has a moderate fullness, suggesting an optimal blood volume being pumped with each heartbeat.
6. **Taction:** The pulse is neither too soft nor too hard when felt, indicating a balance in the bodily fluids and humours.
7. **Period of Pause:** The interval between beats is regular, indicating a balanced cardiac rest and rhythmic heartbeat.
8. **Synchronicity of the Pulse/Equality and Inequality:** It maintains a uniform tempo across successive beats, signifying systemic harmony.
9. **Rhythm of Pulse:** The rhythm is consistent, aligning with a normal, healthy physiological state.
10. **Comparison of Duration of Movements and Pause of the Pulse:** The balance between the active and rest phases of the pulse is equal, indicating a healthy cardiac cycle.

Equal pulse - pulsus aequalis (Nabd mustawi)

Nabd Mustawi can also be called a normal pulse (Nabd Tibbi) in terms of balance and rhythm and can be characterised as:

- **Equal in terms of equality and inequality:** The beats are uniform in force and frequency, denoting a stable cardiac and systemic condition.
- **Regular in terms of rhythm:** There is a consistent pattern to the beats, which is indicative of a healthy heart rhythm.
- **Strong in terms of strength:** The pulse conveys good strength, reflecting robust health and vitality.

---

[325] نبض طبعی

- **Rhythmic in terms of measurement (Wazn):** The timing and weight of the pulse are regular and measured, further confirming the equilibrium of the body's functions.

Causes of pulse (Asbab nabd)

These factors generate the pulse, known as causes or factors of the pulse (Asbab Nabd). They are categorized based on their role and impact on the pulse generation and its characteristics. They have been classified into two types:

1. **Retentive/Intrinsic Causes or Factors of Existence** (Asbab Masaka ya muqawwima[326])

   These fundamental factors are crucial for the generation of the pulse. Without their presence, the creation of a pulse is not possible. The retentive causes include:
   a. **Vital Power of the Heart:** This is the intrinsic energy within the heart that initiates the movement of the pulse.
   b. **Artery (Device of the Pulse):** The physical structure through which the pulse propagates.
   c. **Regulation of Body Heat:** This involves several processes:
      - **Hajat-i-tarweej (Demand for Invigoration/ Need for Activation):** This represents the body tissues' active request for essential elements, primarily oxygen and nutrients, which is especially evident during increased physical activity.
      - **Hajat-i-tatfiya (Demand for Extinguishing/ Need for Neutralisation):** This process complements the demand for invigoration (Hajat-i-tarweej) and refers to the elimination of waste products and the replenishment of tissues with oxygenated blood to maintain homeostasis.

   No changes in the pulse's inherent characteristics occur unless influenced by either Asbab Lazima (Essential factors) or Asbab Mughayyara (Non-essential factors) that accompany these retentive causes (see below).

2. Factors of Non-existence (Asbab Ghayr muqawwima[327])

   These factors do not directly create the pulse but affect its behaviour and characteristics:
   a. **Asbab Lazima**[328] **(Essential factors):** Although not directly involved in the formation of the pulse, certain factors are crucial as they bring about variations in the pulse by altering its foundational principles. These factors include:

---

326 اسباب ماسکہ یا مقومہ
327 اسباب غیر مقومہ
328 اسباب لازمہ

- Air: The quality of air and breathing patterns can significantly affect the pulse.
- Food and Drinks: Nutritional intake has a direct impact on blood quality and pulse dynamics.
- Physical Movement and Rest: The level of activity can influence the circulatory system and pulse rate.
- Mental Activity and Peace: Psychological states can alter the pulse rate and rhythm.
- Sleep and Wakefulness: The circadian rhythm affects cardiac function, thus influencing the pulse.
- Bathing and Exercise: These activities can modify body temperature and circulatory demand, affecting the pulse.

b. **Asbab Mughayyara**[329] (**Non-essential factors**) These non-essential factors refer to abnormal or atypical conditions that can influence the pulse. Although they are not regular contributors to its formation, they can affect the pulse during pathological states. This group includes disease conditions, where illnesses can cause significant deviations in the pulse's nature from the established norm, and emotional disturbances, where stress, joy, and other emotions can transiently alter the pulse characteristics.

Causes of pulse types

These are factors that influence and maintain the pulse parameters. In disease conditions, when the retaining capacity of the pulse is disturbed, we observe an altered pulse. Earlier, we listed different pulse types, and now, we will discuss the causes of each pulse type.

Causes of long pulse (Nabd Tawil)

Remember that the length of a pulse is not the length of the artery itself but rather the length of the artery segment that pulsates when touched by the fingers. When the pulse is felt beyond the fourth finger and resists the pressure of all four fingers, it is called a Tawil pulse (lengthy pulse).

The length of the pulse is determined by many factors, which can be divided into two causes: Haqiqi (essential causes) and Ghayr Haqiqi (unessential causes).

Haqiqi (essential causes) are the ones that create length in the pulse, provided the vessel is rigid. However, due to the rigidity of the pulse, the width of the pulse cannot increase, so it affects the length, and the pulse becomes longer. Thus, the causes of the long pulse are the strong demand for moderation of vital Ruh (pneuma), the strong vital power of the heart, and the rigidity of the vessel of the pulse.

---

[329] اسباب مغيره

Ghayr Haqiqi (unessential causes) appear as though they are due to anatomical changes around the arteries; however, the pulse is not actually long, for example, thinness.

Causes of Short pulse (Nabd Qasir)

Short pulses differ from long pulses because their underlying causes are also different. Short pulses may occur due to various reasons like low demand to regulate the heat of the vital pneuma (Ruh Haywaniyya), weak heart, or hard arteries. In some cases, thickness can also cause short pulses rather than thinness.

Causes of Broad pulse (Nabd 'Arid)

There are two possible reasons for a broad pulse. The first reason could be due to empty arteries or decreased blood volume, which might occur in cases of significant blood loss or dehydration. The second reason could be a softening of the arteries, which can lead to a broader and more diffuse pulse.

Causes of Narrow pulse (Nabd Dayyiq)

A narrow pulse often signifies a reduced flow of blood, as might be seen in states of shock or severe dehydration. It can also result from conditions like convulsions where arterial constriction occurs.

Causes of Elevated pulse (Nabd Mushrif)

The elevated pulse is often a result of increased body temperature or fever, causing the heart to work harder to regulate internal temperature.

Causes of Low pulse (Nabd Munkhafid)

Psychological impacts that lead to an increase in the internal movement of blood and Ruh (pneuma) while cooling the external organs can result in a low pulse. Fear or anxiety can induce such a state, deepening the pulse beneath the palpating fingers.

Causes of Large pulse (Nabd 'Azim)

When the vessels are pliable and the heart's vitality is robust, the pulse becomes strong and bounding, which can be observed in individuals with a healthy constitution or during certain inflammatory states.

Causes of Small pulse (Nabd Saghir)

A small pulse can indicate a weak heart or a heart not under duress. Unlike a weak pulse, a small pulse does not necessarily indicate a lack of strength but rather a balance or moderation of the vital forces.

Causes of Rapid pulse (Nabd Sari')

In conditions of acute need or illness, the pulse may race, striving to meet the body's demands. The rigidity of an artery can also lead to a rapid pulse if it inhibits the proper expansion and recoil that would otherwise regulate the pulse's tempo.

Causes of Frequent pulse (Nabd Mutawatir)

A frequent pulse is often a compensatory mechanism when the heart's faculty is weakened. The pulse quickens its beats to maintain equilibrium and ensure the body's tissues receive sufficient blood.

Causes of Infrequent pulse (Nabd Mutafawit)

The infrequent pulse is characterized by a heart that can generate strong beats but does so at a slower rate, often due to extreme cold or an impending decline in the body's vital forces.

Causes of Strong pulse (Nabd Qawi)

The strong pulse indicates a healthy heart that pumps blood forcefully through the arteries.

Cause of Weak pulse (Nabd Da'if)

A weak pulse can indicate that the heart struggles to perform its tasks. This may be due to several factors, such as lack of sleep, exhaustion, poor health, excessive physical labour, the accumulation of toxic humour around the heart and all types of dissolutions (Tahleelat), which may cause dissolution of the ruh, also make the pulse feeble/weak.

Causes of soft pulse (Nabd Layyin)

A soft pulse can indicate hydration or disease states such as oedema.

Causes of hard pulse (Nabd Sulb)

A hard pulse may indicate dryness within arteries, increased tension or blood pressure, or constriction due to cold.

Causes of Irregular pulse (Nabd Ikhtilaf)

An irregular pulse can be the result of congestion within the body, whether due to overindulgence in food or an imbalance in humors. There are two types of irregular pulse. Therefore, there are two different types of causes of an irregular pulse.

- **Causes of an Irregularly regular pulse (Nabd Mukhtalif Muntazim)**: When the causes of the irregular pulse are weak, i.e., there is less heaviness and congestion in the pulse, then the pulse is irregularly regular.

- **Causes of an Irregularly irregular pulse (Nabd Mukhtalif Ghayr Muntazim):** When the causes of the irregular pulse are strong, i.e., the congestion and heaviness in the pulse increase with disturbs the regularity of the pulse, then the pulse become regularly irregular pulse.

Causes of Normal/Natural pulse (Nabd Mustawi)

The ideal, regular pulse is a testament to the absence of such congestive forces, allowing the heart to beat in a rhythm consistent with health and balance.

Causes of pulse with abnormal rhythm/dysrhythmic pulse (Nabd Radi al-Wazn)

There are two forms of a dysrhythmic pulse:

- Decrease in the duration of the pause between two beats. This decrease will disturb the rhythm of the pulse and this is because the need is extreme and this decreases the duration of the pause.
- Increase in duration of the pause between two beats. It is because the weakness increases and the need decreases.

Causes of Warm Pulse

The hot nature of the touch of the artery is due to the flow of hot humour in it or the spread of Sue Mizaj mada (deranged temperament of humour) from the heart.

Causes of Cold Pulse

This is due to the coldness in the arteries, caused by the flow of cold Mizaj humour.

Causes of Full Pulse

A full pulse arises when the heart's faculty is vigorous, effectively pumping blood through well-nourished arteries. This can result from a state of optimal hydration, robust health, or an excess accumulation of blood or one of the humours in the body, possibly due to dietary habits or a lack of metabolic balance.

Causes of Empty Pulse

An empty pulse occurs when there is a deficiency in the body, such as a reduction in blood volume or essential fluids. This can be due to various factors, including dehydration, significant blood loss, malnutrition, or chronic diseases that impair the absorption or retention of nutrients and fluids.

Causes of compound pulse

Causes of Intermittent Pulse (Nabd Dhu'l Fatra)

When the body is overextended and needs rest, it may experience an intermittent pulse. This erratic pulse rhythm could result from the body's preservation mechanism that momentarily redirects energy to critical healing processes. As a compensatory reaction, the pulse may pause.

Causes of Dicrotic Pulse (Nabd Dhu'l Qar'atayn)

A dicrotic pulse occurs when the strength of the heartbeat is too strong for the vessels to expand immediately to accommodate it. Some believe that if the arteries are rigid and cannot efficiently handle blood flow, a strong heart may cause an additional beat. Conversely, another perspective is that a secondary pulsation can be felt due to backflow or reverberation of blood in the artery when there is a weaker cardiac output combined with highly compliant arteries.

Causes of Mouse-tail Pulse/Decurtate Pulse (Nabd Dhanab al-Far)

It is believed that the decurtate pulse indicates initial weakness in the heart's function, which later improves and leads to a transition from a soft, low-tension pulse to a more robust and high-tension pulse. This change in the pulse reflects the dynamic changes in the heart's pumping ability.

Causes of Deer-leap Pulse/Jerking Pulse (Nabd Ghazali)

A jerking pulse may occur due to overstimulation of the heart caused by excessive emotional or physical stimuli leading to exaggerated contractions.

Causes of Wavy Pulse/Bounding Pulse (Nabd Mawji)

The bounding pulse typically occurs when there is a strong cardiac output, and the arterial wall is highly flexible, allowing for more pronounced undulations of the pulse wave.

Causes of Millipede/Vermicular Pulse (Nabd Dudi) and Ant-like Pulse (Nabd Namli)

These pulses indicate a weak and slow rhythm, possibly due to systemic weakness. The artery subtly expands with each beat, resembling the movement of a millipede or ant.

Causes of Saw-teeth like Pulse/ Pulsus serratus (Nabd Minshari)

An uneven condition within the arteries may lead to the development of a saw-tooth pulse. This could be caused by variable consistency of substances within them or due to medical conditions like meningitis or pleurisy, which can create inconsistent arterial tension and result in a serrated pulse pattern.

Causes of a Spasmodic Pulse (Nabd Mutashannij)

In a spasmodic pulse, inconsistent vessel structure and irregular cardiac actions cause an unpredictable pulse.

Causes of Trembling Pulse (Nabd Murta'ish)

A trembling pulse can occur due to several reasons. It could be because of a strong cardiac output, a rigid vessel, and the body's high demand for circulation. On the other hand, it can also be due to weak pulsations resulting from a reduced force of the heart's contraction or when a soft vessel wall and a feeble heart function are present together.

Effects of age on the pulse

Infant's pulse

Children have a larger amount of moisture in their bodies, making their pulse softer, weaker, and faster than adults. Although their heat is strong, their overall strength is weaker due to their immature development. However, children have a larger pulse in proportion to the smaller size of their organs because their arteries are softer, and their need for oxygen is greater than that of adults. Moreover, their pulse is not as weak as expected from the smaller size of their organs. It is, of course, not as large as that of adults. It is important to note that although children's pulse is larger due to greater need, it is also quicker in speed and more rapid in rate. The greater need in children is because they eat more frequently and consume relatively more food. As a result, they have larger accumulations of vaporous products that require aeration and elimination with the help of natural/innate heat (Hararat Ghariziyya).

Pulse of young people

The pulse of youth is generally elevated, but not rapid. It decreases in frequency, with relatively stronger pulses in early youth.

Differences between the pulse of children and young people

The amount of heat in children is almost the same as in young people, so their vital signs are also similar. However, because young people have a stronger constitution, their pulse rate increases enough to reduce rapidity and frequency. In children, although the demand is higher and their arteries are softer, their pulse does not increase, but rather, they experience rapidity and frequency.

Pulse in the age of decline

Due to a weak faculty, the pulse rate is small, resulting in reduced rapidity. The low demand is another reason for decreased rapidness, leading to an infrequent pulse rate.

Pulse in advanced age

In the elderly, the pulse becomes slow and small, with a softness resulting from extrinsic rather than intrinsic moisture.

Differences in the pulse of men and women

The male pulse tends to be slower and less frequent compared to that of females. This can be attributed to their heightened vigour, greater strength, and higher metabolic demands, necessitating a larger pulse. However, any pulse with consistent strength and frequency will eventually accelerate, with speed preceding frequency. Thus, while men may have a lower pulse rate, it also exhibits a higher frequency.

Effects of temperament on the pulse

The pulse of the hot temperament people

For people with hot temperaments, their need for moderation of vital pneuma (Ruh Haywaniyya) is greater. If the heart's strength and the condition of the arteries are favourable, the pulse becomes more elevated.

The difference between innate heat and corrupted heat

The difference between innate heat and corrupted heat is that in natural/innate heat (Hararat Ghariziyya), the temperament is normal, the faculty is strong and the pulse is elevated. In the corrupted heat produced by Su'-i-Mizaj (morbid/impaired temperament), the faculty becomes weak, the innate heat is reduced, and the Ruh (pneuma) weakens.

The increase in strength of the Ruh (pneuma) is caused by both an increase in innate heat and the strength of respiration. However, an impaired temperament intensifies the heat formed in the body, leading to a weakening of the faculty. The severity of the impaired temperament further exacerbates the issue.

Pulse of cold temperament people

When someone has a cold temperament, their pulse may become depressed. This means that their pulse may become smaller and slower than usual. The smallness of the pulse is an important factor to consider. If the vessel wall is soft, the pulse may become broader and slower in both rate and speed. However, if the artery is hardening, these pulse features may not be as noticeable.

Excessive heat and cold can both cause weakness, but there is a difference in their effects. According to Ibn Sina, the weakness caused by Barid Su'-i-Mizaj (Cold impaired temperament, i.e. chronic condition) impairment is greater than that caused by Harr Su'-i-Mizaj (Hot impaired temperament, i.e. acute condition). This is because cold has a stronger ability to produce weakness than heat. Heat, on the other hand, is more easily accepted by the body's natural healing processes, making its impact less severe.

Pulse of moist and dry temperament people

The pulse of individuals with a moist temperament has a wide range and greater breadth. On the other hand, individuals with a dry temperament have a narrow and hard pulse. However, if the faculty is strong and the need is severe along with dryness, the pulse becomes Dicrotic (mutadakhil), spasmodic (mutashannij), and tremulous (murta'ish).

Effects of seasons on the pulse

Pulse of spring

During this season, the pulse is balanced in all aspects except for being slightly stronger.

Pulse of the summer

During summer, the pulse tends to be faster and more rapid due to the increased 'need' of the body. The excessive heat in the surrounding atmosphere can disperse the vital force and weaken the strength, causing the pulse to become smaller and weaker.

Pulse of the autumn

The pulse feels weaker in the autumn due to the frequent and significant changes in the morning, evening, and night winds. These changes have opposite effects on the body, leading to irregularities in the pulse. Additionally, autumn's weaker heat and excessive dryness oppose the natural state of life, leading to a weakened pulse.

Pulse of the winter

During the winter season, the pulse becomes slow, weak, and infrequent because the heart's faculty weakens due to a decrease in the moderation of vital Ruh (pneuma). This is particularly true in colder climates and for individuals with a colder and weaker temperament who struggle to endure the severity of the cold. However, in some people, the body heat builds up deep inside during winter, making the heart stronger instead of weaker. This only happens when the person's temperament is dominated by heat and is not affected or overcome by cold.

Pulse between seasons

The pulse between seasons is determined by the preceding and succeeding seasons.

Effects of a country's climate on the pulse

The climate of a country is similar to its weather conditions. For instance, in some countries, the climate is moderate and resembles that of the spring season, while in others, it is dry and similar to the autumn season. As a result, a person's pulse in those countries will be affected by the seasons that are similar to those countries, which have been described above.

Effects of food and drink on the pulse

Food and drink have an impact on the pulse in terms of both quantity and quality. The temperature of food and drink, whether hot or cold, can affect the pulse. Furthermore, the amount of food and drink consumed can also influence the pulse.

A moderate amount of food and drink can cause a balanced pulse to become larger and more frequent, increasing the body's temperature. This effect can last for some time. However, consuming a large amount of food can lead to irregularities without order in the pulse due to the exhaustion of the digestive system. If less food is consumed, the pulse irregularity follows a certain pattern. Moreover, the pulse becomes smaller and slower if even less food is consumed. This effect does not last long because the amount consumed is small and is quickly digested.

The pulse becomes small and slow when the digestive system is weakened due to overconsumption or underconsumption. However, when the digestive system is strong, the pulse returns to its normal state.

Effects of alcohol on the pulse

Alcohol, when consumed in excess, can cause an irregular and unstable pulse rate. Drinking it cold can cause the pulse rate to slow down, and the cooling effect disappears as soon as it's absorbed. On the other hand, drinking warm alcohol doesn't result in significant disruption. People who are sensitive to cold substances tend to suffer more if they consume cold alcohol because it weakens the body. Alcohol acts as a tonic and stimulant for healthy individuals. However, the hot or cold quality of alcohol can be harmful to most people.

Effects of water on the pulse

Water plays a crucial role in strengthening our body by aiding in food absorption. It has a similar effect as alcohol, but unlike alcohol, it cools down the body and reduces the need for moderation of vital Ruh (pneuma).

Effects of exercise on the pulse

During moderate exercise, the pulse becomes large and strong as the innate heat increases (Hararat Ghariziyya) and strengthens. It also becomes fast and frequent due to the body's energy needs. However, if the exercise is prolonged or intense, the pulse becomes weak due to the dissipation of innate heat. The pulse can become fast and frequent for two reasons: excessive need or weakness of the innate heat to induce a large pulse. As the innate heat declines, the pulse speed and frequency increase. This can lead to fatigue, and the pulse becomes Namli (Ant-like) due to weakness and intense frequency. Extreme exercise that brings a person close to death can cause a Dudi (Millipede/vermicular) pulse that is irregular, slow, weak, and small.

Effects of bathing on the pulse

Taking a bath in hot water initially increases the body's strength, causing the pulse to become large. However, as the strength disperses, the pulse becomes weak, small, slow, and infrequent. If the bath is taken in cold water, there are two possible outcomes:

1. If the coldness of the water is absorbed into the body, this can cause weakness, slowness, and irregularity in the pulse.
2. If the coldness of the water closes the pores and holds the body heat inside, this increases the body's strength, causing the pulse to become large while decreasing speed and frequency.

Effects of pregnancy on the pulse

The need is greater in pregnant women because the baby also inhales the same air as the mother. It is as if two needs are associated with the two lives from the mother's breath. The faculty strength, without a doubt, does not increase, or it may decrease slightly according to the fatigue of the pregnancy. Due to these reasons, the pulse of a pregnant woman is large, rapid and frequent due to high need and weak faculty.

Effects of pain on the pulse

When pain first sets in, the immune system (Quwwat-i-Mudafa'at) is activated and body heat increases. As a result, the pulse becomes large and fast but also very irregular due to the body's need for a quick response. However, if the pain is so severe that it weakens the body, the pulse becomes progressively smaller and more frequent until it becomes Ant-like (Namli) and Millipede/vermicular (Dudi).

Effects of swelling on the pulse

Swellings in the body can affect the pulse differently depending on their characteristics and the body's response to them.

Overall Impact:

Large swellings, especially those in vital organs, can induce fever and affect the systemic pulse. Even those not associated with fever can still impact the pulse locally or through pain-induced changes.

Hot Swellings:

Hot swellings can produce a rapid, trembling pulse, known as a saw-like pulse (Nabd Minshari). When no moisturising factor exists, the saw-like pulse can transition to a wavy pulse (Nabd Mawji).

Soft Swellings:

Soft swellings can create a wavy or bounding pulse (Nabd Mawji). Very cold, soft swellings may lead to a slow and irregular pulse.

Hard Swellings:

These swellings intensify the saw-like pulse characteristics.

Pustules and Pus Accumulation:

Pustules can soften the pulse, shifting from a saw-like to a wavy pulse due to the moisturising effect of pus. They also contribute to an increased variability in the pulse and a decrease in speed and frequency as the abscess matures.

Phases of Swelling:

In the initial phase, a hot swelling can cause an increase in the saw-like pulse and associated signs. At full maturity, the pulse may exhibit all signs intensively except those related to the faculty, leading to a weakened pulse with increased frequency and speed. As the swelling subsides or ruptures, the pulse strengthens due to the release of faculty pressure, and its trembling reduces due to pain alleviation.

Size and Location:

Large swellings amplify pulse disturbances, whereas smaller ones may have a lesser effect. Swellings in nervous organs often increase the hardness and saw-like quality of the pulse. Vascular swellings, especially those involving dominant arteries, can render the pulse larger and more unequal.

Effects of emotions on the pulse

Anger:

The pulse will become large, full, quick, and rapid. The abrupt expansion of the vital force during anger causes an immediate increase in pulse strength. The pulse will remain regular unless compounded with emotions such as fear or guilt.

Pleasure:

Pleasure can cause a gentle external movement of pneuma and faculty. This can lead to a possibly elevated pulse, sometimes slow and infrequent. When the body's need is met without the necessity for rapidness, the pulse will reflect a more relaxed state.

Joy:

Joy can also gently encourage the external movement of vital forces. This will cause the pulse to become large, soft, and slow. The pulse reflects a state of contentment and is not as demanding in its rhythm.

Grief:

Pulse will become small, weak, and slow. Grief internalizes and weakens innate heat, and the pulse mirrors this inward turning and diminution of energy by becoming more restrained in its expression.

Fear:

Initially, fear causes a rapid, bounding pulse that is regularly irregular. The sudden shock of fear to the system leads to an erratic pulse. If fear is prolonged, the pulse can resemble that of grief. As fear becomes a sustained state, it dampens the innate heat, causing the pulse to slow and weaken, echoing the effects of grief.

Impending death

Certain indications may suggest impending death by observing the pulse. These signs may include a soft and deformed pulse, which lacks its usual form and may indicate the loss of life forces. In combination with diminished mental responsiveness, dilated pupils, and a faltering faculty, this may signify the approach of death. Other pulse types that may indicate imminent death include the ant-like pulse (Nabd Namli) and millipede pulse (Nabd Dudi), which are characterized by their small and frequent beats. Another sign is an exceedingly rapid, frequent, and irregular pulse, especially with extreme intervals. A pulse that ceases abruptly after three strikes is considered a grave indication and is often associated with near death. A bounding or spasmodic pulse, especially one that shows irregular intervals, can signify the body's final struggle.

Condition and diseases of body and their pulses types[330]

Following is the list of specific pulses of different conditions and diseases of body that are mentioned in the authentic medical books.

Category	Condition	Pulse types
Pulse of temperaments	Normal Hot Temperament (Mizaj Harr Tab'i)	Large (Azim) and Strong (Qawi)
	Abnormal Hot temperament (Mizaj Harr Ghayr Tab'i)	Small (Qasir), Fast (sarii), and Frequent (Mutawatir)
	Cold Temperament (Mizaj Barid)	Small and Slow (Bati)
	Moist Temperament (Mizaj Ratb)	Bounding (Mawji) or Broad ('Arid)
	Dry Temperament (Mizaj Yabis)	Small and Hard (Sulb)
	Hot Bilious Temperament (Mizaj Harr Safrawi)	Small, Fast, Frequent and Hard
	Hot sanguineous Temperament (Mizaj Harr Damawi)	Large, Strong and Soft (Lin)
	Congestion of bilious substance (Imtila Safra madda)	Fast, Frequent and Full (Mumtali)
	Congestion of melancholic substance (Imtila Sawda madda)	Small, slow, Infrequent (Mutafawit) and Hard
	Congestion of phlegmatic substance (Imtila Balgham madda)	Small, slow, Infrequent, Soft, Ant-like (Namli)
Pulse of age and gender	Child	Fast and Frequent
	Age of decline	Small and Slow
	Adulthood	Large and Strong
	Advanced age	Small and Strong
	Male	Large and Strong
	Female	Small, Weak and Fast
	Pregnant	Large, Fast and Frequent
Pulse of physique	Thin	Large and Slow
	Obese	Small and Slow

[330] Pulse table amended from Usool-e-Tibb by hakim Kamaluddin Husain Hamdani

Pulse of psychological illness	Anger and rage	Large and Elevated (Shahiq/Mushrif) or Fast and Frequent
	Sudden panic, dread and sadness	Fast, Feeble and Trembling (Murta'ish - pulsus tremulus), Variable (Mukhtalif) and Infrequent, irregular (Ghayr Muntazim)
	Panic, dread and sadness (Not sudden)	Small and Weak
Pulse of sleep and wakefulness	Start of dreams	Small, Weak and Infrequent
	End of the dreams	Small, Weak and Slow
	Excessive dreams	Small, Weak and Slow
	Sleeping on an empty stomach	Small, Slow and Infrequent
	Natural awakening after dream	Large and Fast
	Waking suddenly	Weak then Large, Fast, Feeble and Trembling and Variable
Pulse of food and drinks	Food taken in moderate quantity	Large, Strong, Fast and Frequent
	Food taken in large quantity	Variable, Irregular
	A small amount of food taken	Large, Strong and Fast
	Congestion of food in the stomach	Variable
	After the digestion of food	Large, Strong and Fast
	No food taken	Small, Slow, Low and Frequent
	Drinking a moderate amount of alcohol	Large, Strong, Fast and Soft
	Drinking water	Strong
	Refreshing drinks and foods	Soft
Pulse of exercise	Start of exercise	Large, Strong, Fast and Frequent
	Moderate exercise	Large and Strong
	High-intensity exercise for a long duration	Small, Weak, Slow and Infrequent
	Exercise that exceeds moderation	Small, Weak, Slow and Infrequent
	End of exercise	Fast and Frequent
Pulse of bath	Moderate bath	Large, Strong, Soft, Fast and Frequent
	Excessive hot bath	Small, Weak, Infrequent and Slow
Pulse of seasons	Spring	Large and Strong

Summer	Small, Fast, Frequent and Weak
Autumn	Weak and Variable
Winter	Infrequent, Slow and Small

Disease conditions as seen through the pulse

Category	Condition	Pulse types
Conditions of the Head	Hot headache (Suda' Harr)	Fast and Frequent
	Cold headache (Suda' Barid)	Slow an Infrequent
	Bilious headache (Suda' Safrawi)	Small and Fast
	Sanguineous headache (Suda' Damawi)	Large and Soft
	Phlegmatic headache (Suda' Balghami)	Weak and Slow
	Melancholic headache (Suda' Sawdawi)	Small, Slow, and Hard
	Headache related to eye socket/pupil pain (Suda' hadqa)	Fast
	Acute meningitis (Qaranitus)	Large and Soft
	Hot/Acute meningitis (Sarsam harr)	Large, Fast and Frequent
	Meningitis due to predominance of yellow bile (Sarsam Safrawi)	Small, Fast, and Hard
	Cold meningitis (Sarsam barid)	Slow and Infrequent
	Meningitis due to predominance of black bile (Sarsam Sawdawi)	Small, Hard, Weak, Frequent and Variable
	Cerebrospinal meningitis (Sarsam Mukhkhi Nukh'i)	Fast
	Vertigo due to predominance of yellow bile in brain (Duwar Safrawi)	Small, Fast and Hard
	Vertigo due to predominance of phlegm in brain (Duwar Balghami)	Slow and Soft
	Vertigo due to predominance of black bile in brain (Duwar Sawdawi)	Small, Weak and Hard
	Coma (Subat)	Fast, Weak, Infrequent and Full
	Coma from anaesthetic drugs	Small, Weak, Frequent and Hard
	Amnesia (Nisyan)	Large, Weak, Slow, Infrequent and Soft
	Atony/Flaccidity (Istirkha)	Slow and Infrequent
	Hemiplegia (Falij)	Slow and Infrequent
	Facial Palsy (Laqwa)	Hard
	Apoplexy (Sakta)	Small, Weak and Infrequent

	Sanguineous melancholia (Malankhuliya Damwi)	Small, Infrequent and Hard
	Phlegmatic headache (Suda Balghami)	Frequent pulse
	Epilepsy due to predominance of black bile (Sar' Dimaghi Sawdawi)	Small and Hard
	Unconsciousness (Sakta)	Small, Weak, Slow and Infrequent
	Muscular spasm (Tashannuj)	Sinking and Fast
	Congestion in brain (Imtila Dimagh)	Slow, Full and Infrequent
	Acute coryza/catarrh (Zukam Harr)	Large, Fast, Frequent
Conditions of the Thorax	Bronchial asthma due to heart vapours (Rabw Dukhani Qalb)	Large and Full
	Pleuritis (Dhat al-Janb)	Saw-teeth like (Minshari - Serrate), Fast, Small, Frequent and Hard
	Pneumonia (Dhat al-Ri'a)	Weak, Fast, Soft and Bounding
	Phthisis (Sill)	Small, Fast, Frequent and Hard
	Morbid Hot temperament of the heart (Su'-i-Mizaj Harr Qalb)	Large, Fast and Frequent
	Morbid Cold temperament of the heart (Su'-i-Mizaj Barid Qalb)	Small, Weak, Slow and Frequent
	Morbid Moist temperament of the heart (Su'-i-Mizaj Ratb Qalb)	Slow, Soft and Variable
	Morbid Dry temperament of the heart (Su'-i-Mizaj Yabis Qalb)	Small, Weak, Frequent
	Palpitations (Khafaqan)	Fast
	Sanguineous palpitations (Khafaqan Damawi)	Large, Fast, Full
	Palpitations due increased sensitivity of heart (Khafaqan Hissi)	Large and Strong
	Syncope (Ghashi)	Small and Weak
	Endocarditis (Waram baatin Qalb)	Small, Fast and Variable
Conditions of the stomach	Stomach congestion related to food or a humour	Variable
	Stomach illnesses related to a cold humour	Small, Weak and Slow
	Weak digestion and expulsion	Weak, Soft and Full
	Diarrhoea with vomiting/food poisoning (Hayda)	Weak and Infrequent and towards end becomes Fast
	Hot (Acute) swelling in the stomach cardia (Warm Harr Fam-i-Mi'da)	Small, Weak, Frequent and Hard
	Cold (Chronic) swelling in the stomach cardia (Warm Barid Fam-i-Mi'da)	Small, Weak, Slow, Infrequent and Hard

Category	Condition	Pulse
Conditions of the Liver, spleen and gallbladder	Stomach discomfort with nausea (Karb Mi'da wa Ghathayan)	Small, Weak and Frequent
	Hot (Acute) inflammation of the liver (Waram al-kabid harr)	Large, Fast and Frequent
	Oedema (Istisqa')	Small, Weak, Frequent and Hard
	Jaundice (Yarqan)	Frequent and Hard
	Leukaemia (Ibyaz al-Dam)	Fast and Frequent
	Anaemia (Faqr al-Dam)	Fast and Frequent
Conditions of the urinary and reproductive organs	Renal ulcers (Quruh al-Kulya)	Fast, Hard and Full
	Renal colic (Qulanj Kulwi)	Small
	Cystitis (Waram al-Mathana)	Weak
	Anaphrodisia (Du'f al-Bah)	Weak, Soft and Slow
	Hot swelling of the uterus (Awram Harr Rahim)	Frequent
	Amenorrhoea (Ihtibas al-Tamth)	Slow and Infrequent
	Blood clotting inside the bladder (Jamood al-Dam fi'l Mathana)	Small
Inflammation/Swellings	Initial stage of hot (acute) swelling (Ibtida Awram Harr)	Large, Strong, Fast and Frequent
	Initial stage of hot (acute) swelling (Ibtida Awram Harr)	Fast and Frequent with Saw-teeth like and tremulus (Feeble and Trembling)
	Cold (chronic) swellings (Awram Barid)	Slow and Infrequent
	Phlegmatic swellings (Awram Balghami)	Small, Slow, Infrequent and Hard
	Melancholic swellings (Awram Sawdawi)	Small, Slow, Infrequent and Hard
	Hard swellings (Awram sulbah)	Small and Hard
	Eczema (Nar Farsi)	Fast
Pains	Pain (Waja')	Fast expansion and slow contraction
	Start of pain	Strong, Fast and Frequent
	Severe pain	Small, Weak, Fast and Frequent
	Last stage of severe pain	Ant-like
	Internal pain	Small and Weak
	Plague (Ta'un)	Fast
Fevers	Ephemeral fever/ short term fever (Humma al-Yawm)	Large and Frequent
	Ephemeral fever due to excessive anger and joy (Humma al-Yawm Ghadabiyya wa Farhiyya)	Large and Long

Ephemeral fever due to excessive hunger and thirst (Humma al-Yawm Ju'iyyah o Atashiyyah)	Small, Weak and Hard
Ephemeral fever due to insomnia, grief, and fright (Humma al-Yawm Sahriyya wa Ghamiyya Wa Faz'iyya)	Small and Weak
Ephemeral fever due to unconsciousness (Humma al-Yawm Ghashiyya)	Small and Infrequent
Ephemeral fever due to inflammation (Humma al-Yawm Waramiyya)	Large and Fast
Synochus (Continuous fever) due to Ephemeral fever (Humma al-Yawm Sunukhus)	Large, Strong, Fast, Frequent and Full
Sanguineous (where infection is intravascular) fever (Humma Mutbiqa)	Large, Frequent and Fast
Bilious fever (Humma Safrawi)	Variable
Pure bilious fever (Humma al-Ghibb Khalis)	Small, Weak and Infrequent
Phlegmatic fever (Humma Balghami)	Small, Weak and Soft
Quartan intermittent fever (Humma al-Rib' Da'ira)	Small, Slow, Infrequent and Hard
Initial occurrence of quartan fever (Ibtida Nawbat Humma al-Rib')	Slow and Infrequent
Sanguineous quartan fever (Rib Damawi)	Large and Soft
Phlegmatic quartan fever (Rib Balghami)	Slow and Soft
Bilious quartan fever (Rib Safrawi)	Fast and Frequent
Melancholic quartan fever (Rib Sawdawi)	Fast and Hard
Hectic fever (Humma Diqqiyya)	Small, Weak, Frequent and Hard
Emaciation (Dhubul)	Small, Weak, Fast, Frequent and Hard
Senile emaciation due to dryness (Diqq al-Shaykhukha)	Small, Weak, Frequent and Hard
Tertian/bilious intermittent fever (Humma Ghibb Da'ira)	Initially, the pulse is variable, then large and fast. According to Ibn Sina, during the initial period, variable, and towards the end, fast with tension. Moreover, the pulse becomes strong, rapid, and frequent when the fever rises.
Quotidian/phlegmatic intermittent fever (Humma Muwaziba)	According to Samarkandi, the pulse starts small and infrequent but becomes more frequent as the fever progresses. The pulse remains less frequent compared to in Tertian fever.

	Enteric fever/Typhoid fever (Humma Mi'wiyya)	Fast, Full, Soft and Dicrotic (Pulse with two beats)
	Epidemic fever (Humma Waba'iyya)	Frequent and Weak
	Measles (Hasba)	Fast
	Smallpox (Humma Judariyya)	Large
	Fever with delerium (Humma Ghamiya Hadhayaniyya)	Alongside the increase in heat due to the fever, the pulse becomes fast, but as the fever rises, the pulse becomes weak and small and in extreme cases, the pulse is not detectable.
During crisis period of disease	During absolute crises (Buhran Mutlaq)	Hard
	Secondary crises (Buhran Ardi)	Soft
Diseases of skin	Leprosy (Judham)	Small, Weak and Frequent
	Lepromatous leprosy (Judham Khadri)	Infrequent and Slow
	Vitiligo/Leukoderma (Baras)	Slow, Soft and Broad
Toxins/Poisons	All poisons and anaesthetic	Fast expansion and Slow contraction
	All crushed types	Slow
	Opium	Fast expansion and Slow contraction

Urine

It is understood that various diseases can impact the nature of urine, leading to abnormalities in its characteristics, including its colour, consistency, taste, and sediment components. In such cases, the analysis of urine can be of great assistance in the diagnosis of the underlying disease. Therefore, in these cases, examination of urine helps to diagnose the disease.

Conditions for examination of urine (mu'ayana qarura)

When examining urine, according to Ibn Sina, the following conditions should be considered:

- Collecting the urine sample first thing in the morning
- Ensuring the urine has not been left out for an extended period of time
- It is overnight urine
- Patient should refrain from consuming food or drink before providing the urine sample
- The patient should avoid eating foods that can alter urine colour, such as saffron, pomegranate, certain vegetables, and condiments like Murri[331], which can make urine black.
- The patient should also avoid applying anything on their skin or body that could change the colour of urine, such as henna, which sometimes makes urine black.
- Patient should not have taken any substances that could alter the urine, such as yellow bile and phlegm purgatives
- The patient should avoid engaging in abnormal activity before urinating that can raise the body temperature and affect urine colour, like hard work or walking in the sun, which can alter urine colour.
- It is important to wait until the urine settles in the container before examining it, allowing any sediments to settle down.
- It is important to keep the urine stored in a place where it is not affected by sun and heat.

By following these guidelines, the accuracy of the urine examination can be ensured.

Some out of the ordinary external states change the urine colour, such as fasting, lack of sleep, fatigue, hunger, and anger, which all change the colour to yellow or red. Intercourse markedly increases the oiliness of the urine. Also, vomiting and evacuation change the original colour and texture of urine.

---

[331] A type of fermented condiment, a mixture of salt, vinegar, ginger, black pepper, and water, is fermented to create a sour liquid, which is then strained and used.

It is important to examine urine when it is fresh. After six hours, the indicators become weak, the colour changes, and the density dissolves, changes, or becomes thicker. However, examining it within an hour is recommended to get the most accurate results.

Collecting all of the urine in a large bottle without pouring any of it out is important. After collection, the examination should be delayed until it has settled in the bottle, away from sunlight, wind, and cold. It should be recognized that not all urine will settle or be fully matured. The bottle should not be reused until it is cleaned thoroughly.

Children's urine has fewer indicators, especially that of infants because it is affected by the milk and the persistence of colouring material within it due to their weakness and prolonged sleeping; therefore, it lacks indicators of maturity.

It is important to use a transparent and pure container, such as clear glass or crystal, to examine urine. Keep in mind that the closer you look at the urine, the thicker it may appear, while from a distance, it is clearer. This is a distinguishing property for adulterated specimens that physicians look for. Once the urine is collected in a bottle, it should be protected from cold temperatures, sunlight, and wind. It should be examined without direct exposure to sunlight.

Indications from urine (dala'il bawl)

Indicators of urine include the following things.

1. Colour of the urine
2. Consistency of urine (thick or thin)
3. Clearness and turbidity
4. Sediments
5. Quantity in terms of scarcity and abundance
6. Odour
7. Froth

Initial indications of urine can be linked to the health of the liver, urinary tract, and blood vessels. Urine could indicate other medical conditions when these organs are in good health.

Clearness and turbidity are related to how visible light can penetrate a liquid. The difference between thick and thin urine and clear and turbid urine is that urine can sometimes be thick yet clear, similar to the white of an egg. On other occasions, it can be thin but turbid, like murky water.

Sediment and turbidity differ because sediment appears distinct, while turbidity particles are mixed throughout the urine.

Finally, colour and turbidity differ because the colour is evenly distributed throughout the substance, while turbidity consists of raw components that are not mixed in this way.

Indications from colours of urine (dala'il alwan al-bawl)

The colour of urine can give a clue about a person's health. Urine can appear in shades of yellow, red, white, green, and black, which can be helpful in diagnosis.

Shades of yellow urine

1. Straw-yellow urine (Bawl Tibni): This urine resembles fodder-soaked water and suggests less heat than normal urine.

2. Citron-yellow urine (Bawl Utruji): This colour is similar to that of a citron peel and is considered normal.

3. Reddish-yellow urine (Bawl Ashqar): This urine indicates some degree of heat compared to normal urine.

4. Orange-yellow urine (Bawl Asfar Naranji): This urine resembles the colour of an orange peel but has a more prominent red hue. It suggests a higher degree of heat than reddish-yellow urine.

5. Fire-Colored Urine (Bawl Nari): The color resembles that of a fire flame, indicating extreme heat.

6. Saffron-yellow urine (Bawl Za'frani): This urine appears like filaments of saffron and indicates the highest degree of heat of all the yellow urine shades.

Ibn Sina notes that from orange-coloured urine onward, all shades are indicative of heat, with the degree of heat increasing progressively. Orange-coloured urine is considered a sign of moderation, while straw-yellow urine suggests a colder state. All other types fall into the category of increased heat, often caused by intense exercise, pain, hunger, or dehydration.

Shades of red coloured urine

There are four types of red coloured urine.

1. Yellowish-reddish urine (Bawl Ashab): It is yellowish red.
2. Rose-red urine (Bawl Wardi): It is red like a rose.
3. Intense-red urine (Bawl Ahmar Qani): Very red.
4. Blackish-red urine (Bawl Ahmar Aqtam): Red dusty or blackish red.

All of these types generally indicate the predominance of sanguine in the body.

If saffron colour dominates, it indicates the dominance of bile. More blackness and turbidity in the urine indicate the dominance of sanguine.

Fire-coloured urine indicates even more heat than blackish-red urine. This is because the former is derived from yellow bile humour, which is hotter than blood humour.

In very hot diseases and ardent continued fevers, the urine is predominated by saffron and a fire colour. When it is thin, it indicates that some form of concoction is present in the urine, but the concentration is left. Bright red urine (Ahmar Nasi), indicates extreme heat.

Jaundice causes the urine to become yellow, making it blackish due to its intensity. This type of yellow urine is better because it proves that the substance is being excreted in large quantities and the body is being quickly cleansed of the morbid substance.

If the urine is white or has less yellowness in jaundice, and the jaundice is still present at its peak, then there is a risk of oedema. Hunger makes the colour of the urine darker and sharper as the substance of the disease accumulates in the body and produces oedema.

Shades of green coloured urine

There are five types of green coloured urine.

1. Pistachio-green urine (Bawl Fustuqi)
2. Verdigris-green urine (Bawl Zanjari)
3. Sky-green coloured urine (Bawl Asmanjuni)
4. Emerald-green coloured urine (Bawl Nilji)
5. Leek-green urine (Bawl Kurrathi)

Generally, shades of green-coloured urine are a sign of coldness, except for Verdigris-green and Leek-green, which indicate intense combustion/charring. However, the leek-green is safer than Verdigris.

After strenuous exercise, Verdigris-green urine can signify muscular spasms/cramps (Tashannuj). If a child has green-coloured urine, it is also a sign of spasms.

Sky-green and Emerald-green urine are indicators of intense coldness, and some believe they can indicate poisoning. In cases where there is sediment present in the urine, the patient is expected to survive; otherwise, death may prevail. Verdigris-green urine, in particular, is very dangerous.

It is worth noting that some physicians include olive-coloured urine (Bawl Zayti) in the green-coloured urine category due to the melting of fats and oily substances in the body.

Shades of black coloured urine

Jaundice may turn urine saffron-yellow colour and appear dark due to the concentration of bile or its conversion into black bile (Sauda). If there is a dark red shade in the urine, it may suggest that blood is combusting within the body. If the urine transitions from green or purple to a dark colour, it could indicate the presence of pure black bile.

A history of yellow or red urine, symptoms of bodily heat, combustion, unstable suspension of particles in the urine, and urine that is dark red or yellow instead of purely dark may indicate excessive combustion.

Severe cold may turn urine greenish or bluish, with possibly some coarse sediment settled at the bottom. The urine may appear scanty in amount and exhibit a pure dark shade.

When urine has a strong smell, it suggests a hot temperament. In contrast, a faint odour indicates a cold temperament.

The failure of innate heat indicates weakened bodily functions. It may occur alongside critical evacuation of dark, toxic matter during certain conditions such as quartan fever or after relief from specific organ diseases.

Dark urine can occur with the return of missed periods or relief from obstructed hemorrhoidal bleeding, often following diuretic or emmenagogue use.

Preceding pale and watery urine, relief after urination, and the passage of a large volume of urine are indicators of crisis or elimination.

Dark urine without critical evacuation in acute conditions may signal a poor prognosis due to excessive heat-induced humour destruction. Turbidity worsens the prognosis, while clarity suggests better outcomes. Dark-red urine post-wine consumption does not necessarily indicate a poor prognosis. The presence of dark urine can sometimes signal recovery.

Uniformly dispersed sediment found in dark, thin urine correlates with headaches, insomnia, deafness, and mental confusion. A foul odour and scanty dark urine during fever warn of cerebral disturbances.

Thin, dark urine signals potential kidney stones. Dark urine is generally positive for kidney and bladder diseases, except during acute illnesses. Very thin, dark urine with signs of excessive combustion in kidney or bladder diseases suggests a poor prognosis.

In older adults, dark urine often indicates serious underlying issues and a poor prognosis.

Dark urine after physical exertion may foretell spasms. Early febrile illness stages with dark urine are concerning. Dark urine at the fever's end, without signs of crisis or improvement, is unfavourable.

Shades of white-coloured urine

White urine can have two meanings. The first refers to light and transparent urine or white transparent urine (Abyad Majazi), which is thin and transparent. The second meaning of white urine is when the urine is 'true white' (Abyad Haqiqi). In this case, the urine is white-coloured and viscous, resembling milk and light rays cannot pass through it.

Transparent white urine generally indicates coldness and a lack of maturation. If the transparent white urine is also thick, it signifies phlegm. 'True white' urine is always thick.

Types of White-Coloured Urine:

1. Mucilaginous-Like Urine (Bawl Mukhati): This type of urine denotes an excess of immature phlegm in the body.
2. Oily-Like Urine (Bawl Dasmi): This type of urine contains emulsified fat derived from tissues, indicating the metabolism of fats.
3. Waxy-Like Urine (Bawl Ihali): This urine is as white as ghee and indicates the liquefaction of phlegmatic substances. It also suggests a bad prognosis in acute fevers and a possible future attack of emaciation.
4. Champagne-Like Urine (Bawl Fuqqa'i): When urine is mixed with pus, it indicates ulceration of the urinary tract. Without pus, it indicates the presence of partially matured phlegm or stone in the bladder.
5. Semen-Like Urine (Bawl Manwi): Semen-like urine is produced by the crisis of diseases derived from vitreous phlegm. If the urine is produced without the disease crisis, it indicates the upcoming attack of apoplexy or hemiplegia. If the urine remains white throughout the fever, it indicates it has shifted towards quartan fever.
6. Lead-White Urine (Bawl Rasasi): This urine is greenish-white, and it is considered deadly if it has no sediment in it.
7. Milky-White Urine (Bawl Labani): Milky-white urine in acute disease has a fatal prognosis. It indicates that the diversion of bile is towards some organs, which will become inflamed or will be expelled through faeces. If the urine remains white for some time in the state of health, it indicates the absence of a concoction.

Complex urine colours

These are colours of urine which are a mixture of different colours such as:

Raw Meat Washings Like Urine (Bawl Ghusali): This type of urine is like washings of fresh meat or blood-stained water. This indicates either a hepatic insufficiency or excess blood in the body but primarily due to hepatic insufficiency, irrespective of the dominance of any type of Su'-i-Mizaj (morbid/impaired temperament). Poor digestion and low vitality are common symptoms associated with liver weakness. However, if the various faculties are strong enough, this type of urine may result from excess blood, which might be so high that the body cannot differentiate between water and blood.

Olive oil colour urine (Bawl Zayti): This urine is yellow with a translucent oily tinge. It appears clear, sticky, and moderately dense, giving off an oily sheen, and is considered a bad sign. In rare cases, it may be caused by the critical evaluation of fatty matter from blood, and if so, the symptoms of the disease are expected to subside. Olive-coloured urine, which is oily, scanty, and foul-smelling, is of poor prognosis, especially if mixed with material that looks like meat washings. This type of urine usually appears in ascites, consumption, and severe types of colic. If this type of urine is passed after previously being dark, it is a sign of improvement. If olive-coloured urine is passed on the fourth day of some acute disease, the patient is likely to die on the seventh day. The oily translucence may be diffused throughout the whole sample or confined to the top or bottom of the urine. Sometimes, urine has the colour of oil, as in tuberculosis, especially during the early stage of the disease. In some cases, urine may have an oily texture, and when it has an oily texture and colour, it could indicate kidney disease or a terminal stage of tuberculosis.

Purple urine (Bawl Urjuwani): Urine that points towards a fatal prognosis as it is an indication of the combustion of yellow and black bile, producing abnormal humour.

Flame-red urine (Bawl Jamri): Urine with a red colour tinged with black, a sign of any complicated fever or fever occurring due to thick humour. However, if this colour is present only in the top layers of urine, it may signify pleurisy.

Urine density (qiwam al-bawl)

Urine texture is light, thick, or medium

Thin consistency urine

Thin urine can indicate various health conditions. It may be due to the lack of concoction of morbid matter (Mawad) in the body, an obstruction in the blood vessels, or weakness of the kidneys and urinary tract. In such cases, the urine may appear light or watery, with only the thin products being excreted, while the heavier matters are left behind. It may also occur due to excessive water drinking or a dry, cold temperament. In acute diseases, thin urine may indicate weakness of the digestive faculty, lack of maturation, and weakness of all other faculties. Due to weak faculties, there is unhindered excretion of fluids in such cases.

Urine in children is typically dense due to their moist body and need for ample nutrition to grow and develop. Therefore, thin, watery urine during acute illnesses can indicate a severe abnormality in childhood. Persistent thin urine is a fatal sign in children.

Even during acute fevers, thin urine is a bad sign unless the general condition and other symptoms are favourable. This kind of urine can also indicate abscess formation. The liver's convexity is the most likely site of an abscess. If a seemingly healthy person complains of pain in a particular organ and continually passes thin, watery urine, there is likely swelling in that organ. Pain in the kidney region is a sign of swelling in the kidneys. If pain and heaviness are felt throughout the body and not in any particular organ, it may indicate the development of smallpox or another systemic pustular disease. If urine suddenly becomes thin during the crisis, the disease is likely to relapse.

Thick consistency urine

Thick urine consistency can be an important indicator of one's health. Extremely thick urine can be a sign of concoction or the thick consistency of humours excreted after concoction, as seen in the last stages of humoural fevers. It can also indicate that mature swellings have ruptured, causing the consistency of urine to become thick.

Thick consistency urine in acute diseases: In acute diseases, thick consistency urine indicates the following:

- Putrefaction of substance and its excessiveness
- The digestion that produces consistency in urine
- No concoction in the substance has occurred, which may result in the separation of the substance to settle it down in the urine as sediment.

It is sometimes observed that a patient's urine is white even when they have a hot and bilious temperament or red when they have a cold and phlegmatic temperament. This is because bile, when it is separated from urine, does not mix with it, resulting in white-coloured urine. In cold or chronic diseases, the urine may turn red for various reasons, such as the severity of pain in chronic colic that dissolves the bile and incites it, causing it to mix with urine and make it red. Phlegmatic obstruction can produce phlegm in the duct that connects the gall bladder to the duodenum. In such a condition, the bile may not be secreted into the duodenum but instead be excreted and mixed with urine. Hepatic insufficiency can also cause the faculty to not distinguish between bile and blood, which is common in chronic oedema. If the urine has a slightly sweet odour, it indicates the dominance of blood. The pungent stench in urine indicates the dominance of bile, while the acidic/sour character, along with this stench, indicates the dominance of black bile. Smelly urine in otherwise healthy people indicates fever caused by infections. In acute diseases, if there is no smell, it indicates the loss of faculty.

Urine froth (zubada al-bawl)

During micturition, froth may occur due to the air (rih) mixed with the liquid urine. However, some air can already be present in the urine before it is voided. This is particularly the case for patients who experience excessive distension, which can form large bubbles in the urine.

The colour, size, amount, and time of dissolution of froth can indicate various properties of a substance. For example, black or reddish froth can indicate jaundice, with black froth being a sign of black jaundice. The froth's size can indicate the substance's viscosity, while excess froth can indicate an abundance of gas. A small amount of froth can indicate the opposite. If the froth takes time to dissolve, it can indicate the substance's adhesiveness. In kidney diseases, persistent froth bubbles can indicate disease persistence, and eliminating sticky substances in kidney disease can be a bad sign. The sticky substances can indicate deathly black bile and phlegmatic humours, coldness, turbidity, or Su'-i-Mizaj (morbid/impaired temperament) of kidneys.

Urine sediments

Physicians use sediment to identify materials denser than water, regardless of their position or buoyancy. Sediment can be identified by its characteristics, including its nature, quantity, quality, shape, location, time of appearance, and affinity.

Normal/Natural sediments (Rasub Tabi'i Mahmud)

Natural urine sediments indicate the natural digestion and concoction process in the body. The sediments are white, smooth, round, regular, light, and delicate. They settle at the bottom and consist of uniform particles, similar to the precipitation of rose water. The natural sediment indicates the ratio of concoction in the whole body.

The difference between pus and sediment:

The main difference between pus and sediment is that pus is malodorous, whereas sediment has no odour.

The difference between raw phlegm and pure sediment is that the components of raw phlegm are dense. If the flask is shaken, the components of phlegm will not disperse quickly, whereas the components of sediments will disperse in the urine very quickly. The pure sediment differs from the pus and phlegm in softness and lightness. The sediment is soft and light, whereas pus and phlegm are heavy.

Abnormal sediments (Rasub Ghayr Tabi'i)

They are as follows:

1. Flaky sediments (Rasub Khurati/ Qushuri): These are large red or white sediments that usually come from urinary system organs. There are different types of flaky sediments, such as:

- Wheat husk-like flaky sediments (Nukhali): These are small and thick scales that indicate bladder disorder or wasting of organs.
- Pea-like flaky sediments (Karsani): These are yellowish-grey/earthy sediments.
- Gritty sediments (Dashishi): These are red and dark yellow sediments that are produced due to burning blood.
- Barley-like sediments (Sawiqi): These sediments are reddish when they denote the burning of blood and dark when they show excessive destruction of blood.

- Flat peel-like sediments (Safa'ihi): These are flat and large white or red sediments that generally arise from the immediate urinary tract.

Whether flaky sediments are white or red, they indicate injuries and ulcers of urinary organs.

2. Fleshy sediments (Lahmi): These are similar to meat and indicate the catabolism of the kidney muscles.

3. Fatty sediments (Dasmi): These oily sediments indicate the catabolism of fats and flesh.

4. Purulent sediments (Middi): These sediments with pus indicate the flow of wound/ulcer, especially when the ulcer is in the urinary tract.

Even if thick, flaky sediments are at the bottom of the urine, its indication will be more towards ulcers.

5. Mucoid sediments (Mukhati): These are phlegmatic sediments that indicate thick and raw humour.

6. Fermented sediments (Khamiri): These are like pieces of yeast and indicate gastric and intestinal insufficiency and abnormal digestion in urinary organs.

7. Sandy sediments (Ramli): These sediments, like sand, indicate the presence of calculus. Red sandy sediments are from the kidney.

8. Ash-like sediment (Rasub Ramadi): Ashy sediments indicate raw phlegm or pus.

It is important to note that flaky sediments, whether white or red, indicate injuries and ulcers of urinary organs.

Haematuria (bawl al-dam)

According to Hippocrates, blood in urine without any known cause indicates a vessel rupture in the kidney.

When a patient has splenomegaly and passes red clots in their urine, their spleen's size may decrease afterwards.

In most bladder diseases, there is increased bleeding due to the complex network of blood vessels in the bladder.

Women's urine may appear thicker, whiter, and less clear than men's urine due to possible contamination from vaginal discharge.

When urine is shaken, it becomes murky or turbid in men, and the turbidity is more concentrated towards the top. However, female urine does not become turbid when shaken because the turbid components are distinct and separated. A round froth may also be found in the upper part of female urine.

After intercourse, threads are present in men's urine, which are joined to one another.

Urine of pregnant women

During pregnancy, urine is typically described as being clear with a small cloud at the top. However, there may be variations in colour such as lentil water or trotter's stock. Additionally, there may be cotton wool-like substances or grain-like particles floating and moving in the urine. It's also worth noting that the colour of the urine can indicate the stage of pregnancy. A bluish tint suggests the beginning of pregnancy, while a reddish hue indicates the later stages of pregnancy, with turbidity upon shaking.

Conditions and diseases of the body and their urine[332]

Urine of different ages and genders	Urine
Infancy	White
Childhood (Beyond infancy)	Thick
Age of decline	Inclined towards a thin consistency with whiteness and thickness
Advanced age	Thin and white with blackness. If the urine of an older adult is very thick, this can indicate calculus.
Men	When urine is shaken, men's urine appears cloudy, and the cloudiness is more noticeable towards the top of the urine. In contrast, women's urine is usually not cloudy, and any cloudiness can be seen more towards the bottom when shaken. Additionally, the foam formed on the surface of women's urine tends to be round in shape.
Women	White and thick and less lustrous

Urine during pregnancy

Start of pregnancy	The urine is clear but contains a heavy cotton-like substance with a grain-like object floating up and down. The urine is bluish and does not become turbid when shaken.
Late pregnancy	The urine is red and becomes turbid when shaken
Second and third month of pregnancy	Thin and clear
Fourth month of pregnancy	Towards reddish in colour
Fifth month of pregnancy	Unclear urine
Miscarriage	Extremely unclear urine

---

[332] Pulse table amended from Usool-e-Tibb by hakim Kamaluddin Husain Hamdani.

Colours of urine and related condition and diseases

Colour	Types of urine	Conditions and diseases
Yellow	Straw yellow (like straw-soaked water)	Low temperature, renal insufficiency, diabetes, anaemia
	Orange coloured	Fever
	Reddish yellow coloured	Excess dissolution of matter, yellow fever, diabetes, fever, anaemia, dominance of heat and yellow bile, True dysentery (a type of dysentery occurring due to pouring of yellow bile or saline phlegm on rectum, acute inflammation of rectum, exposure of anus to cold or intake of things having cold temperament), Malaria, diseases of liver and gall bladder, jaundice, obstruction in cystic duct, fistula, use of Revand Chini (Chinese Rhubarb), senna and picric acid etc.
	Fire coloured	Dominance of heat and bile, kidney and bladder stones, jaundice, hot rih (air), severe dominance of heat and bile or bilious remittent fever.
	Saffron, like the colour of the saffron leaf	Dominance of severe heat and bile, and bilious remittent fever.
Red	Yellowish red (onion yellowish red)	Sensory hemiplegia, use of any medicine or dye (in form of desert or food), diseases of liver
	Rose red	Especially the production of blood congestion or fibrous structure in the liver.
	Intense red	Haematuria, hemiplegia, anaemia with hypoproteinaemia (Su' al-Qinya, i.e., Inability of liver to produce normal humour; a morbid state caused by the deranged temperament of liver whose debility is characterized by pallor and oedema of extremities), colic.
	Blackish red	Haematuria, Myoma (tumour in uterus, prostate gland and gastrointestinal tract)
Green	Pistachio	Jaundice, cold temperaments, use of carbolic acid gas etc.
	Verdigris-green	Dominance of black bile, severe oxidation/combustion, spasm
	Sky-green	Cold dominance, poisoning
	Emerald-green	Severe cold, poisoning
	Leek-green	Dominance of black bile, severe combustion, poisoning
Black	Blackish urine	Blackish discolouration of the skin due to various factors such as the impaired spleen (Yaraqan Aswad), spleen diseases, quartan fever crisis, uterine diseases, blood retention, fatigue and convulsions, haematuria, delirium, and mental crisis.

White	Milky urine	Ulcers of urinary tract, bladder stones, indigestion, crisis of phlegmatic inflammation, acute diseases, hectic fever.
	Watery urine	Cold and phlegm dominance, asthma, chronic gout, diabetes, urinary incontinence, hepatic impaired temperament, obstruction of cystic duct, indigestion, gastric, hepatic and kidney insufficiency, ulcers of bladder and urinary tract, phlegmatic crisis.
Other	Like washed flesh water	Inflammation of the bladder, hepatic insufficiency and dominance of blood.
	Olive	Oedema, double malarial fever and pleurisy

Urine smell and Mizaj (Temperament)

Smell of Urine	Mizaj
Odourless	Cold temperament
Strong smell	Hot temperament
Sweet smell	Hot and moist temperament with predominance Dam (blood) humour
Bitter/Acidic smell	Hot and moist temperament with predominance Sufra (yellow bile) humour

Urine sediments and diseases

Urine sediments	Disease
White flaky sediments	Heat and ulcers of bladder
Red flaky sediments	Kidney heat and ulcers of kidney
Wheat husk-like flaky sediments	Bladder heat
Raw Meat Washings Like Urine	Liver and kidney diseases
Brownish to black sediments	Intense heat of urinary organs
Barley-like sediments or Fatty sediments	Catabolism
Purulent sediments	Ulcers of urethra
Mucoid sediments	Congestion of raw humour in the body or cold temperament or crisis, sciatica, polyarthritis.
Sandy red sediments	Kidney stones
Sandy white sediments	Bladder stones
Bloody sediments	Hepatic insufficiency and injuries of urinary organs
Fermented sediments	Gastric insufficiency, high intake of milk and fermented products
Black sediments, cloudy black	Excess movement or excess cold

Blue sediments	Cold temperament
Reddish sediments	Predominance of blood, indigestion of food, raw substance affecting disease.
Olive coloured sediments	Phthisis and hectic fever
Yellow sediments	Congestion of bile, jaundice, overheating

Urine types and diseases

Urine	Disease
Citron-yellow	Headache due to excessive heat
Thick urine	Congestive headache
White and thick urine	Phlegmatic (Balghami) headache
Urine is white and thin, but it becomes black and thick after a complete concoction.	Melancholic (Sawdawi) headache
Urine is white, raw, turbid and thick	Hemiplegia
Thick urine	Muscular spasm due to infiltration of causative matter (Tashannuj Ratb)
Urination may stop, but there may be instances of uncontrollable leakage or blood in the urine due to excessive tension and pressure causing vessel rupture.	Tetany (Kuzaz)
Urine is red and small in quantity	Acute pleurisy
Decrease in quantity of urine	Gastritis
Urination stops	Food poisoning
Urine is black, blackish in colour	Hot morbid temperament of spleen (Su' Mizaj Al-Tihhal Harr)
Blackish white urine	Chronic splenitis Phlegmatic (Waram-o-Salaba al-Tihhal Balghami)
Turbid urine	Splenic Abscess (Taqayyuh al-Tihal)
Blood mixed urine	Leukaemia (Abyad-i-Dam)
Yellow or red urine	Hot morbid temperament of kidney (Su'-i-Mizaj Kulya harr)
White urine	Cold morbid temperament of kidney (Su'-i-Mizaj Kulya barid)
White urine	Renal atrophy cold (Huzal al-Kulya)
Urine like washed water of flesh	Renal Insufficiency

Blurry or dark red or black sediment	Acute nephritis
Small quantity of thin urine	Fatty kidney
Bloody urine and purulent mixed red flakes	Ulcers of kidney
Large amount of urine and light-yellow colour	Diabetes
Urine white and thin. Stones white or blackish	Cystolithiasis
Thick urine, mixed with blood or phlegm	Acute cystitis
Pus mixed urine. Dust type substance found mixed in urine i.e., wheat husk-like flaky sediments	Ulcers or irritability of bladder
Blood mixed urine	Clotting of blood in bladder (Jamud al-Dam fi'l Mathana)
Flatus mixed urine	Bladder gas (Rih al-Mathana)
Yellow urine	Dribbling of urine (Taqtir al-Bawl) due to fullness of urine
White urine	Dribbling of urine due to weak bladder
White urine	Urinary incontinence due to coldness
Urine like washed water of flesh	Haematuria
Coloured urine. Cast and pus are also excreted in urine	Burning micturition (Hurqa al-Bawl)
Pus is excreted in urine which is slightly blue.	Gonorrhoea (Sozak)
Frequent urination	Leucorrhoea (Sayalan al-Rahim)
Excess urination	Amenorrhoea
Frequent urination but in small quantity	Hysteria (Ikhtinaq al-Rahhim)
Small in quantity, dark red in colour, acidic.	Polyarthritis

Urine and fevers

Urine	Fevers
Urine thick and red	Sanguineous fever with increased viscosity of blood (Humma Muttbiqa Ghalayaniyya)
Urine thin like water and of colour of bile or black bile	Epidemic fever
Some patients suffer from haematuria which is a bad sign	Small pox
Urine is reddish fire coloured and thick	Measles
Urine is small in quantity but is deep in colour	Fever with delirium (Humma Ghamiya Hadhayaniyya)

Diseases with their pulse and urine signs[333]

DISEASE	MIZAJ OF DISEASE	PULSE	URINE
Epilepsy	Cold and dry	Uninterrupted	White and thin
Apoplexy	Cold and moist	Very Uninterrupted	White turbid
Insanity (Melancholia)	Cold and dry	Very Uninterrupted	White turbid
Dementia (Humq)	Cold and moist	Intermittent	White turbid
Atony/Flaccidity	Cold and moist	Very Uninterrupted	White turbid
Catalepsy (Jumud / Shukhus)	Cold and moist	Fast	White turbid
Coma	Cold and moist	Fast	White turbid
Insomnia	Hot and moist	Healthy	Healthy
Convulsions	Cold and dry	Very Fast	White turbid
Facial Palsy	Cold and moist	Very Uninterrupted	White turbid
Amnesia	Cold and moist	Healthy	White turbid
Hemiplegia	Cold and moist	Very Uninterrupted	White turbid
Numbness	Cold and moist	Healthy	Healthy
Vertigo and giddiness	Hot and moist	Very Fast	White
Delirium	Cold and dry	Very Fast	White and thin

---

[333] From the 'Selected work of Galen - Hakeen Ashfita Lucknowi, Nizamiya Tibbi College, Hyderabad' as mentioned in Usool-e-tibb by Hakeem Hamdani

Confused state of mind (Ikhtilat al-Dhahn)	Hot and dry	Very Fast	Healthy
Migraine (Shaqiqa)	Hot and dry	Very Uninterrupted	Bright red saffron
Concussion	Cold and dry	Uninterrupted	Healthy
Alopecia with loss of a layer of skin	Cold and moist	Healthy	Healthy
Alopecia areata	Cold and moist	Healthy	Healthy
Vertigo	Hot and moist	Fast	Turbid red
Cold headache	Cold and moist	Very Uninterrupted	White turbid
Hot headache	Hot and dry	Very Fast	Intense red (red is predominant)
Headache due to heat of the sun	Hot and dry	Uninterrupted	Bright red (Saffron)
Headache	Cold and dry	Very Fast	Red and thin
Headache due to moisture	Cold and dry	Very Uninterrupted	White turbid
Coryza	Hot and moist	Uninterrupted	Intense red (red is predominant)
Epistaxis	Hot and moist	Healthy	Healthy
Catarrh	Hot and moist	Healthy	Healthy
Tinnitus	Cold and moist	Millipede/vermicular	White turbid
Ear diseases due to heat	Hot and moist	Healthy	Healthy
Ear diseases due to cold	Cold and moist	Healthy	Healthy

Ear diseases due to dryness	Cold and dry	Healthy	Healthy
Ear diseases due to moisture	Cold and moist	Healthy	Healthy
Mouth ulcers	Hot and moist	Healthy	Healthy
Trachoma	Hot and dry	Healthy	Healthy
Conjunctivitis	Hot and moist	Healthy	Healthy
Pannus	Cold and dry	Healthy	Healthy
Thirst	Hot and dry	Healthy	Bright red
Inflammation of muscles of larynx	Hot and moist	Very Fast	Intense red
Diaphragmitis	Hot and dry	Very Uninterrupted	Bright red
Meningitis	Hot and moist	Very Uninterrupted	Bright red
Pleuritis	Hot and dry	Very Uninterrupted	Bright red
Intercostal pain	Hot and moist	Very Uninterrupted	Bright red
Chronic cough	Cold and dry	Uninterrupted and Full	White and thin
Acute cough	Hot and moist	Very Uninterrupted	Intense red
Syncope	Hot and dry	Very Uninterrupted	Bright red
Flatus	Cold and dry	Healthy	Healthy
Food poisoning	Hot and dry	Uninterrupted	Bright red
Fatigue	Hot and dry	Uninterrupted	Bright red

Liver causes due to heat	Hot and dry	Very Uninterrupted	Intense red
Liver causes due to cold	Cold and moist	Fast	White turbid
Liver causes due to moisture	Cold and moist	Fast	White turbid
Liver causes due to dryness	Cold and dry	Uninterrupted	Intense red
Sprue/ malabsorption syndrome	Hot and moist	Fast	Intense red
Ascites	Cold and moist	Fast	White turbid
Cachexic oedema/anasarca	Cold and moist	Fast	White turbid
Ascites succatus (abdominal distension due to the accumulation of gaseous matter)	Cold and moist	Intermittent	White and thin
Jaundice	Hot and dry	Uninterrupted	Bright red
Spleen causes due to cold	Cold and moist	Very Uninterrupted	Melancholic white
Spleen causes due to dryness	Cold and dry	Intermittent	White turbid
Spleen causes due to moisture	Cold and moist	Full and Thick	White turbid
Renal pain	Cold and moist	Healthy	Clear white
Nephrolithiasis	Cold and dry	Healthy	White
Cystolithiasis	Cold and dry	Healthy	White
Inflammation of uterus	Hot and dry	Very Uninterrupted	Bright red

Gout	Cold and dry	Healthy	Healthy
Arthritis due to heat	Hot and dry	Uninterrupted	Healthy
Arthritis due to moisture	Cold and moist	Healthy	Healthy
Arthritis due to dryness	Cold and dry	Healthy	Healthy
Inflammation of reproductive organs caused by heat	Hot and dry	Healthy	Healthy
Inflammation of reproductive organs caused by cold	Cold and dry	Healthy	Healthy
Sciatica	Hot and dry	Healthy	Healthy
Venous insufficiency	Cold and dry	Uninterrupted	White
Haemoptysis	Hot and moist	Intermittent	Healthy
Empyema thoracis	Cold and dry	Intermittent	Healthy
Urinary stones	Cold and dry	Very Uninterrupted	Healthy
Bloody diarrhoea	Hot and dry	Full	White turbid
Pneumonia	Hot and moist	Fast	Intense red
Large intestinal colic	Cold and dry	Very Uninterrupted	Thin and white
Persistent vomiting	Hot and moist	Healthy	Intense red
Stomach pain	Cold and moist	Healthy	Healthy
Dysentery	Cold and dry	Healthy	Healthy
Haemorrhoid	Cold and dry	Healthy	Healthy

Scabies	Hot and moist	Very Uninterrupted	Healthy
Pruritus	Hot and dry	Healthy	Healthy
Leprosy	Cold and dry	Intermittent	Black
Pityriasis	Cold and dry	Healthy	Healthy
Vitiligo	Cold and moist	Healthy	Healthy
Cancer	Cold and dry	Slow	Turbid black
Eruptions on body	Hot and dry	Healthy	Healthy
Ulcers on body	Hot and moist	Healthy	Healthy
Hard swelling	Hot and dry	Fast	Turbid red
Elephantiasis	Cold and moist	Healthy	Healthy
Small pox	Hot and dry	Uninterrupted and Fast	Intense red
Measles	Hot and dry	Very Uninterrupted	Intense red
Folliculitis	Hot and moist	Healthy	Healthy
Herpes zoster	Hot and dry	Uninterrupted	Intense red
Swelling of the face	Cold and moist	Uninterrupted	Thin and white
Inflammation due to collection of thick blood	Cold and dry	Uninterrupted	Thin and white
Dermatophytosis (ringworm)	Cold and dry	Healthy	Healthy
Ringworm that is contagious	Hot and dry	Healthy	Healthy

Cancrum / gangrenous Ulcer	Hot and moist	Dudi (Millipede/vermicular)	Intense red
Carbuncle	Hot and moist	Very Uninterrupted	Turbid red
Burning ulcer	Hot and dry	Healthy	Healthy
Sloughing ulcer	Hot and moist	Healthy	Healthy
Joint flaccidity	Cold and moist	Healthy	Healthy
Red swelling	Hot and moist	Very Uninterrupted	Intense red
Urticaria	Hot and moist	Healthy	Healthy
Fistula	Hot and moist	Healthy	Healthy
Abrasion/Enteritis	Hot and dry	Healthy	Healthy
Gas-filled blisters	Hot and dry	Healthy	Healthy
Malignant ulcer	Hot and moist	Healthy	Healthy
Thrombus	Hot and moist	Fast	Intense red
Ankylosing arthritis	Hot and dry	Healthy	Healthy
Abscesses	Cold and moist	Healthy	Healthy
Erotomania	Cold and dry	Healthy	Healthy
Obstructions of liver	Cold and dry	Healthy	Healthy
Lienteric diarrhoea	Cold and moist	Healthy	Healthy
Ephemeral fever	Hot and dry	Fast	Intense red
Malarial double fever	Hot and moist	Very Uninterrupted	Intense red

Bilious fever	Hot and dry	Fast	Red and thin
Quartan fever/ melancholic intermittent fever	Hot and moist	Intermittent	Black
cachexic fever	Hot and dry	Millipede/vermicular	Red and thin
Ulcers of intestine	Hot and moist	Millipede/vermicular	Clear red
Night fever	Cold and moist	Healthy	Healthy
Bleeding	Hot and dry	Healthy	Intense red
Excessive thirst (due to subacute inflammation of brain of children)	Hot and moist	Healthy	Healthy

Stool

It is also necessary to understand the form of stool for the diagnosis of a disease.

Which is based on the following things:

1. Quantity of stool

The amount of stool produced can be judged by the amount of food consumed. Large stools indicate an abundance of humours, while scanty stools indicate deficiency. Stools are retained due to obstruction in the caecum, colon or small intestine as a prelude to colic. Sometimes, the stools may be scanty due to the weakness of the expulsive faculty.

2. Consistency of stool

A more liquid form of the stool as compared to the normal indicates either any obstruction, indigestion, weakness of absorptive faculty of mesenteric vessels, increased fluid secretion of intestines or the use of any substance which causes thinning of stool or catabolism of any organ or that any adhesive drugs have been taken in a large amount.

Frothy stool indicates that either ebullition has been produced due to severe heat or flatus has been mixed with it in large amounts.

Dry stool indicates either tiredness, fatigue and dissolution or an increase in the secretion of urine, abnormal fiery heat of the body or dry foods. Stools become dry due to exhausting illnesses or strenuous work, causing dispersion.

Hard and dry stools with mucus indicate a delay in the passage of stools or lack of irritative bile. When there is no evidence of delay in the bowels and no sign of excessive mucus, the cause is likely to be some thin, purulent material or irritating humour expelled by the liver into the neighbouring organs being hurried out with the stools.

3. Colour of the stool

The normal colour of the stool is slightly golden. If the stool is more yellowish/golden, it indicates a high amount of bile. It indicates either raw food or a lack of concoction if it is less than this.

If the stool colour is white, it may be due to an obstruction in the bile duct, which indicates jaundice. When associated with pus and pus odour, it signifies the rupture of an abscess.

If the golden colour increases in stool in the last stages of diseases, it indicates concoction.

Black faeces may indicate severe oxidation, the concoction of melancholic disease, intake of any black substance, or the intake of alcohol, whose substances are excreted through stool. In later cases, oxidation is very harmful. Expulsion of black bile is always considered dangerous and lethal in every case. However, the expulsion of black chyme (humour that has turned black after mixing with black bile) is regarded as a good and positive healthy sign. Pure black bile is only excreted when there is severe oxidation in the body or the humour has transformed into black bile due to a lack of moisture, which is a warning sign. If the stool is swollen like the faeces of a cow, then it indicates flatulence. If the sound is produced during defecation, then it proves flatulence.

Properties of an Ideal Stool:

- It should be solid, with all components having the same thickness and consistency.

- Defecation should not cause any pain in the anus.

- It should be light yellowish, not very smelly, but not completely odourless.

- No grumbling or gurgling sounds should be produced during defecation.

- It should be produced on time and relative to the amount of food taken.

- Normal consistency stool that is relatively thin and has no excess flatulence is considered normal.

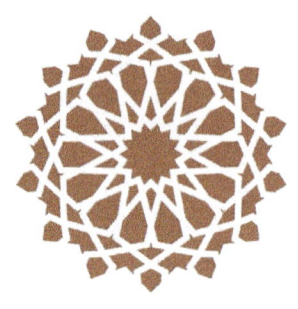

SECTION 4

COMPENDIUM OF DRUGS

'Leave your drugs in the chemist's pot if you can heal the patient with food.'

– Hippocrates

Drug, Diet And Zulkhassa

Definition of a Drug

According to the World Health Organization, a drug is defined as 'any substance or product that changes the pathological condition and cures the disease after being consumed.'

A drug is a substance used to treat a disease. It induces a new condition within the body that mitigates the diseased state and promotes health.

To understand the definition of a drug, it is useful to understand its lexical and terminological meanings:

Lexical meaning of Drug

- A medical substance used for the treatment of diseases.
- Any substance, excluding food, used in preventing, alleviating, treating, or curing diseases.
- A compound that enacts an effect within the body due to its inherent properties.

Terminological meaning of Drug

Ibn Sina Says, 'Anything that enters the body and is affected by the heat and moisture of the body, according to its composition, and then is expelled without integrating into the body is termed a drug'. Each substance that enters the body has three distinct effects:

- Related to its Properties/quality.
- In relation to its substance.
- Concerning its essence.

Drug Classifications

- **Properties/Quality:** These are four conditions a drug might have[334].
   a. Harr (Hot)
   b. Barid (Cold)
   c. Ratoobat (Moist)
   d. Yaboosat (Dry)

---

[334] In Arabic Harr/Barid/Ratoobat/Yaboosat in Urdu Garam/Sard/Tar/Khusuk, respectively.

- **Dietary Substances:** These are substances that, when entering the body, get influenced by its internal heat and moisture, breaking down into smaller constituents like proteins and carbohydrates that integrate into the body.
- **Difference between Drug and diet:**
    a. **Diet**: Nourishment that affects the body after transformation and metabolism, integrating into the body.
    b. **Ghida' Dawa'i**[335] (nutritious drugs) or **Dawa Ghidai**[336] (medicinal diets): Substances used for nourishment and treatment. Their classification (as nutritious drugs or medicinal diets) is based on their dominant effect.

It is difficult to establish a division between drug and diet, therefore rarely, does a thing exist that is only used for diet or only used for treatment and no component of diet or drug is present within it.

Zulkhassa

Zulkhassa refers to drugs whose mechanisms of action may or may not be understood.

- The drug whose mechanism of action is known. For example, Asal Alsoos (Glycyrrhiza glabra - liquorice roots) is beneficial for coughs as it is an expectorant, that is, increases the expulsion of phlegm from the lungs and dilates the airways.
- Some drugs are known to be beneficial through their effects but their mechanism of action is unknown. These types of drugs are called Zulkhassa. For example, the mechanism of action of toxins, theriacs, virucide, or purgative drugs is not known. According to physicians, these drugs have natural functions and effects that are related to their mode of action and their nature.

However, it's worth noting that even for the first group, our understanding is primarily through their mode of action. For instance, if someone were to question why liquorice root functions as an expectorant or why it dilates the pulmonary arteries, the deeper reasons remain a mystery.

---

[335] It is that drug in which the nutritional components are more than the medicinal components. E.g.: Egg, fish and chicken.
[336] It is that drug in which the medicinal components are more than the nutritional components. E.g.: kidney beans, coriander and mint.

Temperament of Drugs

Temperament

Definition of Temperament: Temperament refers to the new condition formed as a result of the interaction of four properties: hot, cold, dry, and moist. This condition is further influenced by factors such as function, reaction, division, and refraction.

Drugs can be classified based on their temperaments:

A. First type of temperament of drugs

Dawa Mu'tadil (Normal drug): A drug that, when reacting with the body's innate heat (Hararat), produces a quality (kefiyat) similar to the body's natural temperament (mizaj).

Dawa Ghayr Mu'tadil (Abnormal/Change causing drug): These drugs, when interacting with the body's heat, produce conditions contrary to the body's moderate temperament. The conditions can be categorized as:

i. **Dawae Haar (Hot Drug):** a drug that produces abnormal heat in the body after being affected by the innate heat.
ii. **Dawae Barid (Cold drug):** a drug that is the cause of abnormal coldness in the body after being affected by the body heat.
iii. **Dawae Ratib (Moist drug):** a drug that is the cause of abnormal moisture in the body after being affected by the body heat.
iv. **Dawae Yabis (Dry drug):** a drug that is the cause of abnormal dryness in the body after being affected by the body heat.
v. **Dawae Haar-Yabis (Hot-dry drug):** the drugs that produce abnormal heat and dryness in the body after being affected by the body heat.
vi. **Dawae Haar-Ratib (Hot-moist drug):** the drugs that produce abnormal heat and moisture in the body after being affected by the body heat.
vii. **Dawae Barid-Yabis (Cold-dry drug):** the drugs that produce abnormal coldness and dryness in the body after being affected by the body heat.
viii. **Dawae Barid-Ratib (Cold-moist drug):** the drugs that produce abnormal coldness and moisture in the body after being affected by the body heat.

(Refer to the chart below for a visual representation of these classifications).

ABNORMAL DRUG TEMPERAMENT IN UNANI MEDICINE

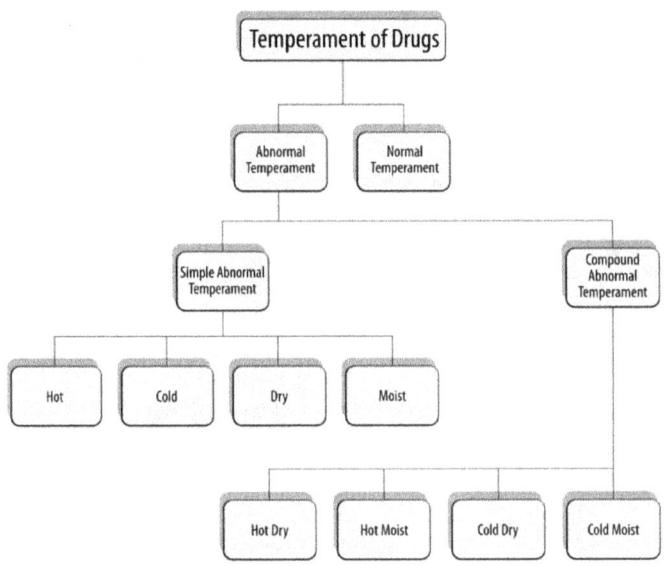

B. Second type of temperament of drugs

1. Mizaj Awali (Primary temperament)

It is that particular mizaj which is produced from the mixing of a few basic elements. It is also called or mizaj-e-Tabaee [337] (natural temperament) or mizaj-e-asli (original temperament). The drugs that possess this mizaj are called mufrad-ul-quwwa (single power) drugs, though they are rare.

2. Mizaj Thanawi (Secondary temperament)

Secondary temperament is produced by the interaction of two or more primary temperaments, function and reactions, division and refraction. In other words, the temperament produced by the combination of a few simple components is called a secondary temperament. The drugs with secondary temperament are called Murakab al-Qawi (strong compounds).

---

[337] In transliteration, words may be written differently, such as "mizaj-e-Tabaee" and "mizaj-i-Tabaee." These variations refer to the same term.

DRUG TEMPERAMENT STABILITY IN UNANI MEDICINE

```
                    Temperament of Drugs
                    /                  \
          Secondary                    Primary
         Temperament                 Temperament
              |
       -------|-------
       |             |
   Unstable        Stable
  Temperament    Temperament
       |
   ----|----------------
   |        |          |
Absolute  Strongly   Loosely
Unstable  Unstable   Unstable
```

In Ibn Sina's words, 'When physicians say regarding some drugs that 'its faculty is a complex of some opposite faculties', it does not mean that its single component is responsible for heat and coldness and that component issues both functions separately, but this (a single component responsible for two opposite functions) is not possible. However, both these functions are related to two different constituents.'

Jawhar Fa'al[338] **(Active parts of drug):**

The dominant effect of a drug is attributed to its main constituent, known as the Jawhar Fa'al. For instance, opium (Affiyun), derived from the secretion of the poppy plant (Papaver Somniferum), contains numerous constituents. One of these constituents has hypnotic and analgesic properties, and because of this specific effect, Affiyun is used. Hence, this particular component of Affiyun represents the Jawhar Fa'al (active principle).

Both plant and animal drugs consist of various constituents and essences. These constituents can be isolated through different resolution and analytical methods. For example, ghee is derived from milk, while sugar is extracted from sources like sugarcane, grapes, and dates.

Similarly, mineral drugs comprise several components. They are purified through different processes.

---

[338] i.e., the constituent responsible for the drug's main action.

Types of Secondary Temperaments:

There are two types of secondary temperament in terms of stability.

1. Stable Secondary Temperament (Mizaj Thani Mustehkam):

A secondary temperament is deemed stable if its components remain intact even after being subjected to intense heat, such as boiling. Gold serves as an example of this.

2. Unstable Secondary Temperament (Mizaj Thani Ghayr Mustehkam):

If the secondary temperament is not stable, it is further divided into three categories:

- Absolute unstable (Rakhu Mutlaq): This type of temperament sees its components separate upon direct heating. For instance, Chamomile has a Qabiz (astringent) component and a Muhallil (resolvent) component. When Chamomile is heated in water, both constituents dissociate from each other.
- Strongly unstable (Rakhu Judda): In this case, the drug's composition is fragile. When exposed to hot water, one component detaches from the other. Lentils, with an astringent and a resolvent component, serve as an example. Upon heating, both components dissolve separately in water.
- Loosely unstable (Rakhu ba Farat): This temperament is so delicate that even washing in water can disrupt its composition. Chicory, for instance, has multiple constituents, including a Mufattih (deobstruent), an astringent and a Mulattif[339] (demulcent). When Chicory is washed, these constituents dissolve in water, especially since they are present on the outer surface of the leaves.

It is vital to consider the stability of secondary temperament in complex substances. Some compounds are sensitive to minor heat or sunlight, causing them to spoil and their components to disintegrate.

Composition of drugs

Nearly all plant origin (nabati) and animal (haiwani) drugs are naturally murakkab-ul-quwwa[340] (compounds). Following different characteristic constituents are found in different quantities in drugs:

1. Tursh mawad (Sour/acidic components): This component is usually found in plant origin drugs and some fruits like lemon, tamarind, dried plums, sour pomegranate, etc.
2. Namkiyath (Salty components): obtained from ashes of burned plants.

---

[339] An agent which liquefies thick and viscous matter.
[340] A particular mizaj which is produced from the mixing of components that have Mizaj Awali (Primary temperament). The drugs which possess this mizaj are called murakkab-ul-quwwa.

3. Shakariya (Sugar components): This component is usually found in plant origin drugs like grapes, sugar cane.
4. Lehmiya (protein components): This component is usually found in animal origin drugs and sometimes from plant origin drugs. E.g., Fish
5. Gondh /Simaghiyath (Gum components): This component is usually obtained from plants and can be dissolved in water. E.g., Simagh[341] arabi (Acacia arabica gum), Simagh kateera (Cochlospermum religiosum)
6. Ra'al (Resins): that gum-like substance that does not dissolve in water, However it can be dissolved in alcohol for example, Saqmonia (scammonia resins). Gondh and ra'al are used as a base in the preparation of murakkabath (compounds) like aqras (distillates) and huboob (pills). e.g., Ushaq (Dorcus ammonicum gum), Usara Rewand (Rheum palmatum), etc.
7. Shehmiya (Fatty components/oils): This component is a fatty substance found in volatile oils such as of Camphor (Kafoor - Cinnamomum camphora), Roghan Bedanjeer (Castor oil) and other fats from animal source.
8. Khashbiya (Wood components): This component is a woody substance or matter that is found in branches, roots, and stem of the plant, such as Burada-e-sandal (sandalwood), Burada-e-Aabnoos (Diospyros ebenum - wood).
9. Launiya (Colouring components): For example, the substance that produces green colour in leaves, red, saffron yellow in flowers and black in cassia.
10. Jauhar-e-faal (Alkaloid components): This component is the active principle of the plant origin medicines, For example, the essence of Azraqi/Kuchla Mudabbar (Strychnos nux-vomica), the essence of Affiyun (Papaver Somniferum -opium) the essence of besh (aconite).
11. Khameer (Fermented components): This component produces fermentation. For example, 'Arq-e-Gaozaban' (Borage distillate) contains fermented components.

Potency variations in drug temperaments

Properties of drugs

Dawa Motadil[342] (Normal/Moderate drug):

This refers to drugs that, when acted upon by the body's innate heat, produce moderate effects. It doesn't mean the drug's essence is inherently moderate but rather its effects on the body are moderate. Consider the pharmacological effects of green tea (Camellia sinensis). Its active constituents impart a subtle stimulant effect, analogous to that of a moderate drug, without the pronounced stimulatory effects of stronger agents such as Coffee.

---

[341] Simagh means Gum.
[342] Drug that does not cause any substantial change in body even when used repeatedly or in higher dose.

Dawa Harr (Hot drug) or Dawa Barid (Cold drug):

When physicians use the terms 'hot' or 'cold' to describe certain drugs, they are not referring to the drug's essence, nor are they comparing it to the temperature of the human body. Instead, what they mean is that the drug has the ability to produce sensations of heat or coldness in the body that exceed the normal range of temperature.

For example, capsaicin, an active compound in chili peppers, exemplifies a 'hot' drug due to its ability to induce a warming sensation. Conversely, menthol, derived from mint, epitomizes a 'cold' drug owing to its cooling properties.

It is not uncommon for a drug to be too 'hot' for one patient but not hot enough for another. If a drug does not prove effective in treating a condition, then another drug from the same class may be prescribed.

Moreover, a patient's response to a particular drug may diminish over time, or another drug from the same class may prove more effective. It is well-known that different people may respond differently to the same medication, and the reasons for this are not always clear.

Drug Potency Levels

The impact of drugs on the human body varies. While some drugs can produce rapid transformations and metabolism in the body, others have a slower effect. A gram of one drug may not have any impact, while the same amount of another drug could be toxic. That is why physicians have created drug potency grades or levels based on the strengths and weaknesses of the drugs' actions, which we will explain shortly.

Guidelines for Determining Drug Potency Levels:

The potency of drugs is discerned primarily through empirical observations, specifically examining both the quantity administered and the resultant efficacy. In the process of categorizing drug potency levels, medical practitioners have delineated several essential criteria:

- The drug dosage should remain within its therapeutic range, avoiding any excess.
- Repetitive administration of the drug should be avoided unless clinically indicated.
- The physiological state of the recipient, particularly concerning the Ruh (pneuma), should be moderate and conducive for the drug's action.
- Environmental factors, especially temperature, play a crucial role in modulating the drug's impact. For instance, a drug with inherent heat properties may have intensified effects during hot weather, while a typically cold drug will have a potent effect in the winter.

Classification of Drug Potency: A Four level Framework

Physicians have demarcated drug effects into distinct levels, moving beyond the standard categorization of the moderate or normal drug (Dawa Motadil). These levels are systematically delineated based on the drug's inherent qualities and resultant physiological manifestations:

First Level:

- **Manifestation**: Drugs within this category introduce a distinct quality (kefiyat, i.e., cold, hot, moist, or dry) into the physiological system. While this effect is more pronounced than the Dawa Motadil's, its presence may not be immediately perceptible.
- **Implications**: Over prolonged consumption, the cumulative effects may become discernible, marking subtle changes in the body's equilibrium.

Second Level:

- **Manifestation**: These drugs, when administered, induce a quality in the body that supersedes the effects of the Dawa Motadil. This newfound quality is prominent enough to be recognized by the individual.
- **Implications**: Despite its perceptibility, the drug's effects do not impede routine functions such as sleep patterns, appetite, or physical activity. These drugs primarily target the body's fluidic systems. For instance, a drug with hot and dry attributes might lead to diminished appetite and sporadic insomnia, whereas a drug characterized as cold and moist can enhance sleep and appetite. Should a disruption in bodily functions arise due to intrinsic causes, a slightly mushil[343] (purgative) hot drug from the second tier can restore balance.

Third Level:

- **Manifestation**: Drugs classified under this category bring about pronounced physiological changes, far surpassing the norm. The effects are immediately evident and can potentially disrupt daily routines.
- **Implications**: Chronic exposure or consumption of these drugs can be detrimental. While they influence the body's fluid and fatty components, they remain non-lethal.

Fourth Level:

- **Manifestation**: This category encompasses drugs that induce extremely potent changes within the body to the point of being life-threatening.

---

[343] Mushil drug which help in the expulsion of morbid humours in the form of loose motions by intestines. This mode of treatment is generally adopted for the evacuation of bad humours of stomach, intestines, liver and joints.

- **Implications**: Many substances within this tier are deemed poisonous and are thus categorized as 'simmi advia' (poisonous drugs).

Differences between Toxic Drugs (simmi advia) and Absolute Poisons (simm-e-mutlaq)

Toxic Drugs (simmi advia):

- **Definition**: Toxic drugs are substances that induce an overwhelmingly potent quality (kefiyat) capable of causing harm.
- **Characteristics**:
    - Their inherent properties can disrupt the natural equilibrium of the body. For example, opium introduces an excessive cold property, whereas arsenic instils an excessive heat.
    - Though inherently harmful in their raw form, their deleterious effects can be mitigated through detoxification processes, known as 'mudabbir'.
- **Examples**:
    - **Opium (affiyun)**: When administered without proper preparation or in excessive amounts, it can overly cool the body's natural mechanisms.
    - **Arsenic trioxide (Sammulfar)**: It can cause harmful heating effects in the body if not appropriately treated or administered.

Absolute Poisons (simm-e-mutlaq):

- **Definition**: Absolute poisons possess inherently detrimental properties with minimal or no therapeutic benefits.
- **Characteristics**:
    - These substances cannot be rendered harmless or therapeutic, regardless of preparation or quantity.
    - Ingestion typically leads to severe physiological consequences such as syncope (loss of consciousness), pronounced weakness, and profuse perspiration.
- **Example**:
    - **Potassium Cyanide**: An archetypical absolute poison, it offers no medicinal advantage and poses grave risks upon ingestion.

Nuanced Understanding of Dosage:

Understanding that the distinction between a therapeutic drug and a poison often lies in the administered dose is pivotal. An excessively high dose of a normally therapeutic drug can manifest poisonous attributes, whereas a significantly reduced dose of a known poison might potentially offer therapeutic properties. This underscores the ancient aphorism, 'The dose makes the poison'.

Effects of drugs

The term 'effects of drugs' refers to the changes that drugs cause in the human body, whether in a healthy or unhealthy state. When we talk about the 'function of drugs', we are referring to the results observed when these substances are administered under normal and healthy conditions.

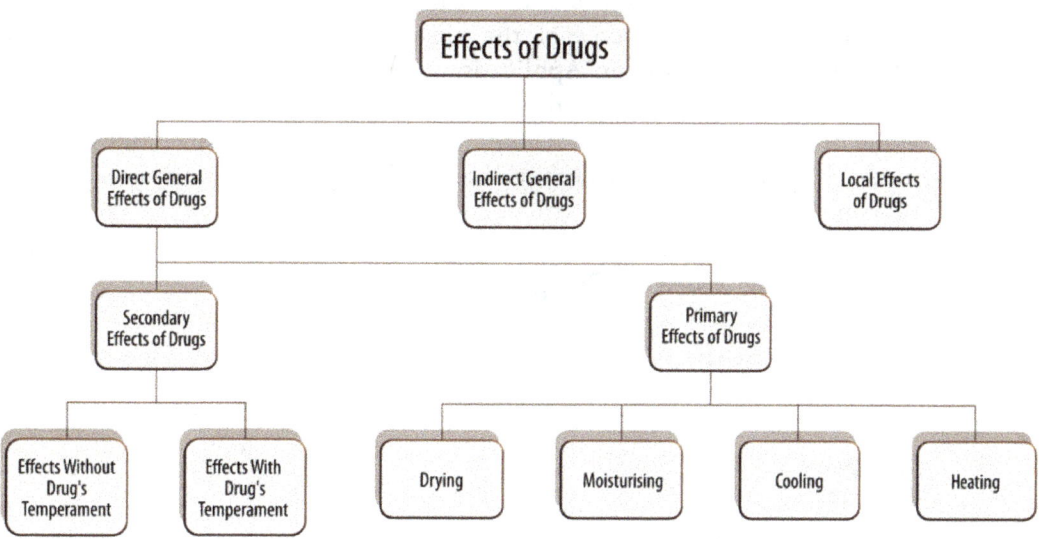

Drug Effects in Terms of Transformation and Metabolism

Drugs can manifest their effects through two primary mechanisms of action:

1. **Taseerate Awal (Primary Effect):** This refers to the immediate impact of a drug upon administration before the body has had a chance to metabolize or alter its composition. An example of this is the immediate effect elicited by acids.
2. **Taseerate Saanawi (Secondary Effect):** Secondary effects arise post-metabolism. Once the body processes and transforms the drug, its subsequent

effects can be different from its primary ones. An example would be acidic medications. These drugs may convert into salts upon entering the bloodstream, leading to varied effects on organs such as the kidneys. To illustrate, ingesting acidic saline can augment the alkalinity of urine.

Differences between the Internal and External Effects of Drugs:

1. **Externally Effective Only**: Some drugs only work when applied externally and not when consumed internally. For example, onions can affect the skin when applied as a paste (Zimad). However, consuming onions does not affect the stomach lining similarly.
2. **Internally Effective Only**: Conversely, some drugs are only effective when ingested and have no notable impact on the skin when applied topically. Zinc oxide (Safeda Kashgari) can be safely applied to the skin but can be dangerous if ingested.
3. **Consistent Effects Regardless of Application**: Some drugs have consistent effects, whether used internally or externally. Drinking water cools the body, while its external application cools the skin.
4. **Opposite Effects Based on Application**: It is important to note that certain drugs can have varying effects depending on how they are used. For example, coriander can reduce hard swellings when applied externally. However, if ingested, it may increase the density of certain bodily fluids or substances instead of reducing them.

Varied Effects of Drugs Based on Dosage:

Drugs can exhibit diverse effects depending on the quantity administered. A few examples are:

1. **Camphor**:
    - In small doses, it acts as an aphrodisiac, enhancing sexual desire.
    - It serves as an anaphrodisiac in larger doses, reducing or inhibiting sexual desire.

2. **Rewand Chini (Chinese Rhubarb - Rheum emodi)**:
    - When taken in minimal quantities (0.2-0.35 grams), it functions as a tonic for the stomach.
    - In higher doses (2-2.5 grams), it serves as a purgative, helping to clear the bowels.

Dual and Unique Effects of Drugs:

Certain drugs can demonstrate dual or opposing effects based on their inherent components:

- **Rewand Chini's Dual Action:** Rewand Chini, when taken in higher doses, can cause diarrhoea initially, but later it leads to constipation. According to Ibn Sina's theory, this does not suggest that a single component is responsible for both reactions. Instead, different constituents in the drug may exhibit their effects successively. In the case of Rewand Chini, it initially shows its purgative properties, followed by its astringent qualities. This makes it a good example of a compound-potent drug.
- **Diaphoretics (Muarriqat):** Some drugs, like diaphoretics, initially elevate body heat (offering relief) and later reduce it.

Physical properties of drugs

Understanding a drug's physical properties is crucial in determining its function, characteristics, and mode of action. These properties encompass smell, colour, taste, weight (referring to the heaviness or lightness of a drug), form, and shape.

It is possible for two drugs to have similarities in some specific properties such as colour, taste, or smell. However, it is important to note that no two drugs will be exactly the same in all physical properties. According to physicians, even if two substances' attributes appear identical, their modes of action and compositions are likely to be different.

Moreover, the external and internal characteristics of all manufactured substances, including drugs, are shaped by their modes of action. When a substance's composition or temperament alters, its mode of action inevitably changes.

Additional properties for drug identification

Beyond the aforementioned properties, several other characteristics can aid in recognising a drug, for example, smoke, heat, melting, freezing, moisture absorption, dryness, dissolving, changes when mixed with something, crystallisation, sedimentation and mixture, etc.

Vaporisation:

Vaporisation is a process in which some drugs turn into smoke and rise when exposed to heat, sunlight, or fire. For instance, camphor (Cinnamomum camphora), purified sulphur (Gandhak), frankincense, rose, pandanus (kewda), aniseed (Pimpinella anisum seed), etc., exhibit such properties.

Based on these properties, the essences of some drugs are evaporated according to their composition. For example, the smoke of purified sulphur, frankincense, and agarwood (ood) is given, while the essence of some drugs, such as rose, aniseed, cardamom, etc., is extracted.

Burning:

Some drugs start to burn from a little or strong heat, such as Gandhak (purified sulphur).

Melting:

Some drugs melt when heated and become thin, and their volume increases. For example, due to porosity, the volume of fats, wax, ghee, Gandhak (purified sulphur), etc. increases.

Freezing:

Instead of being thin and liquid, some drugs become hard and frozen when heated, such as egg white.

Moisture absorption :

Some drugs can absorb the moisture from the atmosphere and are called hygroscopic—for example, saline drugs.

Weather and Drugs: Drugs absorb water vapours from the atmosphere in the rainy season and dissolve.

Drying:

Many drugs have watery moisture that dry when heated, changing their external shape, colour, smell, etc.

Growing:

Some drugs grow when they absorb atmospheric moisture, for example, limestone.

Dissolving:

It is important to note that different drugs dissolve in different substances. For instance, salt and sugar can dissolve in water but not in oil, whereas Gandhak (Sulphur) and camphor can dissolve in oil but not in water. The process of determining which substances can dissolve in which solvent is carried out through experiments.

Crystallisation:

Some drugs take the shape of crystals/grains. For example, Sankhya (Purified Arsenic trioxide) and Raskapur (Calomel)[344], the essence of Darchikna[345] obtained through their sublimation, are crystallised in grain forms.

Sedimentation of the dissolved part:

Although usually liquid, some substances can transform into a thicker, semi-solid state and settle as sediment when mixed with certain agents. A prime example of this is egg whites. When egg whites are mixed with water, they dissolve completely. However, when a small amount of Phitkri (alum) is added to the mixture, the dissolved components in the egg white solidify. Consequently, these solidified particles sink to the bottom, forming aggregates that resemble cotton balls.

Mixture:

Some drugs can interact with each other, either physically or chemically. However, certain drugs, such as oil and water, cannot mix at all.

Hypothesis and experiments

It is clear from the works of Ibn Sina and other pioneering physicians that the properties of drugs can be determined through hypothesis and experimentation.

Experiments

Ibn al-Nafis[346] explains that to determine a drug's effects, it must first be introduced to the human body externally or internally and then observed. Historically, drugs have been first tested on animals such as monkeys and horses. Once a drug's properties have been observed in animals, it can then be cautiously tested on humans to check whether the same effects are reproduced. This is because a drug might produce a particular effect in animals but not in humans or even have the opposite effect due to the distinct temperamental differences between species.

---

[344] A compound of Mercury, Alumina, Armenian bole and Sodium chloride also known as Calomel.
[345] A compound of Mercury and Arsenic.
[346] Ibn al-Nafis (1213–1288) Arab polymath whose areas of work included medicine, surgery, physiology, anatomy, biology, Islamic studies, jurisprudence, and philosophy. He is known for being the first to describe the pulmonary circulation of the blood. The work of Ibn al-Nafis regarding the right sided (pulmonary) circulation pre-dates the later work (1628) of William Harvey's De motu cordis.

Hypothesis

Ibn al-Nafis defines a hypothesis as an assertion about the concealed features of a drug based on its known characteristics. It may or may not be confirmed or refuted by experimentation. It should be noted that a hypothesis does not necessarily have to be correct.

Other means of discovering drug properties:

1. **Through Chance:** Many significant discoveries were made by chance. For instance, an individual visits a new place and consumes an unknown food or drug, leading to symptoms such as diarrhoea, vomiting, sweating, or excess urination, ultimately curing their ailment. As a result, that drug's or diet's properties and functions become known and are later confirmed through additional experimentation.
2. **Mental Inclination:** Sometimes, the choice to use a medication arises from an individual's impulsive desire or inclination. An instance of this is the story of someone with oedema who ate salted fried locusts while in a state of distress and was cured as a result. Their recovery was not from extensive research but rather a simple personal instinct.
3. **Malicious Intent:** For example, using Arsenic trioxide (Sankhya), a toxic substance, in an attempt to harm an individual who was prediagnosed with syphilis and instead of causing harm, the ingestion of Arsenic trioxide resulted in the cure of their syphilis.
4. **During Famine or Travel:** While travelling or in cases of famine, people may consume unfamiliar types of fruits, stems, flowers, root vegetables, etc. This has led to the discovery of these foods' medicinal properties and characteristics. For instance, the medicinal properties and characteristics of Chob Chini (Smilax china root) and tea were discovered through this process.
5. **Intuition:** There have been times when beliefs regarding a drug's efficacy or its potential benefits in managing certain conditions have been perceived as divine or supernatural revelations.
6. **Inspiration:** There are instances where patients feel an innate drive to consume a particular substance, believing it will alleviate their symptoms. When this belief proves true, it can further our understanding of that substance's medicinal properties.
7. **Through Dreams:** Some individuals have reported receiving insights about treatments in their dreams, which, when acted upon, led to their healing.
8. **Observation of the Animal Kingdom:** Observing animals and their natural remedies can provide valuable insights. Galen's[347] knowledge about enemas, believed to be inspired by observing a bird, is a great example. This observation

---

[347] Galen of Pergamon, was a Roman Greek physician, surgeon and philosopher. Considered to be one of the most accomplished of all medical researchers of antiquity.

is why enemas are called Amal-e-Ta'ir, which means 'the action of a bird'. Moreover, the observation that snakes rub their eyes with fennel leaves after hibernation has helped us understand the properties of fennel leaves. This observation also inspired the preparation of kohl using antimony dissolved in anise water, which is now known as an eye tonic.

Experiments vs hypothesis

Experiments are a direct and reliable way to determine the effects of drugs. They differ from hypotheses, which serve as foundational assertions that guide the course of experimentation. Ibn al-Nafis emphasized the distinction and interrelation between the two.

According to Ibn al-Nafis:

1. The true effects of drugs are ascertained through experimentation rather than mere hypothesis. This is because hypotheses can often be erroneous, leading to inaccurate conclusions about a drug's effects.
2. The methodologies and techniques involved in experimentation are universally recognized and can be practised by medical professionals and laypeople. In contrast, formulating a hypothesis is a specialized skill, primarily within the domain of scholarly physicians.
3. Experimentation has the advantage of revealing a drug's primary and secondary effects. Hypotheses, however, can only shed light on primary effects and the conditions under which they manifest.

Principles for experiments on drugs:

1. **Experiments on humans:** It is essential to primarily conduct experiments on humans because physiological responses between humans and animals differ. What may be safe for an animal may be harmful or toxic for humans. For instance, birds can consume Shokran (Conium maculatum seed) without any harm, but it can be toxic to humans. Similarly, substances like almonds or dates can affect animals differently than humans.
2. **Purity of the Drug:** Drugs undergoing testing must be pure and free from external influences or temporary conditions. This is necessary to ensure that the observed effects are solely attributed to the drug itself. For instance, when opium is heated, it causes dilation of blood vessels; however, when it is cooled, it results in vasoconstriction. Such external factors can alter the inherent properties of the drug, which can impact the results of the testing.
3. **Diverse Testing:** In order to identify which diseases, benefit from a drug and which do not, it is important to test the drug across a range of diseases. Administering the drug in varying doses to different age groups, during different

seasons, and through various routes can provide a more comprehensive understanding of its effects.
4. **Simplicity in Diseases:** Drugs should be trialled on simple diseases rather than compound ones for clear and concise results. This approach facilitates understanding the drug's inherent properties without interfering with multiple disease factors.
5. **Dose Proportionality:** A drug's dosage should be proportional to the disease's severity. The further the disease deviates from a state of equilibrium or moderation, and the more potent the drug should be in terms of its properties and weight.
6. **Immediate Effects:** The primary effects of a drug should manifest promptly upon administration. Complex drugs, having multiple essences, might exhibit sequential effects. For instance, Rewand Chini (Rheum emodi) has a purgative essence that acts initially, followed by an astringent essence inducing constipation.
7. **Duration of Effects:** For a drug's effects to be considered primary and natural, they should be prolonged and persistent. Transient effects are usually incidental and not the drug's fundamental properties.

Precautions in Drug Experiments:

1. **Sensory Assessment:** It is important to conduct a preliminary evaluation by smelling or tasting the substance before experimenting with it. If a drug has an unpleasant smell or taste, it could be an indicator of potential harm. It is crucial to keep in mind that some substances can be fatal, even in small amounts.
2. **Animal Testing:** Before human trials, drugs should be tested on animals with similar physiological characteristics to humans, such as monkeys. By observing the effects on these animals, researchers can understand the drug's properties and potential impact.
3. **Selection of Human Subjects:** After the animal testing, human trials should be conducted with utmost care. The first human tests should involve young, healthy, and strong individuals who are deemed ideal candidates. Individuals who are vulnerable, such as children, elderly people, and those with weakened health, should be excluded from initial experimental stages to reduce any potential risks.

Hypothesis

When trying to understand the properties of a drug, its various characteristics, such as taste, smell, colour, consistency, and others, can help us form a hypothesis. According to physicians, the weakest hypothesis is based on the drug's colour, while the one based on its smell is considered stronger, and the strongest is based on its taste.

However, experimental testing is the only way to truly confirm the properties of a drug.

Taste Categories:

Taste is the most important factor used in the hypothesis of the effects of drugs. A total of nine types of primary tastes are mentioned.

- **Pungent/Spicy (Hirrif)**: Examples are pepper and chilli.
- **Bitter (Murr/Talkh)**: Examples are Aloe vera.
- **Salty (Maleh/Namkeem/Shor)**: An example is table salt.
- **Sour (Hamiz/Tursh/Khatta)**: Examples are dried plums, lemons, and Tamarind.
- **Astringent (Ufisa, Kasela)**: An example is Aleppo oak.
- **Mild Astringent (Qabiz)**: An example is Betel nut.
- **Oily (Dasm, Chikna)**: An example is ghee.
- **Sweet (Huluu, Shirin, Meetha)**: Examples are sugar and honey.
- **Tasteless (Masikh, Pheeka)**: An example is water.

Properties of Drugs Based on Taste:

1. **Pungent/Spicy (Hirrif) - Adwiya Hirrif**: Causes dilation of vessels, softening and thinning of substance, resolution, and heating.
2. **Bitter (Murr/Talkh) - Adwiya Murr/Talkh:** It shares properties with spicy/pungent drugs, but some, like opium, are astringent. Some bitter drugs are also antiseptic.
3. **Salty (Maleh/Namkeem/Shor) - Adwiya Malih/Namkin:** Exhibits deobstruent (Mufattih), demulcing, cutting, resolving, heating, and antiseptic properties.
4. **Sour (Hamiz/Tursh/Khatta) - Adwiya Hamiz**: It is characterized by demulcing, cutting of substance, diffusion, and deobstruent properties for ducts and vessels.
5. **Astringent (Ufisa, Kasela) - Adwiya Ufisa**: It often constricts the ducts due to its deterring and inhibiting nature, produces hardness and thickness in organs, acts as a refrigerant (Mubarrid), and can cause blood retention and diarrhoea.
6. **Mild Astringent (Qabiz) - Adwiya Qabiz**: Their characteristics often align with those of bitter drugs.
7. **Oily (Dasm, Chikna) - Adwiya Dasm**: Generally, acts as a moisturizer for the body, softener, relaxant, lubricator, flatulent, and Musakhkhin (warming agent).
8. **Sweet (Huluu, Shirin, Meetha) - Adwiya Hulu/Shirin**: Often detergent, relaxant, concoctive (munzij), softening, lubricating, and Musakhkhin.
9. **Tasteless (Masikh, Pheeka) - Adwiya Masikh/Phiki**: When moist, it often relieves heat and thirst.

All the mentioned rules are hypotheses, as exceptions may be found in each category.

Properties and Taste:

1. **Har kefiyat (Hotness)**: Associated with strong/hot and oily tastes.

2. **Barid kefiyat (Coldness)**: Found with bitter tastes, followed by sweet, and then, to a lesser extent, oily taste.
3. **Ratib kefiyat (Wetness)**: Present with a bitter taste, then sweet, and after that with an oily taste.
4. **Yaboosat kefiyat (Dryness)**: Corresponds with pungent, saline, astringent, and sour tastes.

Smell:

The properties of drugs can be explained by their smell, which is due to the lighter particles that produce vapours reaching our noses. The dense constituents of drugs do not form fumes nor do they evaporate, and their colours don't reflect and reach our sight. By sniffing drugs, we can identify whether they are hot or cold, as the odorous constituents evaporate in fumes and contain some heat. Strong-smelling drugs usually generate heat in the human body, such as Saffron, Amber, Musk, Cloves, Cinnamon, and Cumin. On the other hand, drugs that soothe the brain through their fragrance are cold in temperament.

According to Ibn al-Nafis, heat is necessary for the odorous components to evaporate, whether it comes from air, sun, or fire. Therefore, when the odour is faint, it can become more potent when cooked or heated, indicating that heat carries the scent to our nostrils.

All components of drugs do not need to be hot. Some constituents of the drugs can be cold and odourless. For instance, Sankhya (Purified Arsenic trioxide) has no odour. However, it is hot and a potent Musakhkhin (produces heat in the body), whereas Camphor (Kafoor), despite having a strong odour, is considered cold by most physicians. Therefore, the hypothesis that smell determines the nature of a drug cannot be considered a universal law, as several other factors may influence the nature of a drug.

Colour of the drug:
When discussing the properties of a drug, relying solely on its color is the weakest hypothesis; it is similar to calling something white 'cold'.

Consistency and weight of a drug:

The term 'consistency' in the context of drugs refers to the physical state of the drug, whether it is in a solid, liquid, or gaseous form. Solid drugs may be either hard or soft, and their constituents may be crimped, making them easy to disperse. Liquid drugs can be either similar to water, mucinous, or semi-liquid. Similarly, a drug may be light or heavy depending on the weight. A light drug is called Khafeef[348] and a heavy drug may be called Thaqil[349].

Different Degrees of Consistency and Weight:

1. **Dawa Latif (Light Drug):**
    a. Easily disintegrated and absorbed by the body over a short duration.
    b. Examples: Zafran (Saffron - Crocus sativus Linn.) and alcohol.
2. **Dawa kasif (Dense/Heavy Drug):**
    a. It disintegrates slowly and requires more time for absorption.
    b. Fast-digesting foods are termed dawa latif, while slow-digesting foods are referred to as dawa khatif.
3. **Dawa Jaamid (Solid Drug):**
    a. Characterized by structural rigidity and resistance to changes in shape or volume.
4. **Dawa Hush (Brittle Drug):**
    a. A solid drug that easily disintegrates under gentle pressure or when rubbed lightly.
    b. Examples: Aloe vera and mushroom.
5. **Dawa Lazij (Viscous Drug):**
    a. It spreads easily and possesses adhesive and sticky qualities.
    b. Example: Honey.
6. **Dawa Sayyal (Liquid Drug):**
    a. A fluid drug that assumes the shape of its container.
7. **Dawa Lu'abi (Mucilaginous Drug):**
    a. Produces mucilage when immersed in water.
    b. Examples: Quince seed and marshmallow seeds when soaked in water.
8. **Dawa Duhni (Oily Drug):**
    a. Contains oil content.
    b. Examples: Almonds, walnuts, and other nuts.

Other physical and chemical properties

When developing a hypothesis, the properties of drugs, both physical and chemical, can be useful. As Ibn Sina wrote, the functions and effects of drugs we already know can guide understanding their unknown effects through hypotheses and experiments.

Ibn Sina suggests that while we know certain drug properties, others may remain unknown. Examining the drug's taste, smell, colour, and nature can guide us in discovering the unknown effects through hypothesis. Similarly, we can use the known effects of drugs to establish a hypothesis about the unknown effects. For instance, if a

---

[348] A drug weighing relatively less than another drug of the same origin.
[349] Drug weighing more as compared with another drug of the same origin

drug has an astringent effect on the mucous membrane of the mouth and tongue, we might hypothesise that it can stop epistaxis or be beneficial in leucorrhoea.

In such cases, we can hypothesise by comparing it with other astringents, assuming that they contain astringent constituents since these drugs have an astringent effect on mucous membranes. This leads to a strong hypothesis that the astringent component can constrict blood vessels and stop nosebleeds. Its astringent power affects the mucous membrane of the vagina, thus decreasing the secretion of fluid as other astringents do.

Issues in hypothesis

Our above stated hypothesis does not always apply. There is a possibility of encountering misconceptions when dealing with compounds and potent compound drugs. This is because even after the development of the secondary temperament, the dominating properties such as the odour, colour, and taste of any of the components of the compound persist.

However, the effect of heat and cold on these components, as compared to the odour, colour, taste, etc. is weak and recessive, making it difficult to identify the second property. This means that the odour, colour, and taste dominate one component of the compound, but their significant effects are subsidiary to other constituents.

For instance, if 10 grams of farfiyun (Cactus latex - spurge) are added to half a kilogram of milk, the resulting mixture's effects and temperament will be related to the dominating effect of farfiyun, making it hot. However, the colour will remain white due to the colour of milk.

Similarly, if potent drugs like Sankhya (Purified Arsenic trioxide), Beesh (Aconitum nepallus root), Azraqi/ Kuchla Mudabbar[350] (Strychnos nux-vomica), and khushta[351], which are strongly effective even in small amounts, are mixed with drugs whose taste, odour, and colour differ from them, and these toxic drugs become indistinguishable in them, then relying solely on colour, odour, and taste can lead to dangerous consequences.

Effects of drugs on organs

The human body is composed of organs of the nervous system, vital organs and digestive organs. Therefore, the effects of drugs on these organs are explained in detail below to explain the principle of treatment for the diseases of these organs.

Effects of drugs on digestive organs

Drugs affecting the stomach

---

[350] Drug subjected to certain treatments for the purpose of cleaning, purification or detoxification in order to improve efficacy and reduce toxicity.
[351] Farsi word which literally means burning of drugs of metallic, mineral or animal origin into their ash.

1. Drugs that strengthen digestion by increasing the gastric juices of the stomach are called Muqawwi-e-Meda (stomachic).
2. Some of them are aromatic, such as aniseed (Anisoon), fennel (Badiyan), Cardamon, Coriander seeds (Kishneez), Sonth (Zingiber officinale – dried ginger), cloves, nutmeg, mint, etc.
3. Some are bitter, such as Chamomile flowers, Orange peel, and pakhanbed (Bergenia ligulata) etc.
4. Some are spicy, for example, red chili and Kabab Chini (Piper cubeba – tailed pepper), etc. Some astringent drugs also act as gastrotonic.
5. Also, there are some substances that are not included under the above headings, such as alcohol.
6. Some drugs reduce the gastric juice of the stomach (Muzayyif-e-Meda - stomach depressants), such as Suhaga/Tinker (borax), Jawakhar (Potassium Carbonate), Noshadar (Ammonium Chloride), etc. These types of alkaline drugs reduce the secretion of gastrium.
7. Some drugs increase the acidity of the stomach, such as acids, Gandhak (purified sulphur).
8. Some drugs prevent the formation of yeast in the food in the stomach, such as Ajwain (Carum capticum seed).
9. Some drugs dilate the vessels of the stomach, such as aniseed, fennel, dried ginger (Sonth), clove, mint, Suranjan (Colchicum leutiun root), etc.
10. Some drugs constrict the vessels of the stomach, such as acid, Gandhak (purified sulphur) and Phitkri (alum).
11. Some drugs affect the nerves and muscles of the stomach and increase the rotatory movements of the stomach, such as Kuchla Mudabbar (Strychnos nuxvomica seed), Gandhak (purified sulphur) and camphor oil, etc.
12. Some drugs affect the nerves and muscles of the stomach and weaken the rotatory movements of the stomach, such as Yabruj (Atropa belladonna root), opium and Ajwain Khurasani (Hyoscyamus niger), etc.
13. Some drugs expel flatus from the stomach and intestines and increase the movements of the stomach and intestines. These types of drugs are called carminatives (Kasir Riyah). For example, asafoetida, fennel, mint, dried ginger, aniseed, Kabab Chini (Piper cubeba – tailed pepper), black pepper and rye, etc.
14. Some drugs cause vomiting by directly affecting the stomach, while others do so by affecting the vomiting centre[352]. Examples are rye, Phitkri (alum), Indian squill (Urginea Indica), Tootia (Copper sulphate); these are called emetics.
15. Some drugs are anti-emetics, e.g. opiates and alcohol (in small amounts).

Drugs affecting the intestines

---

[352] located in the medulla oblongata of the brain.

These are drugs that affect the intestine and cause defecation. Following are the types according to their effect:

1. **Mullaiyinath**[353] **(Laxatives):** Drugs that stimulate the muscles of the intestine and improve their expulsive ability, making it easy to pass stool. Some examples of such drugs are castor oil (Roghan Bedanjeer), raisins (Maveez), Shir khest[354] (Cotoneaster nummularia), Almond oil, honey, figs, tamarind.
2. **Mushilath**[355] **(Purgatives):** Drugs that not only strengthen the Quwwat Dafia (expulsive faculty) but also increase the production of moisture, which makes the stool watery. Purgatives can be classified based on their potency:
   - Mushilath Zaif/Daif (mild purgative): Drug of low potency that excretes morbid humours of the body by inducing diarrhoea e.g., Senna (Cassia senna - Cassia angustifolia), Khayarshamber (Cassia fistula), Arand (Butea frondosa pulp)
   - Mushilath Qawi (Strong purgative): Drugs that have high potency and are used to excrete morbid humours from the body by inducing watery stool. These drugs have a severe purgative action, which may lead to dehydration, and in extreme cases, even death. Some examples of these drugs include, Jamal gota (Croton), Turbud (turpeth roots), Saqmonia (scammonia resins), Usara Rewand (rhubarb - extract), Tukhhm-e-neel (Ipomoea nil seeds), Hanzal (Citrullus colocynthis) seeds, Jalapa (Ipomoea purga root).

[There are notable differences between mullaiyin (Laxative) and mushil (Purgative). Laxative drugs move material from the stomach and intestines, while purgatives move matter from the stomach and intestine and the whole body. Therefore, laxatives only clean the stomach and intestines, while purgatives clean the whole body.]

3. **Mushilath Balgham (Phlemagogue):** These drugs cause the evacuation of balgham (phlegm) through the intestines and stools. Examples are Turbud (Ipomea turbathum), Khayarshamber (Cassia fistula pulp).
4. **Mushilath Safra (Cholagogue):** Drugs that cause evacuation of safra (yellow bile) from the liver towards the intestines, such as Aloe vera, Rewand Chini (Chinese Rhubarb - Rheum emodi), Saqmonia (scammonia resins).
5. **Mushilath Buraqi (Saline purgatives):** Purgative drugs are saline and they cause excitement and stimulation in the inner layer of the stomach and intestines. This strengthens their expulsive faculty (Quwwat Dafia), increases the rotatory movements, and secretion of watery fluids. This prevents the absorption of fluids in the intestine, thus increasing the pressure in the bowel. This initiates the medicatrix naturae (Tabi'at) to accelerate the expulsive faculty to expel matter—for example, salty sea water, borax, types of salts

---

[353] Mullaiyin (singular)
[354] شیرخشت
[355] Mushil (singular)

6. **Laziyat (Irritants):** Drugs that cause stimulation and irritation in the mucous membrane of the stomach and intestines, causing inflammation and pain in the stomach and intestines and resulting in nausea, vomiting, cramps, haemorrhage and other disorders.
7. **Dafi-i-Taaffun (antiseptic):** Drug that prevents/removes putrefaction. For example, Elaichi (Elettaria cardamomum - Cardamon), Ajwain (Carum capticum seed), etc.
8. **Qatil-i-Didan-i-Am'a (Anthelmintic):** Vermicide, drug that kills intestinal worms, such as Aloe vera, Kameela (Mallotus phillipinensis), Baobarang (Embelia Ribes), Sarakhs (Dryopteris filix-mas).

Drugs affecting the liver

1. Some drugs increase safra (yellow bile humour) and its flow; they are called mudirat safra (cholagogue) or drugs increasing the flow of safra. For example, Saqmonia (scammonia resins), Rewand Chini (Chinese Rhubarb - Rheum emodi), Jalapa (Exogonium purga, Ipomoea purga seeds).
2. Some drugs increase bowel movements and cause diarrhoea. For example, Jamal gota (Croton), Turbud (turpeth roots), Kharbaq (Helleborus niger) and strong Mushilath (purgatives).
3. Some drugs strengthen the liver. They are called Muqawwi-i-Kabid/Muqawwi-i-Jigar (hepatotonic[356]). For example, cinnamon (Darchini - Cinnamomum zeylanicum), Afsanteen (Artemisia absynthium herb), Mastagi (Pistacia lantiscus gum), Raisins, Zarishk (Berberis vulgaris - barberry), Falsa (Grawia asiatica fruit), Gulab Surkh (Rosa damascena flower), Halela (Terminalia chebula), etc.
4. Some drugs regulate liver function back to normal. For example, Aab Berge-kasni sabz (Cichorium intybus leaf juice), Muravvaq Afsanteen (distillates of Artemisia absynthium - worm wood).
5. Some drugs decrease the production of bile, such as Aab Anar Tursh (bitter pomegranate water) and Aab Inab-us-Salab[357] sabz (Solanum nigrum leaf water).
6. Some drugs increase the production of safra (yellow bile humour), such as Rewand Chini (Chinese Rhubarb - Rheum emodi), Suranjan (Colchicum luteum), sibr (aloe vera), Naushader (Ammonium chloride), etc.
7. Some drugs with diverse effects also act on the liver as well as on the stomach, intestines and other organs.

Drugs affecting the urinary organs

1. Drugs that affect the kidneys and increase urine production are called Mudirat-i-Bawl (Diuretics). For example, Shora Kalmi (potassium nitrate – Saltpeter), Jaosheer (Ferula galbaniflua), Tukhme Kharpaza (Cucumis melo seed - melon

---

[356] liver tonics
[357] Inab-us-Salab comes from Arabic, which is two words Inab, meaning grapes and salab, meaning fox. More commonly called Mako in Unani.

seeds), Sheera Khayareen (milky liquid made with cucumber seeds), Sheera Khar-e-khasak/Gokhru (milky liquid made with Tribulus terrestris), etc.

2. Drugs that decrease the secretion of urine, such as Frankincense. The mizaj of these drugs is dry. Eg: Habb-ul-Aas (Myrtus communis Linn.), Khulanjan (Alpinia galanga), Saadkofi/Nagarmotha (Cyperus rotundus), Kundar / Lobaan (Boswellia Serrata - Frankincense), etc.
3. Drugs that make the urine acidic, such as Kundar / Lobaan (Boswellia Serrata - Frankincense).
4. Drugs that make the urine Alkaline, such as Shora qalmi (Potassium nitrate/saltpetre), Jawakhar (Potassium Carbonate/potash), Alkaline emetics, etc.
5. Drugs that break down stones in the kidneys, bladder, ureter. The drugs prevent the formation of minute particles in the kidney. E.g., Hajrul yahood (Lapis judaicus), Sang-e-sarmahi[358] (fish stone), etc.
6. Some drugs, such as Rogan e Sandal (sandalwood oil) Kabab Chini (Piper cubeba–tailed pepper), treat urine infections.
7. Some drugs change the colour of the urine vial. For example, the colour of the vial becomes either saffron-coloured or purple with the use of senna and Rewand Chini (Chinese Rhubarb - Rheum emodi), and Sankhya/Sammulfar (Purified Arsenic trioxide), which causes the black colour in the vial.
8. Some drugs sedate the urinary organs and are useful in case of stimulation and pain, such as Affiyun (Papaver Somniferum – opium), Yabruj (belladonna) and datura (Datura metel) etc.

Drugs affecting the reproductive organs

1. **Muqawwi-i-Bah (Aphrodisiacs)**: These drugs enhance the desire for sexual activity. Some strengthen the reproductive nerves and centres, while others stimulate blood circulation in reproductive organs. Examples include Kuchla Mudabbar and Zarareeh/Telni Makkhhi (Cantharides[359]) and most drugs used in fomentation and massage.
2. Certain drugs, like alcohol and cannabis, stimulate the brain's higher centres to increase sexual desire.
3. **Muqawwi-i-ama (General tonics)**: These drugs boost reproductive function by increasing blood production and enhancing overall health.
4. **Qati'-i-Bah (Anaphrodisiacs)**: Drugs that reduce sexual desire by weakening reproductive nerves. Examples include such as Shokran (Conium maculatum seed), opium, Ajwain Khurasani (Hyoscyamus niger), datura (Datura metel), etc.
5. Some drugs act as anaphrodisiacs by decreasing blood flow to reproductive organs, such as Shailam (Lolium termuletum).
6. Drugs like borax reduce sexual stimuli and libido excitement.

---

[358] an isolate from the skull of Channa sp., commonly known as snakeheads - useful in kidney and bladder stones, amongst other things.
[359] Broken dried remains of the blister beetle - Lytta vesicatoria.

Drugs affecting female reproductive organs

1. **Musqit-i-Janin/Mukhrij-i-Janin (Abortifacient)**: Drugs that promote contractions to expel a foetus or placenta. They may also induce menstruation. Examples include Such as Sudab (Ruta graveolens), Abhal (Juniperus communis), Doda Kapas (Gossypium herbaceum fruit)[360], Post Amaltas (Cassia fistula fruit epicarp), Ood-e-Balsan (Commi-phora opobalsamum Linn.). All strong Mushilath (purgatives) Phitkri (Alum), Alsi (Linum usitatissimum seed). All strong diuretics such as Persiaoshan (Adiantum capillus herb), Zaravand (Aristolochia longa, A. rotunda root), Hanzal (Citrullus colocynthis fruit), Zeera Siyah (Carum carvi seed).
2. **Mudir-i-Hez (Emmenagogue)**: Drugs that stimulate or increase menstrual flow. Examples include asafoetida and tukhme karafs (Apium graveolens - celery seeds, Hansraj / Persiyoshan (Adiantum capillus-veneris).
3. Some drugs induce menstruation by improving blood flow or stimulating the uterus, like Aloe vera and Kuchla Mudabbar (Strychnos nux-vomica seed).
4. **Mudif-i-Rahim**: Drugs that decrease uterine contractions, like opium and Qinnab (Cannabis sativa leaf).

Drugs affecting the female breasts:

1. **Mudirr-i-Laban (Galactagogue)**: These drugs boost milk production in the breasts. Examples are aniseed, dill seeds, turnip seeds, onion seeds.
2. **Muqallil-i-Laban (Antigalactic)**: Drugs that reduce or halt milk production, such as Yabruj (belladonna).
3. **Mugheer-i-Laban (Milk-altering drugs)**: Some foods and drugs can change the taste and composition of a lactating mother's milk, affecting the baby. For instance, the consumption of asafoetida and garlic can alter the taste of milk, while the intake of bitter food can cause pain and discomfort in the baby's stomach. Similarly, consuming salty foods can increase the borax component in milk.

Effects of drugs on vital organs

Effects of drugs on Qalib (heart) and Ruh (pneuma)

Ibn Sina has described the following drugs that affect the heart:

Drug Name	Botanical Name	Drug Name	Botanical Name
Aas	Myrtus communis	Marwareed	Pearls

---

[360] Plant origin drugs parts used are root, stem, fruits, flowers, leaves, seed, gum and peel. You will commonly see these words in front of names of plants: Flowers (Gul) and leaves (Barg), Seeds (Tukhm) and fruits (Phal), Roots (Beikh), Branches (Shaakh) and barks (Chaal), Shrubs (Bootiyan) Gums (Gond), shell/outer cover (post).

Abresham	Bombyx mori	Meat soup	
Ambar	Ambra grisea	Mint	Mentha
Amla	Phyllanthus emblica	Momiyaee	Asphaltum
Anar	Punica granatum (Pomegranate)	Musk	Moschus moschiferus secretion
Apple	Malus pumila	Nilofar	Iris Florentina
Armaak/Kewda	Pandanus odoratissimus	Nimam/Kali Tulsi	Ocimum canum sims
Azaryun/Azarboya	Helianthus annuus	Ood Saleeb	Paeonia officinalis, root
Badranjboya	Melissa officinalis	Pista	Pistacia vera
Badrooj	Ocimum basilicum	Rewand Chini	Rheum emodi
Barg-e-Gaozaban	Borago officinalis, leaf	Rose petals	Rosa centifolia
Behman	Centaurea behen	Saad/Nagarmotha	Cyperus rotundus
Coriander (Dry)	Coriandrum sativum	Saleekha/Taj Kalami	Cinnamomum cassia
Darchini	Cinnamomum zeylanicum	Sandal	Santalum album wood
Darunaj Aqrabi	Doronicum pardalianches Linn.	Sausan	Iris - Iris Florentina
Egg yolk of hen, partridge, quail		Sazij Hindi/Tez Paat	Cinnamomum tamala leaf
Elaichi	Elettaria cardamomum	Shaqaqul Misri	Pastinaca secacul Linn
Fizza/Chandi	Argentum	Sumbul-ut-teeb	Valeriana Officinalis Linn.
Franjmishk	Ocimum gratissimum seed	Tabasheer	Bambusa arundinacea
Ghareeqoon	Polyporus officinalis	Tamer Hindi	Tamarindus indica
Gil-e-Malthtoom	Terra sigillata	Ushna/Charila	Parmelia perlata
Guava	Psidium guajava	Ustukhudus	Lavender stoechas
Hajar-e-Armani	Lapis anninium	Utruj/Turanj	Citrus medica
Halela[361]	Terminalia chebula	Yaqoot	Ruby
Jadwar	Delphinium denudatum root	Zafran	Crocus sativus Linn.
Kafoor	Cinnamomum camphora – camphor	Zahab	Aurum
Kundar	Boswellia Serrata	Zaranabad	Curcuma zedoaria

---

[361] Halela – usually refers to Halela Kabuli -Myrobalan.

| Lajwar | Lapis lazuli | Zarnab | Abies alba Linn |

Among the above-mentioned drugs affecting the heart:

1. **Calming, Relaxing, and Strengthening:** Some drugs have a calming, relaxing, and strengthening effect on the heart. Examples include Abresham and Sandalwood.
2. **Strengthening and Contraction:** Some drugs offer the effect of strengthening and contraction. Their contracting ability aids in strengthening. For instance, Amla.
3. **Essence of the Ruh (pneuma):** Certain drugs are suitable for the essence of the Ruh due to their aromatic properties. Owing to their holding power, they bolster the essence of the Ruh and serve as Muqawwi (tonics) for palpitations. These encompass Ushna (Parmelia perlata), Cinnamon, Sumbul-ut-teeb (Valeriana Officinalis Linn.), Cardamom, Amber, and Ood Saleeb (Paeonia officinalis root).
4. **Exhilarating and Strengthening for the Essence of Ruh:** Some drugs possess exhilarating and strengthening attributes for the essence of Ruh. Examples are Saffron and Musk.
5. **Ruh (pneuma) Resplendence:** Certain drugs that render the Ruh resplendent are advantageous in exhilaration and strengthening of palpitations, such as Utruj (Citron), Kahruba (Vateria indica - Yellow Amber), Tabasheer (Bambusa arundinasia), Marvareed (Pearl), and Yaqoot (Ruby).
6. **Strengthening, Exhilaration, and Contracting:** Some drugs have traits of strengthening and exhilaration coupled with contracting capabilities. They drive out the melancholic vapours from the heart's blood through mushil (purgation), inducing strengthening and exhilaration in the heart. Examples include Lavender, Gaozaban (Borago officinalis), Badranjboya (Lemon Balm), Faranjmushk (Basil), Hajre armani/Bura armani (Armenian Bole), and Lajwar (Lazuli).
7. **Theriac (Antidote) Properties:** There are drugs which are not only invigorating and exhilarating but also possess theriac (antidote) properties. Jadwar, Busd (Coral), Abresham, and Musk are such drugs that, in addition to being Mufarreh (exhilarants) and Muqawwi (tonics), are also antidotes to snake bites and other venoms. Also, theriac properties can be found in Ghariqoon (Polyporus officinalis) and Utruj (Citron).
8. **Exhilaration, Strengthening, Refining, and Tightening:** Some drugs, in addition to exhilarating and strengthening the heart, also have refining and tightening capabilities. For instance, Behman (Centaurea behen root), Zarnab (Abies alba), and Zaranabad (Curcuma zedoaria).
9. **Aromatic, Softening, and Contracting:** Certain drugs also carry softening and contracting attributes and aromatic features. Due to these characteristics, these

drugs are beneficial in treating palpitation and acute syncope as heart exhilarants. For example, Gule surkh (Rosa damascena flower).
10. **Innate Energy for Strengthening and Refreshment:** Some drugs are instrumental for strengthening and refreshing the heart and Ruh (pneuma) owing to their innate energy. Examples are Amla, Abresham, and Hajre armani/Bura armani (Armenian Bole).
11. **Mushilath (Purgatives):** Some Mushilath serve to expel a detrimental khilt (humour) from the heart and brain via purgation. For example, Joshanda (Decoction) of Aftimoon (Cuscuta reflexa roxb - Dodder) and shabyar pills made from Aftimoon.

Use of other drugs with Qalib Mufarreh (Heart exhilarants) and Muqawwi (tonics)

Certain therapeutic agents have dual purposes. They are used for purgation and act to purify the blood of the heart, resulting in the formation of a pristine Ruh (pneuma). For example, the combination of Lajwar (Lazuli) and Hajar-e-Armani (Armenian Bole – Lapis anninium) with Saffron (Zafran – Crocus sativa stigma) and Musk (Moschus moschiferus) serves this purpose. These drugs are specifically drawn towards the heart when introduced into the system and actively dispel the melancholic vapours that form within the heart's Ruh.

- **Mushilath (purgatives)** can be harmful to the heart for two reasons:
    a. In addition to eliminating undesirable matter (Mavaad), purgatives also remove beneficial substances essential for the Tabi'at (medicatrix naturae).
    b. Istifragh[362] (evacuation) places undue stress on the body's organs and the (Tabi'at). This is because it draws the humours (Akhlat) from the organs, directing them towards the stomach and intestines. As a result, the Tabi'at, works to absorb these humours and anchor them where they naturally belong. Whereas the Mushilath (purgatives) medicines act as opposite to Istifragh (an evacuation) and do not act until they are able to weaken the vital power.

    Also, purgatives tend to decrease the substance of the Ruh (pneuma) and weaken the temperament of the heart.
- **Mudirrat (diuretics) and Muarriqat (diaphoretics)** are beneficial when the weakness of the heart is due to the fluidity and thinness of blood. However, diuretics and diaphoretics are drying in nature and hence are harmful in agitation and fear because during this state the blood's turbidity and sawda (black bile) increases in thickness.

---

[362] of the six essential factors for maintenance of health; it is necessary for removal of waste products/metabolites through defecation, micturition, menstruation, coitus, sweating and spittle; in case of any imbalance, various disorders may occur; it may also be used for managing certain disease conditions.

- **Mulattif**[563] **(demulcent)** drugs such as Cinnamon and Saffron (Crocus sativus Linn.) are added to the drugs for the heart when the agitated heart is Sawdawi (melancholic) in nature and weak heart due to coldness and density of blood heart and is unable to produce Ruh (pneuma) in sufficient quantities.
- **Mulayyin (resolvents)** drugs, for example, Jund Bedastar (Castoreum).
- **Mufattih (deobstruent)**, such as lavender, and honey, are added to the drugs for the heart to infuse into 'heavy' drugs such as Hajre armani/Bura armani (Armenian Bole) and Amber due to their strong Taftih (dissolving) action.
- **Muqabid (astringent acting)** drugs, such as coral are added to drug for the heart to provide strength to the essence of the Ruh so that it does not dissolve too quickly. They are also more useful in a weaker heart than in agitated heart because a weak heart is often due to dilution of blood and Ruh (pneuma) whereas agitated heart is due to the concentration of blood.
- **Radi**[364] **(matter diverter)** drugs, such as psyllium husk (Ispaghol), are added to heart medications when Su-e-Mizaj har (acute abnormal temperament) causes discomfort to the heart.
- **Mukhaddir (anaesthetic)** drugs such as opium are added to the drugs of the heart to protect them until they reach the heart and to preserve their potency in the heart.
- **Munaqi (detergent/cleaning)** drugs are added to the drugs of the heart to facilitate respiration and promotion of the heart as these drugs provide strength and faculty to the heart.

Adverse Effects of Munaffikh (Gas-Creating) Substances on the Heart

Substances like ginger, black-eyed peas, and garden cress are known to produce gases. These are especially detrimental for individuals with weak or agitated hearts. The reason is that these substances emit vapors that negatively affect the essence of the Ruh (pneuma). The impact of these vapors can be likened to how waste products affect bodily organs. Consequently, they are not recommended for the Ruh since they diminish its functionality, leading to further weakening and agitation of the heart.

The harmful effects of Mulayyin (resolvents) on the heart

Mulayyin (resolvents) generally are not recommended for a weak or agitated heart. Their effects can differ based on the underlying condition:

- **In a Weak Heart**: If the heart's weakness results from a cold and concentrated Ruh (pneuma), resolvents may be detrimental. They can cause the dissolution of

---

[363] ملطّف A drug which liquefies thick and viscous matter into smaller particles.
[364] رادع Drug that diverts matter from one part of the body/organ to another part.

an already dilute or scarce Ruh. This is because substances resembling vapours or flatus (gas) are more susceptible to dissolution.
- **In an Agitated Heart**: Resolvents can be harmful in two scenarios:
    a. If the agitation is due to an insufficient amount of Ruh, using resolvents can further reduce its quantity.
    b. If the agitation stems from a dense and concentrated Ruh, resolvents might dissolve only the softer parts, resulting in an even denser remainder.

For situations where resolvents are necessary, it is important to pair them with drugs that strengthen, accumulate, and protect the Ruh's function. These drugs should also be beneficial for the heart. Examples include Mint and Halela (Terminalia chebula).

Muqawwi (tonics) possessing Tiryaq (antidotal or theriac) properties are often incorporated into heart medications. They are deemed particularly compatible with human nature and since the heart is the core of human nature, these medicines are believed to bolster its strength and safeguard it against toxins. Examples of tonics with antidote properties are Darunaj Aqrabi (Doronicum pardalianches Linn.), Jadwar and Musk (Moschus moschiferus).

Mufarreh (Exhilarants) are a subclass of Tiryaq (antidotal drugs), but it is important to note that not every antidote is an exhilarant.

There are different types of antidotal drugs with varying properties. Some, like Jund Bedastar (Castoreum), have a warm nature, while others, like camphor and parsley (Karafs), have cooler properties. However, the temperature of these drugs is not always linked to their antidotal effects. These drugs are essential because toxins are harmful to the Ruh (pneuma), and Tiryaq (antidote/theriac) drugs help counteract their effects. In certain cases, antidote drugs with increased warmth are necessary to stimulate the powerful movement of Ruh.

When dealing with toxins, the antidotal effects must work quickly to ensure the therapeutic properties can mix with and neutralize the toxin before it reaches the heart. These drugs also warm the essence of Ruh (pneuma) to such an extent that they can eliminate the toxin. At the same time, their antidotal attributes protect the Ruh from disintegration and contamination, which could have otherwise resulted from such intense temperament.

This suggests that the most potent antidotal drugs induce a state in the Ruh (pneuma) that, although not inherently therapeutic, offers resilience and defence against toxins.

Fragrances and sweetness are intrinsically connected with the vital Ruh (pneuma) in the heart and the natural Ruh in the liver, respectively. The reason for this is that fragrances resonate with the soft essence of gases or smoke, while sweetness aligns with a more concentrated, localized essence. In other words, fragrances nourish the pneuma, whereas sweetness nourishes the body.

Therefore, medications designed for the heart generally have low fragrance levels but are high in sweetness. Conversely, liver medications are less sweet but more aromatic. This distinction exists because the heart serves as the source of sustenance for the spirit, while the liver provides nourishment for the body.

Effects of drugs on respiratory organs

1. Drugs Affecting Overall Lung Function:

- **Stimulants:** Certain drugs stimulate sensory nerves to enhance lung function. When inhaled, tobacco is an example, while Kuchla Mudabbar (Strychnos nux-vomica seed) is an example when consumed.
- **Irritants:** The vapours from Lakhlakha (inhalation) and Nashuq[365] (insufflation) are potent. They penetrate vessels, leading to mucous membrane irritation.
- **Depressants:** Some drugs decrease lung function by dampening sensory nerve stimulation. Opium and Shokran (Conium peculator) are examples.

2. Drugs Impacting the Lung Airways:

- **Phlegm Producers:** Some drugs like tobacco, garlic, and liquorice root (Asal Alsoos - Glycyrrhiza glabra) amplify phlegm production in the airways.
- **Phlegm Reducers:** Drugs such as Yabruj (belladonna), Affiyun (Papaver Somniferum - opium), and datura (Datura metel) diminish phlegm production.
- **Infection Expellers:** Kabab Chini (Piper cubeba), mint essence, and Ajwain (Carum capticum seed) essence, along with specific inhalation and insufflation fragrances, help eliminate phlegm infections.
- **Spasm Relievers:** Tobacco, Shokran (Conium maculatum seed), and datura (Datura metel) aid in alleviating airway spasms.
- **Expectorants:** Aroosa (Adhatoda vasica), Asal Alsoos (Glycyrrhiza glabra - liquorice root), Anisoon (Pimpinella anisum seed - aniseed), Ispand (Peganum harmela seed), and Ushq (Dorcus ammonicum gum) facilitate the expulsion of phlegm.
- **Phlegm Consistency Modifiers:** Affiyun (Papaver Somniferum - opium), Yabruj (Belladonna), and Kushta Faulad (Iron Calx) thicken phlegm, making its expulsion more challenging.

Effect of Drugs on Blood Vessels

---

[365] A liquid preparation or powder that is used for insufflations.

There are two primary types of drugs affecting blood vessels:

1. **Vasodilators (Mufattih-e-Uruq)**
2. **Vasoconstrictors (Qabizat-e-Uruq)**

1. Vasodilators:

Vasodilators dilate blood vessels, enhancing blood flow. They also expand capillaries. These drugs can be further classified into:

- **Externally Used Drugs:**
    - Muhammirat (rubeficients)
    - Laza'iyat (irritants)
    - Kawiat (caustics, e.g., borax drugs)
    - Zimadat (pastes)
    - Kimadat (hot fomentation)
    - Hot Natul (irrigation)
    - Examples: Kafoor (Cinnamomum camphora - camphor), Sankhya (purified - Arsenic trioxide), Rai (Mustard - Barassica nigra), cloves, etc.
- **Internally Used Drugs:**
    - Examples: Tea, coffee, besh (aconite), Yabruj (belladonna), datura (Datura metel), tobacco, etc.

2. Vasoconstrictors:

These drugs cause blood vessels to constrict. In cases of haemorrhage, they can close the vessel. Commonly referred to as haemostyptics, they can be:

- **Externally Used Drugs:**
    - Examples: Phitkri (alum), Mazoo (Quercus infectoria), Kath (Acacia catechu), Neela thotha (Copper sulphate), etc.
- **Internally Used Drugs:**
    - Examples: Shailam (Lolium termuletum), Kuchla Mudabbar (Strychnos nux-vomica seed).

Special Categories Based on Action on Capillaries:

- **Kawi (caustic):** Drugs that irritate the skin and increase blood supply due to their burning action. Examples: Tezaab (acids), garlic, hot metals.
- **Munaffit (vesicant):** Drugs that produce blisters. Examples: Beladur (Semecarpus anacardium) and Zarareeh (Cantharides).

- **Mubassir (eruptive):** Drugs that enhance blood supply by producing pus-filled acne. Example: Jamalgota (Croton).
- **Muhammir (rubefacient):** Drugs that irritate and redden the skin, thereby increasing blood supply. Example: Garlic.
- **Akaal (corroding drugs):** Drugs that burn the skin and flesh, like sulphate.
- **Muqarreh (Ulcerative):** Drugs that create ulcers on the skin, affect capillaries, and increase blood flow. Examples: Rai (Brassica alba, B. nigra seed), Choona (Calcium hydroxide - Quick lime), Jamalgota (Croton).
- **Mumalli (scabbing drugs):** Drugs used to reduce pain and swelling by dilating blood vessels of nearby structures through irritation. This process is known as diversion. For instance, Kafoor (Cinnamomum camphora - camphor) is placed on the forehead for headaches, and Rai (Mustard - Brassica nigra) Zimad (Paste) is applied to the skin for liver inflammation.

Effect of drugs on the blood

Drugs can influence various aspects of the blood, from salinity to clotting properties. Here is how different drugs impact the blood:

1. Drugs Increasing Blood Salinity:

Examples: Table salt, Naushader (Ammonium chloride), and saline water from springs.

2. Drugs Reducing Blood Salinity:

Examples: Lemon water, decanted water, tamarind, and bitter pomegranate water.

3. Drugs that Concentrate/Thicken the Blood:

- These drugs reduce the nature of the blood.
- Examples: Drugs that increase flow, such as Muarriqat (diaphoretics) and Mushilath (purgatives).

4. Drugs that Dilute the Blood:

- While they dilute the blood, they enhance its nature.
- Examples: Intake of juicy fruits or increased water consumption.

5. Drugs Increasing the Solid Constituents of Blood (RBCs):

- These drugs enhance the redness in the blood, making them known as blood Muqawwi (tonics).
- Examples: Kushta Faulad (Iron Calx), Sharbat Faulad (liquid Iron), Sankhya (Purified Arsenic trioxide).

6. Drugs Reducing the Solid Constituents of the Blood:

- These drugs result in less vibrant blood colour.
- Example: Excessive use of Sankhya.

7. Drugs Enhancing Blood Clotting Function:

Examples: Sadaf sokhta (Ostrea edulis), Sartan Muharraq (Scylla serrata, ash), Sange Jarahat[366] (magnesium silicate).

8. Drugs Reducing Blood Clotting Function:

Examples: Sour alcohol, Tursh mevajaat (sour dry fruits).

Effect of drugs on the organs of the nervous system (A'da Nafsaniyya)

Effect of drugs on sensory nerves (Asaab-e-Hissiya)

Drugs that affect the nerves either stimulate the nerves or slow them down. Then, this stimulation of nerves either takes place in the sensory nerves or the motor nerves. Similarly, this stimulation occurs in either the nerve axons or its dendrites. These drugs are divided into three groups.

1. **Laziyat (Irritants):** Drugs that irritate the terminal branches of the sensory nerves, due to which the vessels of the diseased part become dilated and red. That is, inflammation and pain occur. For example, Zamad Khardal (mustard paste) in syncope and loss of consciousness and the toxic character of Affiyun (Papaver Somniferum - opium) in stimulating the Tabi'at (medicatrix naturae) are used as irritant drugs.
2. **Musakkinat (Sedatives):** Drugs that decrease the action of the terminal branches of the sensory nerves, and some of their effects reach the nerve centres and relieve pain. For example, besh (aconite), Luffah (Atropa belladonna), Affiyun (Papaver Somniferum - opium), Kafoor (Cinnamomum camphora - camphor), etc.
3. **Mukhaddirat (Anaesthetics):** Drugs, when used externally and applied at a site, make it numb and without sensation are called anaesthetics.

Effect of drugs on the spinal cord (Nukha)

a. Some drugs stimulate the action of the spinal cord, such as Kuchla Mudabbar (Strychnos nux-vomica seed), Affiyun (Papaver Somniferum - opium), etc. When their action increases, it causes spasms in the organs of

---

[366] Sang = wounds, Jarahat = stones.

the body. These drugs are not very effective in the diseases of paralyses/flaccidity of the spinal cord, but taking Kuchla Mudabbar (Strychnos nux-vomica seed), is often useful in hemiplegia.
b. Some drugs weaken the action of the spinal cord, such as Affiyun (Papaver Somniferum - opium), cannabis, Kafoor (Cinnamomum camphora - camphor), Sankhya (Purified Arsenic trioxide), etc.

The initial effect of Affiyun (Papaver Somniferum - opium) is stimulatory, but the secondary effect is depressant, so it has both effects.

Effect of drugs on the brain (Dimagh)

a. **Mufarreh (exhilarants):** Drugs that, along with increasing brain functions, also cause excitation, joy and pleasure, such as alcohol.
b. **Muhziyat (Delirium causing drugs):** Drugs that cause anxiety and delirium.

These stimulate the brain functions so irregularly that it causes apathy, and the person starts talking meaningless and nonsense (delirium), such as cannabis.

Drugs that are Muhzi (**delirium causing drug**) are often also exhilarant, such as cannabis and alcohol, i.e., they cause both excitation and delirium.

a. **Musakkinat (Sedatives):** Drugs that, when used internally, reduce the feeling of pain, irrelevant to the site/organ of the pain, such as Affiyun (Papaver Somniferum - opium).
b. **Mukhaddir (Anaesthetics):** Drugs that nullify brain sensations and cause unconsciousness.
c. **Mushannijat (Spasmodics/convulsants):** Drugs that stimulate the brain's motor faculty to such an extent that they cause convulsions in the body.
d. **Dāfi'-e-Tashannuj (Anti-convulsants/Antispasmodic):** Drugs that weaken the motor faculty of the brain. Such drugs are used to relieve convulsions in uterine asphyxia, epilepsy, etc. For example, Asafoetida, Dawa al-Shifa formula, etc.

Effect of the drugs on the respiratory centre

Two types of drugs affect the respiratory (tanaffus) centre:

a. Drugs that stimulate and increase respiratory movements, which also help in the expulsion of phlegm. For example, Ajwain Khurasani (Hyoscyamus niger), Datura (Datura metel) and Kuchla Mudabbar (Strychnos nux-vomica seed).

b. Drugs that decrease the stimulation, which makes the respiratory movements weak and slow, such as Affiyun (Papaver Somniferum - opium), besh (aconite), etc. These drugs are beneficial in the increased respiratory movements and provide relief to the respiratory organs.

Effect of drugs on the sensory organs

Effects of drugs on the eye and related structures:

1. **Enhancing Eyesight**: Surma/Kohl (collyrium [367]) is applied externally to potentially enhance eyesight. In contrast, Kuchla Mudabbar (Strychnos nux-vomica seed) may be used internally for its benefits on vision.
2. **Hallucinatory Effects**: Some drugs can induce visual hallucinations, causing the user to see things that are not present in reality.
3. **Colour Alteration**: The essence of Dirmana Turki (Artemesia maritima: sea wormwood) is an example of a drug that can alter the perception of colours. Initially, users perceive everything as purple, which later turns to yellow.

Drugs affecting the conjunctiva:

1. **Vasoconstriction**: Drugs like Phitkri (alum), triphala, and Rasoot (Berberis Lycium Royle) can cause the blood vessels in the conjunctiva to constrict.
2. **Analgesic and Anaesthetic Effects**: Affiyun (Papaver Somniferum - opium) can act as a pain reliever or an anaesthetic for the conjunctiva.
3. **Anti-Infective**: Drugs such as surma (collyrium) and Kafoor (Cinnamomum camphora - camphor) can help clear infections in the eye.
4. **Irritants**: Nila thotha (copper sulphate) and gaungchi (Abrus precatorius - jequirity bean) can irritate the conjunctiva.

Drugs affecting the lacrimal gland:

1. **Stimulants:** Some drugs, such as Euphrasia officinalis (Eyebright), can stimulate the lacrimal glands, increasing tear production.
2. **Suppressants:** Drugs like Yabruj (belladonna) can reduce the activity of the lacrimal glands, leading to decreased or blocked tear flow.

Effects of drugs on the iris:

1. **Miosis (Pupil Constriction)**: Drugs like Affiyun (Papaver Somniferum - opium) and general anaesthetics can cause the pupil of the eye to constrict.
2. **Mydriasis (Pupil Dilation)**: The essence of Yabruj (belladonna) can cause the pupil to dilate.

---

[367] Antimony sulphide

Effects of Drugs on the Ear

1. Effects on Hearing:

Some drugs can amplify the auditory capacity. For instance, Azraqi/Kuchla Mudabbar (Strychnos nux-vomica) acts on the auditory nerves, potentially enhancing the power of hearing. And some drugs[368] might lead to tinnitus, a condition where one hears a ringing sound.

2. Drugs Acting on the Ear's Mucous Membrane:

i. Analgesics: For alleviating ear pain, certain remedies like Affiyun (Papaver Somniferum - opium) and Kafoor (Cinnamomum camphora - camphor) can be dissolved in almond oil and then administered into the ear.

ii. Astringents: To treat otorrhoea (ear discharge), which is often associated with infection, astringent drugs are beneficial. They are typically used alongside disinfectants to ensure the infections are treated. A concoction can be made by dissolving substances like Mazoo (Quercus infectoria), Phitkri (alum), and Borah Armani (Armenian Bole - Bolus Armenus) in neem (Azadirachta Indica) leaf, either in water or oil.

iii. Antiseptics: To prevent or combat infections, Kafoor (Cinnamomum camphora - camphor) can be mixed with neem leaf water and administered as ear drops.

iv. Emollients: For a moisturizing and softening effect on the ear, almond oil or rose oil can be used as ear drops.

Effect of Drugs on the nose

Effect on the Olfactory Nerve:

1. **Stimulants:** Drugs like compounds of Choona (Calcium hydroxide - Quick lime) and Noshadar (Ammonium Chloride) stimulate the olfactory nerve and enhance its function.
2. **Depressants:** Asafoetida and Musk (Moschus moschiferus secretion) initially boost the olfactory nerve's function, but with time, they decrease its activity.

---

[368] Such as those that contain a lot of Salicylates such as willow bark.

Effect on the Mucous Membrane:

1. **Errhines**[369]: These drugs induce sneezing and promote phlegm expulsion when inhaled. Examples include Nakchikni (Dregea Volubilis - Sneeze wort), black and red pepper, ginger, and Katki/Kharbaq (Helleborus niger).
2. **Soothing Agents:** Besh (aconite) is cited as a drug that calms irritation in the mucous membranes.
3. **Astringents:** Drugs like Phitkri (alum), dam-al-akhwayn (dragon blood tree), Gero (Ochre - Hematite), and Sange Jarahat (magnesium silicate) exert an astringent effect on the mucous membranes, reducing fluid flow and potentially stemming nosebleeds (epistaxis).

Effect of Drugs on the Tongue:

1. **Fragrant**: Examples include anise and cardamom. These substances have a pleasant aroma that can be sensed when tasted or even smelled.
2. **Bitter**: Drugs such as Sibr (Aloe vera), Azraqi (Strychnos nux-vomica), and Neem Ki Chaal (Azadirachta Indica – bark) are known to impart a bitter taste.
3. **Mucinous**: Arabic gum is an example of a substance with a mucilaginous or viscous texture, providing a thick, gel-like sensation on the tongue.
4. **Spicy**: Substances like black pepper, Rai (Mustard - Brassica nigra), and Kabab Chini (Piper cubeba) are pungent and can produce a burning or warming sensation on the tongue.
5. **Sweet**: Naturally sweet substances include honey, grapes, and raisins, which taste sugary.
6. **Sour**: Items like lemon, vinegar, tamarind, and dried plums are known for their tangy or acidic taste.

Effect of the drug on the skin

1. **Muarriqat (Diaphoretics)**: Drugs that stimulate sweat production.

    - **Kafoor (Cinnamomum camphora - camphor)**, increases sweat production by influencing sweat glands.
    - **Affiyun (Papaver Somniferum - opium)** stimulates nerves in the sweat glands to induce sweating.

---

[369] معطسات – sneezing

- **Hot water and hot air** open the skin pores, leading to sweat release.

2. **Manat-e-arq (Anaphoretics)**: Drugs that inhibit sweat production.

    - **Kushta Faulad (Iron Calx)** reduces or stops sweat production by affecting sweat glands.
    - **Ajwain Khurasani (Hyoscyamus niger) and Datura (Datura metel)** affect the nerves of sweat glands to reduce sweat production.
    - **Cold water and cold air** close the skin pores, inhibiting sweating.

3. **Mughayyar Arq (Sweat modifying drugs)**: Affiyun (Papaver Somniferum - opium) alters the state of sweating.
4. **Murkhiat (Relaxants)**: Agents that soften the skin, widen the blood vessels, and relax its structure. Examples include oils, hot pastes, and hot water.
5. **Mumaddat (drugs that relieve irritation)**: Psyllium husk is an example that soothes skin irritation.
6. **Mubassirat (eruptives) and Munaffith (vesicants)**: Drugs that cause various skin reactions like bumps, blemishes, or even ulcers. Sankhya (Purified Arsenic trioxide), Yabruj (belladonna), and Tezpat (Cinnamomum tamala leaf) cause skin blemishes and bumps. Drugs that ulcerate the skin and form wounds are called Mubassirat (eruptives) and Akkalat (Corrosives).

Drugs affecting hair

Zifit roomi (Roman pitch) is a hair growth promoter that stimulates hair growth. Hair oils are commonly used to nourish and encourage hair growth.

To remove hair, a mixture of Hartal (Arsenic trisulphide) and Choona (Calcium hydroxide - Quick lime) can be applied. This mixture weakens the hair roots and makes it easier for the hair to fall off with slight scratching.

Effect of drugs on metabasis and metabolism of the body

The substances that enter our body through food, water, and air, as well as those already present in our organs and humours (Akhlat), undergo continuous changes, producing different types of suitable substances but also corrupted ones (Fasad Mavaad). These changes are called metabolism (Istihalaat) and involve anabolism and catabolism (Kawwun wa Fasaad), which respectively refer to the processes of creating and breaking down substances. The ancient physicians gave these processes the names of Hazm (digestion) and Nuzj (concoction).

The body is nourished and heat is produced due to the process of metabasis. Excretions are also completed through this process. The food we consume undergoes various processes of metabasis and metabolism before becoming easily absorbable and becoming a part of the body.

Ibn Sina believed that every part of the body and its organs possess a natural power or faculty that enables them to receive nourishment. In addition, it is accepted that four powers are essential for the Quwwat-e-ghaziya (nutritive faculty) to function optimally: Quwwat-e-jaziba (absorptive power), Quwwat-e-masika (assimilative power), Quwwat-e-hazima (digestive power), and Quwwat Dafia (expulsive faculty). Metabolism occurs more or less in every part of the body.

Ancient physicians also said that the real nourisher is blood, as it is a unique composite of different constituents. Every organ absorbs its specific number of constituents from the blood through Quwwat-e-jaziba (absorptive power), and these constituents then remain in the organ for some time due to the Quwwat-e-masika (assimilative power). During this time, metabasis and metabolism are produced in these constituents through the Quwwat-e-hazima (digestive power), through which the organ gets nourished. It then produces different types of waste products, which are expelled out from the structures of the organs to the blood by the Quwwat Dafia (expulsive faculty), which is produced by nature to expel them out so that these excreta do not reach the organs.

The waste matter of pneuma enters the bloodstream and is eventually expelled through respiration. Similarly, urinary waste enters the bloodstream, reaches the kidneys, and is expelled as urine. Some waste matter is expelled through mucous membranes as perspiration and phlegm, while the excreta of food is expelled through the rectum as faeces after passing through the intestine. This process of exchange and metabolism is continuous in all body fluids, including the blood.

Causes that increase or decrease metabolism

Health refers to a moderate level of metabolism. If these changes slow down for some reason, then measures are taken to accelerate and if they are accelerated then measures are taken to slow them down.

Understanding factors that affect metabolism

Each component of the body has a role in influencing metabolism, and this can either help maintain good health or contribute to the development of diseases. A prime example is the balance of the six essential factors (asbab-e-sitta zarooriya). When these factors are in harmony, they create a state of health. Conversely, if there is an imbalance, it can lead to disease.

Apart from the essential factors, there are non-essential factors (asbab-e-ghair zarooriya) that have an impact on the crucial substances of the body, such as blood, pneuma (vital breath), and body heat. This category also includes factors that can disrupt the functions of the excretory organs and those that provide nourishment to the body.

Furthermore, certain drugs play a significant role in influencing metabolism, either by accelerating or decelerating metabolic processes as required. The drugs are mentioned in this chapter.

The Four Pillars of Nutritive Faculty (Quwwat-e-ghaziya)

The functioning of Quwwat-e-ghaziya, or the nutritive faculty, rests upon four essential powers:

1. **Absorptive Power (Quwwat-e-jaziba)**: The ability of the body to absorb nutrients and other essential substances from food and drink.
2. **Assimilative Power (Quwwat-e-masika)**: The body's capability to assimilate these absorbed substances, integrating them into its systems.
3. **Digestive Power (Quwwat-e-hazima)**: The power that allows the body to break down food, turning it into absorbable forms.
4. **Expulsive Power (Quwwat-e-dafia)**: This helps the body expel waste products and toxins, ensuring a clean internal environment.

These powers ensure that both metabasis (transformation of substances) and metabolism (the set of chemical reactions) function harmoniously in every part of the body.

Classification of drugs based on metabolic impact

In relation to metabolism, drugs can be categorized based on their therapeutic impact on metabolic processes:

1. **Drugs that Accelerate Metabolism**: These are administered to stimulate sluggish metabolic processes, aiding in faster nutrient absorption and energy production.
2. **Drugs that Decelerate Metabolism**: These are beneficial in conditions where metabolic activities are overly rapid, helping to stabilize and calm the system.
3. **Drugs that Maintain the Metabolic State**: These drugs ensure that the metabolic rate remains steady, fostering a balanced state of health.

Metabolism Stimulants: Accelerating Metabolic Processes

Characterized by their hot (har) temperament, metabolism stimulants function as heating (Musakhkhin) drugs that primarily raise body temperature either in the whole body or in a specific part of the body.

Types of Musakhkhin (heating drugs):

1. **Local Metabolic Stimulants:** These drugs target specific organs or body parts. Their primary functions include enhancing digestion, absorption, excretion, blood circulation, and the power of nutrients. When a specific body part requires added nutrition, calorific drugs, known as Musakhkhin, are prescribed. This leads to artery dilation and an increase in nutrient supply. Consequently, the Nutrient faculty (Quwwat Ghadhiya) [370] and Digestive faculty (Quwwat Hadima [371] /Quwwat Mughayyira Thaniyya)are enhanced, promoting the expulsion of morbid matter.
2. **General Metabolic Stimulants:** Two sub-categories exist within this:
    a. Drugs that intensify overall body changes, accelerating metabolism to a point where putrefaction might occur.
    b. Drugs that moderate metabolic changes, thereby enhancing organ functions, aiding digestion, increasing appetite, and improving blood health. If needed, they can also help increase body weight. Such drugs are referred to as general tonics (Muqawwiat amma).

Tonics Based on their Function:

- **Muqawwi-i-Mida:** Targets the stomach to enhance appetite and digestion.
- **Muqawwi-i-Dam:** Improves blood health.
- **Muqawwi-e-Aṣab:** Alleviates nerve weakness.
- **Muqawwi-i-Qalb:** Benefits the heart.
- **Muqawwi-i-Kabid/Muqawwi-i-Jigar:** Optimizes liver functions.
- **Muqawwi-i-Dimagh:** Fortifies the brain.

Additionally, there are tonics like Muqawwi-i-Kulya (renal tonic) and Muqawwi-i-Rahim (uterine tonic) that are tailored for specific organs.

Mechanism of tonics

---

[370] Or transliterated as Quwwat-e-ghaziya - One of the types of physical faculties making alteration in the food in such a manner that it becomes temperamentally (mizaj) similar to the body and suitable to replace daily wear and tear.

[371] Or transliterated as Quwwat-e-hazima - Faculty which serves the nutritive faculty and digests the dietary material to make it part of an organ.

According to some physicians, tonics (Muqawwiat) can affect the vital pneuma of organs after their constituents are metabolized, transformed and mixed with the structures and fluids of the organs. This can lead to the treatment of specific functions of the organ.

It is also possible that after absorption, the drug may affect the matter (mavaad[372]) inside the organs, which could have been impaired due to various reasons. The constituents of these drugs can break down the diseased material or change it in such a way that it becomes easier to excrete them from the body, and the organ can then become strong after its expulsion.

Drugs that Decelerate Metabolism

Nature of the Drugs: These drugs are classified as Barid (cold) or Mubarridat (refrigerants). They function to reduce heat production, either locally or across the body.

Types of Metabolic Suppressants:

1. **Local Metabolic Suppressants (Mud'ifat Istihala):**
    - These drugs target specific areas to inhibit assimilation, digestion, and waste excretion. Their effect is achieved by narrowing veins, resulting in decreased blood flow and reduced nutrient delivery.
    - Drugs that constrict local vessels fall under this category. Examples include Hibisaat-e-Dam (haemostyptic) and Qabiz-i-'Uruq[373], which are comparable to the effects of cold substances or ice.
2. **General Metabolic Suppressants (Mud'ifat Istihala):**
    - Upon entering the bloodstream, these drugs influence blood constituents and the body's Akhlat (humours). The result is a slowdown in the functions of the vital pneuma, a significant component of body metabolism.
    - Medications that reduce body temperature during fevers are categorized as general metabolic suppressants. They might function by modifying blood constituents or impacting nerves or nerve centres.

Certain drugs alter the body's Akhlat (humours) and organ structures. The exact mechanism through which they operate remains a subject of study and is not yet fully understood.

Blood purifiers (Musaffiat-i-Dam/ Musaffiat-i-Khun)

There are certain drugs called 'blood purifiers' that help in removing waste products from the bloodstream, thus cleansing it. They work by promoting excretion through urine, faeces, and sweat. However, in cases where the blood contamination level is too high for

---

[372] Mavaad is matter, material substances - depending on the context of the sentence.
[373] The Arabic form is Qabiḍ-i-'Uruq

these methods to work effectively, alternative drugs are used. These drugs cause internal changes in the bloodstream that expel impurities, although the exact mechanisms are unknown. Examples of such drugs include Seemab/Para (Cinnabar/mercury) and Sankhya/Sammulfar (Purified Arsenic trioxide), which not only remove these contaminants but also address their subsequent effects.

There exists a variety of drugs equipped with diverse purification capabilities:

- There is a range of drugs that have different functions when it comes to purifying the bloodstream:
- Some drugs work by improving the functions of the intestines
- others enhance the performance of the kidneys
- Certain drugs stimulate the skin functions to induce sweating, which helps to eliminate unhealthy substances.
- Some drugs interact with the unhealthy components in the blood to speed up metabolism or use other unknown means to remove such substances.

Concoctives (Munzijat)

These drugs instigate changes in both the Akhlat (humours) and organ structures, leading to the expulsion of morbid substances. Either the drug directly triggers this expulsion, or it enhances the organ's inherent Quwwat Dafia (expulsive faculty) to do so.

There are instances when, during the expulsion process, the substance becomes diluted, complicating its removal. In such cases, Munzijat (concoctives) come into play, concentrating the substance to facilitate expulsion. Conversely, there are times when the morbid substance exhibits heightened adhesiveness, risking it becoming anchored to an organ. To counter this, substances that reduce this stickiness are employed.

The overarching impact of concoctives is twofold: they either modify the consistency of bodily fluids—making them either more diluted or concentrated—or they regulate their adhesiveness—either intensifying or diminishing it. Observations have shown that most disease-causing substances are naturally expelled over time. This indicates the active role of the Tabi'at (medicatrix naturae) in processing these substances during this duration, preparing them for easier expulsion and priming the expulsive faculty for this purpose. Concoctives amplify the Tabi'at's efforts in this regard. Therefore, physicians fundamentally advocate for the administration of concoctives several days prior to both Tanqiya[374] (cleansing of morbid Matter) and Istifragh (evacuation).

For a list of concoctives, please refer to the section on the list of drugs.

Antiseptic (Mani-i-Ufunat[375])

---

[374] Induced elimination of morbid material from the body, usually done after proper concoction (Munzij).
[375] Also known as Dafi'-i-Ta'affun / Dafi'-i-'Ufunat - Drug that prevents/removes putrefaction.

Ufunat (Infection[376]) and Takhmir (Fermentation) both fall under the category of metabolic processes, and their operational mechanisms share similarities. Given these resemblances, physicians typically emphasize the concept of infection. Just as external substances can undergo infection and fermentation, internal changes can also manifest within body fluids and Akhlat (humours). Infections can either be localized, such as in ulcers, or more widespread, like blood infections resulting in persistent fevers.

Antiseptic Drugs: These are medicines designed to inhibit the onset of infection and eliminate infectious agents. Notable examples include Neem (Azadirachta Indica) and Tootia (Copper sulphate).

Additionally, certain drugs counteract the malodours of infections, aptly termed Daf-i-Natn (odour removers). For instance, Rai (Mustard - Brassica nigra) oil is commonly for its efficacy in neutralizing unpleasant scents.

Infected ulcers (Muta'affin Qarha)

Historically medical methodologies have advocated the use of camphor-derived medicines in the treatment of infected ulcers. The purpose of these medicines is to decrease the ulcer's moisture content. Medications specifically designed for this are termed Mujaffifat (desiccants /drying agents), and the act itself is referred to as Tajfif (drying).

This approach stems from the understanding that fermentation and infection processes necessitate a specific balance of heat and moisture. Both increase and decrease in moisture can interfere with the process of infection, and it has been observed that objects that remain dry tend to resist putrefaction. Therefore, the effective strategy to reduce the risk of infection is to dry fluids from ulcers.

Action of drugs on parasites

Parasitic infestation has been previously described, and it should be noted that parasites are present both outside and inside the body. In diseases like Hummaat Ajamiyya (infectious fever)[377] and Didan al-Am'a (intestinal worms), the parasites lie within the body, whereas lice, ticks, etc, lie outside the body.

Head lice and nymphs are killed by preparing Gandhak (purified sulphur) and Para (Hydrargyrum -Mercury). According to Ibn al-Nafis, Para has the power to kill worms. The worms of scabies are also killed by Gandhak (purified sulphur) Marham (ointment) and sandal (sandalwood) oil, Balsan (Commiphora opobalsamum) oil and Mia

---

[376] An abnormal change occurring in the humours/ body fluids caused by extrinsic or intrinsic factors; in extrinsic factors there may be morbid bodies, which come from dead bodies and stagnant waters that may be interpreted as microorganisms; due to this change the physiological functions of the humours alter; the other causes are stagnation in blood vessels or obstruction in viscera and irregular diet which is very prone to become septic.
[377] Infectious fevers are caused by the organisms found in the stagnant water. This is characterised by the enlargement of the spleen.

Saila/Silaaras (liquidambar orientalis - Storax). Some worms are also killed by blood purifiers.

Effect of Drugs on Disease Substances (Mawad-i-Marad[378])

Each specific disease substance possesses unique attributes, including its constituents, temperamental conditions, and characteristics. As a result, treatments tailored to these unique substances will also vary.

For example, Gandhak (purified sulphur) may be effective against Jarab (Scabies), but not necessarily against Atshak (Syphilis). Gilo (Tinospora cordifoli) might treat Hummaat Ajamiyya (Infectious fevers) but not necessarily Moti[379] Jhara/ Hummaat Mi'wiyya[380] (Typhiod fever/ Enteric fever). Likewise, while Suranjan (Colchicum luteum) can treat Mafaasil (Arthritis), it might not be effective against Judham/Juzam (Leprosy).

The exact composition and nature of many disease substances remain elusive. Consequently, our understanding of the drugs that impact these substances, including their mechanisms and nature, is often incomplete. This holds true for antidotes for toxic diseases; we may only know that these drugs counteract a specific substance without understanding how.

When confronted with diseases of unknown nature without an identified treatment, the strategy often involves medications that alleviate symptoms and bolster the Tabi'at (medicatrix naturae). For instance, in the absence of a known remedy for Diqq al-Shaykhukha (emaciation due to dryness)[381], drugs beneficial to the body's faculty and nutrition are employed.

Similarly, for inflammation of membranes, Arq Kasni (distilled Cichorium intybus-chicory leaf) and Arq Gilo/giloy (distilled Tinospora cordifolia leaf) are recommended either separately or combined. Distilled Turb (Raphanus sativa leaf) is suggested for Yarqan (Jaundice) while Suranjan (Colchicum luteum) and Azraqi/Kuchla Mudabbar (Strychnos nux-vomica) are used for Arthritis. Chronic cases of Waram al-Kabid (hepatitis) and Hummaat Ajamiyya (Infectious fevers) benefit from Afsanteen (Artemisia absinthium). Additionally, pills made from Karanjwa seeds (Caesalpinia bonducella) and

---

[378] مواد مَرَض
[379] The word Moti means pearl with reference to the marks on the body during this disease.
[380] Mi'wiyya i.e., related to intestines hence enteric fever.
[381] A type of cachexia of the body in which there is massive dryness of the body without fever.

keenaa (Cinchona officinalis – quinine), which contain bark essence (quinine), can help mitigate these fever episodes.

Various other treatment methods focus on symptom relief. In managing Hummaat Ajamiyya (Infectious fevers) and other types of fevers, laxatives are utilized to cleanse the intestines. Drugs like Muarriqat (Diaphoretics) that enhance flow and Mubarrid (refrigerant) are applied to reduce fever temperatures.

Effects of drugs on innate heat

Historical physicians, such as Galen and Al-Razi, posited that innate heat arises from the metabolic processes inherent to the human body.

Physicians recognize the heat produced by the temperament of the elements within the human body. When this heat remains balanced, it is referred to as Hararat Ghariziyya (Innate/Natural heat). However, when this heat surpasses its equilibrium, becoming excessive, it is termed Hararat Ghariba[382] (morbid heat/abnormal heat).

This innate heat generation in humans operates via a distinct system facilitated by pneuma and nutritional components. If the mechanisms responsible for producing and moderating this heat falter, the innate heat may either escalate or diminish.

Heat producing and refrigerant drugs (Musakhkhin [383] wa Mubarrid[384])

Musakhkhinat (Calorifacients/Heat-Producing Agents)

Drugs that augment body heat, either locally or throughout, are termed Musakhkhin. Their warming effect, known as Taskhin, stems from the stimulation and excitement of nerves, leading to the dilation of local blood vessels and enhanced blood circulation. This, in turn, quickens metabolism, boosting heat production. Some Musakhkhin agents, like tea and coffee, can disturb the nervous system, accelerating metabolic processes and thus raising body heat globally. Certain toxins, such as Luffah/Yabruj (Atropa belladonna), also have similar effects.

Mubarrid (Refrigerants)

---

[382] Abnormal increase of heat disturbing body functions.
[383] Drug which produces heat in body.
[384] Drug which reduces body temperature from normal limits.

Mubarrid drugs counteract heat, reducing body temperature either in specific regions or throughout the body. This cooling action, known as Tabrid, directly opposes the effects of Musakhkhinat.

There are two categories of Mubarrid drugs:

1. **Inherently cold agents:** This includes substances like ice or cold water.
2. **Functionally cold agents:** While these drugs are not inherently cold, they produce cooling effects in the body in several ways:

    a. Some induce sweating, leading to cooling through evaporation. As gases evaporate, heat is expelled.
    b. Others, when applied topically, evaporate rapidly, drawing away other gases. For instance, vinegar applied to a patient's forehead via lint can aid in cases of meningitis and fever.
    c. Certain drugs target nerve centres to reduce metabolic activity, resulting in less heat production.
    d. Some agents instigate changes in the body that accelerate heat dissipation. Examples include:

        - Drugs like Alcohol and Besh (aconite) dilate skin vessels, enhancing heat expulsion through diaphoresis (sweating) and evaporation.
        - Drugs that impact internal systems without affecting skin vessels but still reduce heat.

    e. A few drugs lower body heat by combating the root cause, such as a disease that's elevating the temperature. These drugs have a direct impact on the disease, leading to an indirect effect on body heat. Afsanteen (Artemisia absynthium herb) and Neem (Azadirachta Indica) flowers, for instance, target Hummaat Ajamiyya (Infectious fevers) and effectively treat the fever.

Shapes of drugs

Drugs come in various shapes, each designed for a specific use or route of administration. Typically, drugs can be categorized into three main shapes: Jamid (Solid), Sayyal (Liquid) and Bukhare (Gaseous).

Forms of solid drugs are as follows:

Form	Description

COMPENDIUM OF DRUGS | 293

Atus	Snuff
Banadiq	Big pill (Bunduqa [pl])
Barud Kohl	Eye-dusting powder / eye coolant
Dharur/ Zuroor	Dusting powder
Fatila	Medicated wick
Firzaja	Pessary
Ghaliya	Perfumed powder
Ghaza	Face powder
Gulqand/ Gulshakar	Flower conserve
Hab	Pill (Haboob [pl])
Halwa Kushuk	Semi-solid nonmedicated or medicated sweet preparation – dry
Hamul	Tampon
Kabus	Disc-shaped preparation for local application
Kajal	Topical ophthalmic medicament / eyeliner
Kohl	Antimony sulphide – collyrium
Kushta	Prepared metal/minerals
Madugh /Mazugh	Chewable drug
Nafukh	Insufflation
Norah	Hair remover
Qurs	Tablet (aqras [pl])
Rubub kushuk	Dried Extract
Safuf	Powdered drug
Sanun / Manjan	Toothpowder

Forms of semi-solid drugs are as follows:

Form	Description
Anoshdaru[385]	Gooseberry-based electuary
Bershasha	Paste containing opium
Dawa al-Misk[386]	Musk-based electuary
Faludhaj/ Faluda	Starch-containing preparation
Halwa Ter	Medicated sweet preparation – moist
Hasw/Harira	Semi-liquid preparation with high nutrient value
Itrifal[387]	Electuary based on three medicinal fruits

---

[385] Anoshdaru, a Persian word that means digestive. It is made of five ingredients: Haleela, Balela, Amla, Khabsul Hadeed (Ferroso-Ferric Oxide Calx), and honey.
[386] It is used in cardiac, gastric and brain ailments. It acts as an adaptogenic or immunomodulator, e.g., Dawaulmisk motadil.
[387] From the Sanskrit: Triphala, i.e., contains the herbs, Haleela, Balela, Amla.

Jawarish[388]	Digestive electuary
Khameera	Fermented confection
Laboob[389]	Kernel-based electuary
Latukh/ Latookh	Epithem
Lauq/Laooq	Linctus
Lazooq/Lazuq	Adhesive medicine
Majun	Confection/Electuary
Marham	Ointment
Mufarreh[390]	Exhilarant electuary
Qairooti/Qayruti	Ointment made of oils and wax
Usara/Afshurdah	Extract
Yaqooti	Ruby based electuary
Zimad/laip	Paste/balm

Liquid drugs have the following forms:

Form	Description
Ab-kama/Murri	A type of fermented condiment
Abzan	Sitz bath
Arq	Distillate
Daluk	Massage oil
Dayaqoozah	Poppy rind- and seed based medicinal preparation
Fuqqa	Barley beverage
Gharghara	Gargle
Ghasul	Wash lotion
Huqna	Enema
Joshan-da/Maṭbukh/Sulqa	Decoction
Jullab	Preparation of rose water and sugar

---

[388] Jawarish is an Arabic word made from Gawarish, which means digestive. Its consistency is more liquid than majun. Jawarish is made for the digestive system. It acts slowly because its powder is coarse than a standard majun e.g., Jawarish Jalinus (Galen's paste).
[389] This formulation contains dry fruits; therefore, it is called laboob, e.g., Laboob kabir.
[390] Contains scented drugs. Two tymaabqalbhar for those who have a cold temperament and Mufarreh barid for those who have a hot temperament). Also, Mufarreh motadil is for balanced temperaments.

Khidab/Khizab	Hair dye
Khesanda[391]/Naqu	Infusion
Luabat	Mucilage
Madmada/Mazmaza	Mouthwash
Mahlul	Solution
Marukh	Oil-based liniment
Masuh	Oily-liquid preparation
Maul jubn	Whey
Maul baqool	Vegetable juice
Maul-asl	Hydromel/Honey Water
Maul Lahm	Distillate of meat
Ma-ush-shaeer	Barley water
Maal-Fawakih	Fruit Juice
Nabeez/Nabidh	Type of non-intoxicating fermented drink
Naduh/Nazuh	Liquid used to splash on affected part
Nutul	Irrigation
Qatur	Drops
Ruh	Essence
Sakob	Irrigation
Sharab	Wine
Sharbat	Medicinal Syrup
Sheera/Haleeb	Milky emulsified product
Sibgh / Sibgha	Dye
Sikanjbin	Mix of Vinegar and Honey- oxymel
Sirka	Vinegar
Tila	Liniment
Wajur	Throat drop
Zaruq	Liquid used for syringing

[391] Liquid preparation made by soaking crushed/whole drug overnight in water or other suitable liquid and used after straining.

Zulal	Decanted liquid

Bukharart (Vapours) or Hawai (Gaseous) drugs have the following forms:

Form	Description
Bakhur/Dhooni	Fumigation
Inkabab/Bhapara	Vapour bath
Lakhlakha[392]	Inhalation of vapour arising from fragrant drugs
Nashuq	Liquid snuff
Shamum[393]	Inhalation

Overview of Drug Forms in Unani Medicine

Abkama/Murri (a type of fermented condiment): This preparation is also known as Indian vinegar or kanji. It is made by mixing salt, vinegar, ginger, black pepper, and water and allowing it to ferment until it turns sour. The liquid is then strained and used as needed.

Abzan/Hamam/Juloosi (Sitz bath): A Joshanda (Decoction) of liquid or drugs in which the patient is made to sit (Usually for the ailment of urogenital organs).

Atus/Atoos (snuff): (The drug that causes sneezing), which is in powdered form and causes sneezing if sniffed. These may also be solid or liquid as powder of Nakchikni (Sneeze wort).

Bakhur / Dhuni (Incense): Aromatic smoke is any substance burned for fragrance, also known as Tadkhin or Tabkhir.

Bershasha (electuary contains opium): Bershasha is derived from the Syriac word Barasata, which means instant relief. It is a type of Majun that contains Affiyun (Papaver Somniferum - opium) and is beneficial for pain relief, particularly in cases of arthritis and gout.

Burud kohl (Eye dusting powder): Originally called Burud, meaning cold in Arabic, because it used to be made with cold drugs, Kohl is a ground powder that is used to cool

---

[392] Inhalation of fragrance of drugs kept in a wide-mouthed bottle.
[393] Inhalation of drugs which may be in dry or liquid form so that volatile substances reach nasal cavity and respiratory tubes.

and treat eye diseases. It is applied to the eyelids using a stick and may also contain mint and other medicinal ingredients.

There are also eye-dusting powders that are solid and require water to be added before being applied to the eyes.

Daluk (massage oil): Oil containing drugs that is applied to the body and massaged vigorously. Examples are strong massage, light massage, hard massage, and soft massage.

Dayaqoozah (poppy-based medicinal preparation): It is a type of syrup made from poppy rind and poppy seeds. It is a Greek word that means poppy syrup. It is used for throat ailments and coughs.

Dharur/ Zuroor (Dusting powder): A dry crushed medicine, such as Zuroor-i-Qula, is topically applied for mouth ulcers and other ulcerated areas.

Dohan/Adhan/Roghan (Oils): These are different oils that are used externally and internally.

Faluda (starch-containing preparation): A frozen liquid drug which is a food made by mixing starch or starchy ingredients in water or milk. When frozen, it has a texture similar to cuttlefish. To use it, it needs to be in the form of thick vermicelli or barley soup. The preparation involves pouring it through a sieve while hot and then passing it through cold water.

Fatila (Medicated wick): Piece of cotton soaked or dipped in a liquid mixture of certain drugs for application in vagina, rectum or other body orifices

Firzaja (pessary): A solid, roughly conical or cylindrical medicinal preparation, usually the size of a jujube (Ziziphus jujuba), which is inserted through the cervix and into the uterus. A thread is left outside the body so that the pessary can be removed.

Fuqqa (barley beverage): This is a type of wine derived from barley.

Ghaliya (Perfumed powder): Also known as Argajah, Ghaliya is a perfumed mixture. It is typically smelled for its fragrance and can also be scrubbed onto the body for a scented effect.

Gharghara (Gargle): This is a liquid preparation made in different forms, such as Joshanda (decoction), Khesanda (infusion), or a solution. It is designed for gargling to help cleanse the throat and offer therapeutic benefits.

Ghasul (Wash lotion): A liquid solution used to cleanse wounds or affected body parts, with medicinal or antiseptic properties depending on its ingredients and purpose.

Ghaza (Face powder): This powder is applied to the face to improve complexion and may contain ingredients for specific hues and finishes.

Gulqand (flower conserve): This is a semi-solid medicinal concoction made primarily from flower petals. The most common flower used is the rose. Hence the name 'Gul', meaning flower, and 'Qand', signifying sugar. The basic composition is usually rose petals preserved in a dense sugar syrup. However, variations exist where Eglantine (Rosa rubiginosa) replaces rose petals, or honey is used instead of sugar.

Hab (Pill): Derived from the word meaning 'seed-like', a hab is essentially a solid or semi-solid medication shaped like a circle. The term 'haboob' refers to the plural form, meaning pills. Pills come in various sizes, from small grain-sized to as large as a soap nut (Sapindus). Particularly, large pills are equivalent to the soap nut size and are labelled as Banadiq (with the plural being Bunduqa).

Halwa: This refers to a sweet preparation that can be medicated or non-medicated. There are two primary types of halwa: dry and moist. The basic ingredients for a simple halwa include Maida (refined fine flour) or wholemeal wheat flour, sugar or honey, and oil. Optional additions might include almonds, raisins, and coconut. In the medicated variety, other medicinal ingredients are infused. For instance, Halwa Gheekwar is enriched with Aloe vera.

Hamul (tampon): A piece of cloth soaked in a drug mixture for vaginal or rectal use.

Harira/Hasw. A highly nutritious and medicinal semi-liquid dietary preparation made from dry fruits, seed kernels, and milk.

Huqna (enema): The process commonly referred to as colon cleanse or colonic evacuation aims to remove excess waste, harmful toxins, or imbalanced humors from the intestines. This is achieved by introducing warm water, liquid drugs, or other medicinal preparations into the bowel through the anal canal.

Inkibab or Bhapara (Vapour bath): This type of therapeutic treatment involves exposing the body or a specific body part to the steam coming from a hot solution of medicinal drugs like Joshanda (Decoction) or plain hot water. The method is primarily used for its revitalizing and healing effects.

Joshanda /Matbukh/Sulqa (Decoction): Liquid dosage form prepared by boiling one or more plant drugs. The drugs for Joshanda are soaked for a few hours before or overnight. It can also be prepared as a distillate and can be taken orally or applied externally.

Jullab: This is a liquid medicine taken orally and consists of rose water, honey, sugar, and other suitable drugs. The name Jullab comes from the Persian words 'gul' and 'aab'. 'Gul' (and the derivative 'Jul') means flower, while 'aab' means water.

Khamira (Fermented confection): During the Mughal period, a type of Majun was introduced. It is made by mixing a decoction of drugs in a base of purified honey, sugar or jaggery. The mixture is continuously stirred while it is still hot until it becomes thick and white. It contains non-plant drugs and some plant materials in either powder or paste form. This delicious and palatable preparation is mainly used to manage diseases, including those related to the heart and brain. When the Khamira is stirred, air reacts with carbon dioxide, and it swells like yeast (Khamir). This is why it is called Khamira. An example of Khamira is Khameera Abresham.

Khesanda/ Naqu (Infusion): Liquid preparation made by soaking crushed or whole drugs in water or other liquid overnight, then used after straining.

Khizab (Hair dye): Liquid/semi-liquid preparation used as hair dye

Kushta (prepared metals/minerals): These are commonly used in the form of powder and sometimes in the form of tablets.

Lakhlakha (inhalation of vapour arising from fragrant drugs): Fragrant drugs can be inhaled by opening a wide-mouthed bottle containing a liquid mixture of fragrant flowers and other substances. Another method is to grind and tie the fragrant drug in etuis, then dry it. Alternatively, the drug can be dipped in a liquid and inhaled, which is called 'shamum' (see later). These methods allow the volatile substances of the drugs to evaporate and reach the nose and respiratory tubules during inhalation.

Latukh (Epithem): Medicated preparation for external application, such as poultice, which is thinner than Zimad (Paste) and thicker than Tila (Liniment). Solid form, at the time of use, these are heated and changed into semi-solid form and used.

Lauq (Linctus): Also spelt La'uq, it is a drug which is prepared in syrup form. The half-grounded drugs are soaked in water overnight and boiled the next day till the quantity of water is reduced to half. The decoction is then strained and mixed along with some other powdered drugs in a base of sugar. This preparation is used in cough, asthma, and other diseases of the lungs and chest, e.g., Laooq Sapistan.

Lazuq / Lasuq (adhesive medicine): Adhesive drug which is spread over a piece of cloth or paper and pasted on the affected organ or part of the body e.g., Zimad Baboona.

Lu'ab (Mucilage): Mucilaginous liquid obtained by soaking mucilage-secreting drugs in water. Examples are mucilage Behi dana (quince seed - Cydonia oblonga Miller), mucilage Katan (Linum usitatissimum – Flaxseed), etc.

Maal Fawakih (Fruit Juice): Water from juicy fruits obtained by squeezing them. For example, grape juice, pomegranate juice, orange juice, watermelon juice, etc.

Madmada/Mazmaza (mouthwash): Medicated liquid preparation, which may be a Joshanda (Decoction), **Khesanda** (infusion) or solution, used for rinsing the mouth.

Madugh /Mazugh (chewable drug): A powder or chewable tablet (e.g., Bozidan - Pyrethrum indicum) which is chewed to increase secretions in the mouth, which helps in reducing gum and tooth pain.

Mahlul (Solution): Liquid obtained after mixing some plant, animal and mineral drugs which have the ability to become dissolved in water or other suitable liquid.

Majun (Electuary): Majun is a thick mixture made from finely crushed and sieved ingredients, which are then blended with honey or sugar. Its consistency is similar to that of moist halwa. Some examples of Majun include Majun Azaraqi, Majun Falasfa, and Majun Akseer ul badan.

There are different types of Majun, each with its own name and composition. For instance, Dawa al-Misk is a variant that includes aromatic components like Musk (Moschus moschiferus). La'bub is a type of Majun that is enriched with nuts such as almonds, seeds, and walnuts. Zar'uni is a type of Majun that is prepared as a tonic for enhancing kidney function and libido.

'Majun' comes from 'Ajn', which means 'thorough mixing'. It is a concoction of powdered medicinal substances meticulously mixed with a specific consistency of sugar or honey solution. These preparations are often named after their primary ingredients, therapeutic benefits, inventors, or other defining characteristics. For example, Itrifal, Jawarish Anooshdaru, Yaqooti, and Bershasha are all types of Majun, each with its unique name based on their composition, purpose, ingredients, method of preparation, and other inherent traits.

Marham (Ointment): It is a thick mixture which is prepared by mixing one or two ingredients in wax, fat or any oil and applied externally in skin diseases and other ulcerative diseases e.g., Marham Dakhilyun.

Maul asl (honey water): Liquid honey is mixed with water in a 1:4 ratio, boiled, and filtered. When combined with other drugs, it's called Maul-asl Murrakab (honey water compound).

Maul asul: (Root water): This refers to the water obtained from boiling and filtering roots such as Badiyan (Foeniculum vulgare), Kasni (Cichorium intybus), Kabar (Caper - Capparis spinosa), and Karafs (Celery - Apium graveolens).

Maul baqool (vegetable juice): Juice of green vegetables or green herbs such as mako (Solanum nigrum) and Kasni (Cichorium intybus), obtained by crushing and expressing them, or water obtained by boiling some vegetables, for example, green pumpkin water, this type of water is called vegetable juice.

Maul Buzur (Seed water): Water obtained from boiled and filtered seeds such as Kasni (Cichorium intybus), Khayaren (Cucumis sativa – cucumber), Katan (Linum usitatissimum – Flaxseed).

Maul Jubn (Whey): After milk curdles, the solid part is cheese known as 'Jabn', and the remaining liquid is called 'cheese water'.

Maul Lahm (distillate of meat): An extract produced from the distillation of select drugs combined with a meat extract.

Ma-ush-shaeer (Barley water): Barley seeds are initially soaked in water; their outer coating is then removed with mortar and pestle, and the seeds are boiled in water (in a 1:12 ratio) until the water becomes thick in consistency.

Murabba (Fruit Preserve): Fruit preserves are made by cooking and safely storing boiled and pierced fruits, such as apples, quince, pear, tamarind, Halela (Terminalia chebula), and carrot, in sugar or honey to prevent spoilage.

Marukh (Oil-based liniment): Oil or oily preparation applied over the skin as a thin layer.

Masuh (oily-liquid preparation): A liquid preparation made with oil that is applied on the body with gentle rubbing movements.

Nabeez/ Nabidh (Fermented drink): Grapes, dates or other fruits, when fermented, produce a beverage that does not have an intoxicating effect, such as Nabeez tamar (fermented dates).

Naduh/Nazuh (Spray): A liquid medication that is sprayed onto the affected area of the body.

Nashuq (insufflation): A liquid preparation or powder used for insufflation.

Norah (Hair Remover): A hair removal preparation available in paste, powder, and liquid forms. It contains lime as the primary ingredient.

Nutul (Irrigation): A medicinal liquid preparation in the form of Joshanda (Decoction), Khesanda (Infusion), or solution. It is applied to a hot or cold organ, a process also known as irrigation. Based on the temperature of the liquid, it can be classified as hot irrigation or cold irrigation.

Pashoya (Footbath): A footbath in which the feet are soaked to the knees. It is usually done with hot water.

Qairooti (Paste used on thorax): A paste that is a mixture of wax and oil, similar to an ointment, often containing other drugs. For example, Qairooti aarad karsana is used externally in axillae in diseases like pleurisy.

Qars (Tablet): (Plural form is aqraas). Tablets are flattened out, unlike pills, which are circular.

Rubb (Extract): Plant extracts are used to produce a drug that is obtained by soaking or boiling the juice of plants such as fruits, flowers, leaves, roots, etc. The juice is then heated to thicken it. There are various types of plant extracts used for this purpose, such as Rasaut (Berberis aristata extract), Elva (Aloe vera dried juice of leaf), and Rubbussoos (liquorice- Glycyrrhiza glabra extract).

To prepare the dry extract of fruits, fruits like grapes, pomegranates, Jamun (java plum), berries, apples, Zarishk (Berberis vulgaris - barberry), etc., are cooked to around a quarter of their original size. Then, white sugar, half of the weight of the fruit, is mixed to make the extract thicker and semi-solid (thicker than sharbat - syrup).

Ruh (Essence)[394]: Essences are the most concentrated and refined volatile components extracted from aromatic plants and drugs. These essences are primarily obtained through steam distillation.

Safuf (Powder): This type of drug can be taken orally or used externally for various purposes, such as toothpowder (Manjan), dusting powder (Dharur/Zarur), insufflation (Nafukh), snuff (Atus), face powder (Ghaza), antimony sulphide collyrium (Kohl/Surma), among others.

Sakob (Effusion or Decantation): This is a process where a medicated hot or cold liquid, such as (Decoction), Khesanda (Infusion), is poured over a body part from a height. This technique is known as douching. For instance, pouring cold water over the head in cases of meningitis or insanity is referred to as Sakob barid (cold effusion). When using hot water, it is known as Sakob har (hot effusion).

Sanun / Manjan (tooth powder): This is toothpowder used to strengthen loose teeth and gums. For example, Sanoon Post Muqlian can be used for this purpose.

Saut (Nasal drops): is a medication that is applied to the nose drop by drop.

---

[394] Note: this is not the same as the factors of existence, Ruh (pneuma).

Shamum (inhalation/Olfaction or smell): A drug that can be in the form of a liquid or a dry substance. The plural form of Shamum is Shamumaat. When the volatile substance of the drug turns into vapours, it reaches the nose through the nostrils and affects the olfactory centre of the brain by entering the respiratory tubules.

Sharbat (medicinal syrup): Sharbat is a sweet liquid mixture that is made from fruit juices such as grape juice, pomegranate juice, apple juice, grewia juice, etc. It can also be made from drugs that are soaked, boiled, and strained and then mixed with white sugar, rock sugar, or honey to adjust its consistency. For example, Sharbat Banafsha (Viola Odorata syrup), Sharbat Unnab (Zizyphus Vulgaris syrup), Sharbat Senna (Senna syrup) and so on.

In the case of Arqat (distillates), sugar is simply added to the Arq (distillate) to make a Qawam[395] (sugar base). Examples are Sharbat Kewra (Pandanus syrup), Sharbat Gulab (Rose syrup), etc.

Sheera/Haleeb (milky emulsified product): This is a milky emulsified product that can be obtained through different methods. It can be prepared by grinding kernels of dry fruits or seeds with water or any suitable liquid to create a liquid mixture that resembles milk. Alternatively, it can be a white liquid mixture in which oily substances are suspended in a water base. Another method involves using a base of sugar and honey to prepare various medicinal preparations.

Shyaf (Suppositories): Derived from 'Shaffah', Shyaf suppositories are intended for external application. They are made in a conical form and can be dissolved in water or a specified solvent. These suppositories are formulated by blending medicinal ingredients with a base such as cacao butter or glycerinated gelatin and are shaped for insertion into the rectum, vagina, or urethra. Interestingly, the base materials are solid at room temperature but liquefy once inside the body, taking advantage of the body's warmth. To maintain their integrity, it is advisable to store the suppositories in a refrigerator, especially during warmer months.

Applications include:

(i) Ocular use, examples being Shyaf Abyaz, Shyaf Ahmer, and Shyaf Shibb-e-Yamani.

(ii) Wound and Fistula Treatment: Suppositories designed for this purpose are inserted directly into wounds or fistulas. Such Shyaf are typically sized comparably to the seeds of Jau (Hordium vulgare).

---

[395] Sweetened solution of particular consistency that is generally made by adding water, distillate or fruit juice to purified honey, sugar or jaggery and boiled until it attains required consistency.

(iii) Some suppositories are also created specifically for anal applications.

Sibgh/ Sibgha (dye): Dye used to colour skin or conceal discolouration, either permanently or temporarily, e.g., cosmetic camouflaging in vitiligo. It is a liquid or semi-solid that can be used as a form of Tila (Liniment) or Zimad (Paste).

Sikanjbin (Oxymel): This is a syrup made from a combination of vinegar, honey, and sugar.

Sirka (Vinegar): Sirka, is a sharp and pungent liquid that is made by soaking the juice, Joshanda (decoction), or Khesanda (infusion) of sugary or starchy substances in water for a few days until it becomes acidic. This process is called fermentation. Sugarcane, java plum, grapes, and jaggery are examples of substances used to make vinegar.

When vinegar is distilled, it becomes transparent and loses its brownish-white colour. The vinegar produced by the effect of fermentation is called the 'mother of vinegar'. A small amount of vinegar is used as a combining agent in the liquid or dish, which already contains the effects of vinegar. In some cases, vinegar is infused in the walls of a clay pot, which converts the juice to vinegar.

Alcohol can also be easily converted into vinegar since it is made from similar substances.

Tadkhin (Fumigation): Is the process of inhaling or exposing the affected body part to fumes produced by burning drugs. It is also used to repel or kill insects.

Tila (Liniment): refers to a kind of medicated oil or thin medicinal preparation that is applied externally.

Ubtan (scrub): is a drug that is applied to scrub the body and has a fragrant scent. A bath is taken after its application.

Usara (Extract): is the water extracted from plants and dry fruits by squeezing them. The extract has two forms: (1) Liquid obtained by grinding fresh herbs with water and straining, and (2) a collection of crude mixture extracted from different parts of plants. When this extract is dried, it is called Rubb. For example, Usara Revan.

Wajur (Throat drops): Wajur is a medicated liquid preparation that is slowly instilled into the throat, drop by drop. It is used to provide relief for throat irritations.

Zaruq (liquid used for syringing): Liquid preparation used for syringing urethra, vagina, nose, ear, or any other sinus, etc., through syringe or clysma apparatus.

Zimad, laip (poultice): Zimad is a type of poultice made from semi-solid crude drugs that are applied externally on the body. There are two types of pastes: thin pastes that can be applied using a finger, which is known as Tila (Liniment), and thick pastes called Zimad that are made from substances like Brassica alba and B. nigra seed, such as the Zimad-i-rai.

Zulal (Decanted water): Some drugs are soaked in water and not strained; this is called decanted water. For instance, Alu bukhara (Prunus domestica fruit dried) decanted water, Imli (Tamarindus indica fruit) decanted water, etc.

METHODS OF DRUG ADMINISTRATION

There are a number of methods utilised to administer drugs for treating diverse symptoms and diseases.

Broadly, drug administration is categorized into:

1. Internally used drugs
2. Externally used drugs

Internal drugs

Drugs in this category enter the body either through natural orifices (e.g., mouth, nose, anus, urethra, or vagina) or via artificial means, such as puncturing the skin or blood vessels using a syringe.

External drugs

These pertain to drugs applied directly to a specific body part.

Methods of administration of internal drugs

Oral route: Most internal drugs are ingested orally, often accompanied by food or beverages. For example, Haboob[396], Safuf (Powder), Ma'ajen[397], Jawarishaat[398], Itrifalat[399], Khamirajat[400], Laooqat[401], Murabbajaat[402], Gulqand (flower conserve), Sharbat (Syrup), Sikanjbin (Oxymel), Joshanda (Decoction), Khesanda (Infusion),

---

[396] Plural of Hab (Pill).
[397] Plural of Majun (Confection/Electuary).
[398] Plural of Jawarish (digestive electuary).
[399] Plural of Itrifal (electuary based on three medicinal fruits).
[400] Plural of Khamira (Fermented confection).
[401] Plural Lauq (Linctus).
[402] Plural of Murabba (Fruit preserve).

Sheerajat[403], Lu'abat[404], Arqat[405], Sharbat (syrup), Maul-asl (honey water/Hydromel), Ma-ush-shaeer (Barley water), Faluda (starch-containing preparation), etc.

Local drugs of mouth and throat: Examples here include Mazmaza (mouthwash), Gharghara (Gargle), Wajur (Throat drops), Nafukh (Insufflation), Zarur (Dusting powder), Saut (Nasal drops), Sanun (toothpowder), Mazugh (chewable drug).

Through absorption:

The body's ability to absorb drugs largely depends on the drug's composition and nature, as well as its shape. Pills and tablets tend to be absorbed more slowly in the stomach and intestines compared to liquids. It's possible that some pills may not dissolve completely and could be excreted later, especially those with gold or silver foil coverings. In addition, certain drugs are more efficiently absorbed on an empty stomach.

Excretory Route: Rectal drug administration can be a beneficial alternative in cases where oral administration is not possible or may have negative effects. It involves administering drugs like Huqna (enema) or Shyaf (suppositories) into the rectal area to stimulate related regions, such as enhancing uterine contractions during childbirth. Rectal administration may be chosen for various reasons, including the need to target specific areas like the rectum or anus, as well as treating male or female reproductive organs, cleansing intestines to prevent harmful substance absorption, or when there is a risk that a drug may be expelled during vomiting.

Compared to oral administration, rectal drug administration can result in a quicker effect, but the stomach and intestines absorb certain drugs more efficiently than the rectum.

Respiratory Route:

The process of respiration begins with the nostrils, then moves through the throat (talaq), larynx (Hanjara), trachea (Qasaba al-Ri'a), and finally to the alveolar capillaries (Urooq-i-Khashna) throughout the lungs. This pathway is also used to administer drugs in the form of vapours (Bukharat) or smoke (Dukhat). For example, the combined effect of Shamum (olfaction), Lakhlakha (inhalation), and Ghaliya (perfumed powder) impacts all respiratory organs. However, some drugs are only applied locally to the nose, throat, or trachea. Nasal drops and dry drugs that induce sneezing (Atus) are examples of such drugs. Some drugs, like Nafukh (Insufflation), are inhaled, while others are applied in the form of Tila (Liniment) or suppositories. The nasal cavity can also be washed with liquid drugs using a syringe - a process known as Sakob (Nasal Irrigation).

---

[403] Plural of Sheera (milky emulsified product).
[404] Plural of Lu'ab (Mucilage).
[405] Plural of Arq (Distillate).

Inhalation of certain drugs can cause a loss of consciousness. This indicates that even vapours (Bukharat) can be absorbed into the blood and other fluids and can reach the brain or heart, causing a loss of consciousness. This demonstrates the potency of these drugs and their effects through absorption.

Ophthalmic Route:

Typically, medication in liquid or dry form is applied to the eyes using Burud kohl or Kajal, which are, respectively, eye dusting powder and eyeliner that contains Antimony sulphide. Alternatively, dry suppositories can be mixed with water and applied. In addition, the eyes can be washed with liquid medication such as Aab Itrifal (trifala water), ointments can be applied, or dusting powder can be dusted on the eyes.

Ear Route:

Medications that are administered through the ear work by acting on the tympanic membrane. Generally, these drugs are administered as ear drops or sometimes via a medicated wick (Fatila). In certain cases, lukewarm liquid drugs or drugs can be used to wash the ear and remove any buildup, followed by suctioning with a liquid used for syringing (Zaruq). Aural effusion (Sakob) is another technique that may be used to administer medication through the ear.

Urethral Route:

This route can be used in the diseases of the bladder (Mathana/Masana) and urinary tract (Majari-i-Bawl) like Gonorrhoea (Sozak), inflammation of the bladder (Waram-i-masana), urinary calculi (Hasat-i-masana), ulcers of the bladder (Quruh-i-masana), etc. liquid drugs are administered in the urethra through a syringe. In some diseases of the urethra, drugs are inserted in the form of Shyaf (Suppositories).

Vaginal route:

For the treatment of vaginal (Mahbil), cervical (Unuq·al-Rahim), and uterine (Rahim) diseases, medications can be administered using a syringe, and the vagina can be washed using syringing (Zaruq) and effusion (Sakub). Sometimes, a small parcel or a wick of medication is inserted into the vagina. A tampon (Hamul) or pessary (Firzaja) can also be used. An ointment (marham) such as marham dakhilyun can be applied to the vagina, and medications can also be applied in the form of a Tila (liniment) in the vagina.

Methods of administration of external drugs

Drugs that are applied to the body externally are known as external drugs. This includes Tila (Liniment), Zimad (Paste), Khizab (Hair dye), Marham (Ointment), Kabus (disc-shaped preparation for local application), Ghaza (Face powder), and Qairooti/Qayruti (Ointment made of oils and wax).

Other examples of external drugs include Abzan (Sitz bath), Sakub (Irrigation), Hammam (Turkish bath), Pashoya (Footbath), Nutul (Irrigation), and Ghasul (Wash lotion). In some cases, the effects of drugs are produced through Dhooni (Fumigation) and Bhapara (Vapour bath).

Certain drugs are applied on the skin and then massaged, such as Masuḥ (oily-liquid preparation), Daluk (massage oil), and Ubtan (scrub).

For skin ulcers or deep wounds like Nasur (fistula), drugs are administered in the form of Shyaf (Suppositories) and Fatila (wicks). Liquid drugs can also be dropped on the affected area, powdered drugs can be dusted on the skin, or ointment can be applied.

When it comes to wounds of the skin and fistulas, they are abnormal openings in the skin through which the drug effect reaches the organs and nerves.

Collection Of Drugs

The quality and effectiveness of a drug depend on various factors, including its type, cultivation method, collection, storage, and physical properties such as colour, smell, taste, consistency, and weight. If any of these properties are outside the expected ranges, it can lead to changes in the drug's internal properties, constituents, and bio-action, reducing efficacy. Therefore, it is important to ensure that drugs are of good quality and meet the required standards to achieve the desired results.

Ancient physicians believed that the effects of drugs varied depending on where they were grown, whether they were of plant (Nabati), animal (Haiwani), or mineral (Madini) origin. To ensure the effectiveness of the drugs, they recommended obtaining high-quality ones from areas where their beneficial effects had been proven, such as Arabian Senna (Cassia angustifolia) and Chinese Rhubarb (Rheum emodi). The potency of the same drug grown in two different locations was thought to be influenced by the air and water in those areas.

Some plants are more effective when they are young, while others are more effective as they age. For instance, the Rewand Chini tree is mature and ready to use after six years. However, some people use small buds, leaves, and branches, while others prefer mature leaves and fully bloomed-flowers from the same tree. Similarly, for some diseases, raw fruits are recommended, while others require ripened fruits. For instance, raw mango is recommended on hot days for cooling and relief from the heat, and ripened mangoes are beneficial for nourishing the body and gaining weight.

When collecting healthy drugs, it is important to consider the time and season of collection, as they greatly affect the drug's effectiveness.

Typically, flowers and leaves should be harvested when they have matured, but before they change colour or lose their fragrance. They should then be dried in the shade before use. If immature buds or leaves are to be used, they should be collected before they mature.

Similarly, fruits and seeds should be collected when they are fully ripe. If unripe fruits such as mangoes or papayas are to be used, they should be collected before they ripen. Ripe fruits should not be left to fall to the ground but instead should be harvested while still attached to the branch.

To obtain maximum active constituents, roots should be collected after plants have matured but before fruiting. Branches and barks should be gathered in the spring season while they are fresh and not from dry or diseased plants. Herbs, whether on the ground or on shrubs and trees, should be fresh with flower fruits and are typically used as whole herbs. Resin and gum should be collected while the flowers are falling, before the sun rises or after it sets, as the sun's heat can alter the constituents of some products. Some secretions, such as Affiyun (Papaver Somniferum - opium), are obtained in the afternoon. Gums should be collected before they break into pieces, preferably as an entire lump.

Drugs from animal sources: Drugs from animals are typically obtained from young, healthy, and fat animals. However, this principle is not always followed as chicks, young goats, sheep, etc. are also used.

Drugs from mineral sources: Drugs obtained from mineral sources should be free from impurities like mud and stones and retain their colour, shine, fragrance, and other properties.

Storage Of Drugs

To preserve drugs, it is necessary to follow certain instructions. Some of these instructions are:

1. Always store volatile drugs like Mint leaves, Camphor, Saffron, Musk, and Amber in airtight containers to prevent the loss of their volatile constituents.
2. Herbs like Mint, Sumbul-ut-teeb (Valeriana Officinalis Linn.), and Rose flowers should be stored in glass jars to prevent the loss of their fragrance and potency.
3. Store each drug in a separate container to avoid contamination.
4. Keep drugs sealed and protected from moisture as moisture can cause decomposition.
5. Avoid storing fragrant drugs in cloth or tote bags as their fragrant constituents may be lost, and moisture and air may reach them through the pores of the bag.

6. To preserve raw and fresh fruits, animal-origin drugs, gemstones, etc., immerse them in honey or sugary syrups. Glass containers immersed in ghee can also be used to preserve them.
7. Liquid drugs like Arqat (distillates), Sharabats (syrups), Sikanjbin (Oxymel), Jawarishat (digestives), Khamirajaat (Fermented confectionaries), Murabbajaat (Fruit preserves), Gulqand (flower conserve), Roganat (oils), and others should be stored in glass bottles and closed with a cork to preserve them longer. Avoid storing liquid drugs in metal containers as the metal can produce toxins and affect the drugs. If you must store them in metal containers, keep them in cool places during summers and rainy seasons.
8. Dry drugs like Haboob (pills), Qursat (tablets), and Safufat (powders) should be stored in glass jars instead of metal containers.
9. Compound drugs like digestive powder (Churan) and Habbe Kabid Naushadri[406] and sour and saline salts should also be stored in glass containers to protect them from moisture.

Utilisation period of drugs

All drugs have a limited efficacy period. After this time, the natural temperament (Mizaj Tibbi) of the drug, its natural composition (Tarkib Tab'i), and its mode or form of action (Surat Naw'iyya) can change. Heat, sunlight, moisture, and water can easily affect most drugs. However, some drugs are less affected by seasonal changes.

There are two types of drugs based on their stability and weakness of temperament:

1. Drugs with a weak temperament:
   These are the drugs that can be easily affected by the environment and the season, such as air, water, light, etc. They may lose their natural composition, mizaj and medicinal properties due to such factors.
2. Drugs with a stable temperament:
   These are the drugs that do not lose their natural composition, mizaj and medicinal properties easily. They remain stable even when exposed to different environmental conditions.

Expiry period of drugs

Determining the exact expiry period of a drug can be a difficult task, but ancient physicians have made estimations based on their experience. The expiry period of a drug depends on how it has been stored. For instance, fragrant drugs like camphor (Kafoor) have a shorter expiry period when exposed to air. However, if stored in glass and kept in a cool place, it becomes hard to estimate its expiry period.

---

[406] Unani hepatic pills

To calculate the expiry period of a drug, its features, colour, smell, taste, form, weight, and freshness are examined. This principle applies to all types of drugs, whether mineral, plant, or animal-based. The fragrance of drugs like Musk, Saffron, and Amber that have high fragrance indicates that their effectiveness and functions have not declined. Conversely, if their fragrance has decreased, their potency has also decreased. This same principle applies to drugs with bitter, astringent, sweet, sour, or other tastes.

Expiry period of drugs in terms of their sources

In terms of sources, drugs come from three categories: minerals, plants, and animals, and each has its own expiration date.

Mineral drugs

In this, all the metals, stones, and certain types of clays are included. Gold, silver, iron, copper, etc., are metals (Zawil ajsad/ Fili ziyya). Sulphur, Mercury, Arsenic, etc., are non-metals (Zavil arwah), which evaporate on heating and Diamond, Ruby, etc., are stones. Metals play an important role in drugs that provide a cure for diseases and are not as affected by the environment, and because of this, they have a longer life.

Metals drugs:

The expiry period of metals varies. Some metals, for example, gold, silver, etc., are less affected by air and water, but other metals are more affected by them, such as iron, and copper, which tend to rust.

Non-Metal drugs:

Non-metals have a shorter shelf life than metals as they tend to evaporate at high temperatures. Some examples of non-metals are Gandhak (Sulphur), Para (Hydrargyrum - Mercury), Hartal (Arsenic trisulphide), among others.

Stone and Clay drugs:

The shelf life of stones and clay can vary, and it is hard to estimate the exact shelf life of stones as they can last for thousands of years. However, storing finely powdered stones can decrease their lifespan. Clays such as Gile Armani (Arminium bole) and Gile[407] Multani (Silicate of aluminia) can be used for a few years, whereas Safeda Kashgari Powder (Barytes Powder - Zinc Oxide) can last up to six years.

Plant drugs

---

[407] The word Gile means clay.

Samaghiyat (gums): are natural resins that can last up to three years. Examples include Ushaq, Dam-al-akhwayn (Dracaena cinnabari - Socotra dragon tree), Samagh Arabi (Acacia arabica gum), Kateera (Tragacanth - Astragalus gummifer gum).

Usarat (Extracts): These are dry extracts, such as Aqaqia (Acacia extract), Rasaut (Barberry extract), and Rubbussus (Glycyrrhiza glabra root extract). Their estimated expiry period is shorter than that of gums.

Shagufa aur Phool (Buds and flowers): These can be used for up to two years if they have not lost their volatile constituents, such as Gul Banafsha (Viola Odorata flowers), Gul Nilofar (Iris Florentina flowers), Gul surkh (Rosa damascena flowers), Gul Gaozaban (Borago officinalis flowers), Qaranfal (clove - Caryophyllus aromaticum bud), Izkhir (Cymbopogon schoenanthus) and others.

Barg (Leaves): Different leaves like Senna (Cassia senna leaf - Cassia angustifolia), Gaozaban (Borago officinalis), Tezpat (Cinnamomum tamala – Bay leaf), Hansraj / Persiyoshan (Adiantum capillus) have different expiry periods. The expiry period of Saqmonia (scammonia resins) is twenty years, farfiyun (Cactus latex) is forty years, and Affiyun (Papaver Somniferum - opium) is fifty years.

Roghan (Oils): Those oils that are cold and moist oils expire in two to three weeks, while hot and moist ones expire in one to two years. However, the expiry period of Balsan (Commiphora opobalsamum) oil is long, and it is said that the older it is, the more potent it becomes. Similarly, olive oil, Kafoor (camphor) oil, and Izkhir (Cymbopogon schoenanthus) oil retain their potency for two years.

Thmar/Samar (Fruits): It is important to use fresh fruits within one to ten days. However, some fruits can be preserved as Murabba (fruit preserve) and can be used for up to a year. Dry fruits can be stored for one to two years, but if their hard outer coat is removed, they can only last for ten days. Alu bukhara (dried plums) are an exception and can be used for up to a year. Dry fruits that contain oils, such as walnuts, almonds, pistachios and pine nuts, can also be used for up to a year.

Tukhm (Seeds): Seeds can be used for up to two to three years. However, seeds that contain oil have a shorter shelf life than those that do not. For example, cumin seeds, chicory seeds, coriander seeds, lettuce seeds, poppy seeds, sesame seeds, cucumber seeds, watermelon seeds, pumpkin seeds, etc., lose their potency when the oils evaporate.

Shakh (branches), Jar (roots), and Chal (bark): These can be divided into two groups: those that are effective for only one year and those that can last for approximately five years. If there are any changes in the physical characteristics, or if the plant becomes infested with termites within a year of harvest, then the root, bark, or branch of that plant should not be used. Examples of such plants include Asal Alsoos (Glycyrrhiza glabra - licorice roots), Behman (Centaurea behen root), Chob Chini (Smilax china root), Turbud (turpeth roots), Zaranbad (Curcuma zedoaria Rosc.), Zanjabeel (Zingiber officinalis rhizome), Aqarqarha (Pellitory - Anacyclus pyrethrum), and more. On the other hand, there are medicinal plants that can be effective for up to five years, such as Juntiana (Gentiana lutea herb), Darchini (cinnamon - Cinnamomum zeylanicum), Chob zard (turmeric: Curcuma longa), Qust (Sassurea lappa root), and more.

Haiwani Advia (Drugs from Animal sources): Their shelf life varies according to the part used. If the gallbladder of an animal is dried, its potency can last for four to five years. Cheese can last for one to two years, while dried Sartan (crab) can be used for up to two years. Salted fats are good for one year, and Jund Bedastar (Castoreum) can remain potent for up to ten years. Musk (Moschus moschiferus) and Amber (Ambra grisea) can last as long as their fragrance persists. Seep (Ostreoidea - oyster shell) and Marwareed (Pearl- Mytilus margaritiferus) can be effective for five to ten years.

Laban/Shir/Dudh (Dried latex): These dried milky substances can be used for a long period of time. For instance, Affiyun (Papaver Somniferum - opium) can be stored for up to fifty years, Saqmonia (Scammonia resin) can be kept for twenty years, and Ferfiun (Euphorbia neriifolia latex) can be utilized for approximately thirty years.

Drug substitutes (Abdal Advia)

Substituting one drug for another becomes necessary in certain instances. The reasons for such a substitution can be the prohibitive cost of the original drug, its unavailability, potential side effects, or even religious restrictions. Additionally, it is possible that the desired part of a plant used for the drug might be inaccessible, while other parts remain readily available.

In such situations, it is appropriate to choose a drug that shares similar functionalities and characteristics with the original drug. This replacement is often referred to as a second-line or substitute/alternative drug.

Principles of alternative drugs

1. No two drugs are identical in their functions and characteristics. As a result, several drugs lack suitable substitutes. For instance, certain drugs, like Ood saleeb (Paeonia officinalis, root), tobacco, cannabis, and Yabruj (Atropa belladonna root), are deemed irreplaceable.
2. The alternative drug must not be too different from the first-line drug; its Mizaj (temperament) should be the same as the first-line drug or very similar. For example, if a drug is hot and dry in the first degree, then its alternative drug's temperament should also be hot and dry at the same degree. But if the Mizaj of the alternative drug as compared to the first-line drug is hotter and drier, then its quantity should be less, or if it is less hot and dry, then its quantity should be greater than the first-line drug's.
3. It is also possible that if a drug is from an animal source, its alternative drug can be made up from a plant source. According to Al Razi, the second line drug for Jund Bedastar (Castoreum) is black pepper in half the quantity. Similarly, a drug from an animal source can be an alternative for a plant drug, like, for example,

Post Baiza Murgh (hen egg shells) used in half the quantity instead of the plant Kateera (Tragacanth - Astragalus gummifer gum).
4. One variety of drugs can be an alternative to another drug. For example, one variety of mint for another variety of mint.
5. Sometimes, when a specific part of a plant is not available, then another part of the plant can used as an alternative. For example, if Neem (Azadirachta Indica) flower is not available, then Neem leaf and bark can be used, just as Banafsha (Viola Odorata) is an alternative drug for Hansraj/Persiyoshan (Adiantum capillus).

With regards to the drug and its alternative, we need to be sure that both drugs have a similar mizaj (temperament). Next, do both drugs and their alternatives have similar properties and actions, and in which diseases can both drugs be used? Therefore, when the replacement of a drug is selected, it should be understood clearly why the substitute drug is chosen and for which illnesses.

Selecting an alternative drug based on constituents, functions, and mechanism of action.

As discussed previously, when looking for an alternative drug, it is important to assess whether any constituents or functions are similar to the original drug and to check if their mechanism of action and constituents are alike. For instance, pumpkin seeds, watermelon seeds and many other types of seeds contain similar constituents and can serve as substitutes for each other.

The constituents of oysters and pearls have certain similarities, which make them viable alternatives for each other.

Various astringent drugs that constrict vessels with their astringent essence can be used interchangeably.

Dried plums, tamarind, small cardamom (Elettaria cardamomum), large cardamom (Amomum subulatum), and other similar drugs can be substitutes for each other. Although their composition and functions differ, their mechanism of action is similar.

However, it can be challenging to select an alternative drug since the composition of each drug is unique.

It is important to bear in mind that a substitute drug may not always be as effective as the primary drug. For example, the drug Dirmana (Artemesia maritima) is the primary drug for long worms, and its substitutes are Afsanteen (Artemisia absinthium) and Suddab (Ruta graveolens); however, these are not as effective on long worms as Dirmana.

Al Razi[408] has provided a list of drugs and their alternatives, which can be found below:

Drug Unani name (Transliteration)	Botanical name	Alternative Drug Unani name (Transliteration)	Botanical name
Abhal (Juniper berries), ابہل	Juniperus communis	Salikha (Chinese cinnamon/Cassia), سلیخہ	Cinnamomum cassia
Afis/Mazoo (Oak gall), مازو / عفص	Quercus infectoria	Mayeen Kalan/Jhao flowers (Tamarisk), مائیں کلاں / جھاؤ کا پھول	Tamarix dioica flowers
Afsanteen (Wormwood), افسنتین	Artemisia absinthium	Asaroon (European wild ginger) or Halela zard (Yellow myrobalan), اسارون، بلیلہ زرد	Valeriana wallichii, Terminalia chebula yellow
Aftimoon (Dodder)[409], افتیمون	Cuscuta epithymum Linn	Turbud (Turpeth roots), تربد	Ipomoea turpethum Linn
Aqarqarha (Pellitory), عاقرقرحا	Anacyclus pyrethrum	Darunaj Aqrabi (Leopard's-bane), درونج	Doronicum pardalianches
Asaroon/Tagar (European wild ginger), اسارون	Asarum europaeum	Qirdmana (Cuckoo Flower), قردمانا	Cardamine pratensis
Badaward, باذآورد	Amberboa ramose	Shahatraj/Shahatra (Fumitory), شاہترج/ شاہترہ	Fumaria parviflora Linn.
Badranjboya (Lemon balm), بادرنجبویہ	Melissa parviflora Benth	Abresham (Silk pod), ابریشم	Bombyx mori
Baladur (Marking nut), بلادر	Semecarpus anacardium Linn.	Bunduq (Hazel nut), بندق	Corylus avellana Linn.
Barg Balsan (Mecca myrrh leaf), برگ بلسان	Commiphora opobalsamum Linn.	Ood-e-Balsan (Mecca myrrh), عودبلسان	Commiphora opobalsamum Linn.
Behman (Behman Safed), بہمن	Centaurea behen	Tudari (Wallflower), توداری	Cheiranthus cheiri Linn.[410]
Behroza/Qinnah (Chir pine), بہروزہ	Pinus longifolia Roxb.	Sakbinaj (Sagapenum), سکبینج	Ferula persica Willd.
Biranjasif (Yarrow), برنجاسف	Achillea Millefolium Linn.	Babuna (Chamomile), بابونہ	Matricaria Chamomilla
Darchini (Cinnamon), دارچینی	Cinnamomum zeylanicum	Salikha (Chinese cinnamon/Cassia), سلیخہ	Cinnamomum cassia

---

[408] *Maqala Fi Abdal Al-adwiya Al-mustamala Fi Al-tib Wa Al-ilaj* by Al-Razi (translated by CRIUM)
[409] Aftimoon walati (افتیمون ولایتی)
[410] Abu-Asab, Mones - Avicenna's Single Drugs - references this as Sisymbrium officinale - but this is not mentioned as such elsewhere.

Darunaj Aqrabi (Leopard's bane)	Doronicum pardalianches Linn.	Zaranbad/Kachoor (white turmeric/zedoaria) زرنباد	Curcuma zedoaria Rosc.
Elaichi Khurd (True cardamom), الائچی خورد	Elettaria cardamomum	Kababa/Kabab Chini (Cubeb pepper), کبابہ/کبابہ چینی	Piper cubeba
Fadaniya/Ood saleeb (Peony), فادانیا	Paeonia officinalis root	Post Anar (pomegranate skin) or Jaws essarew/sarew (Mediterranean cypress), پوست انار، جوز السّرو (سرو)	Punica granatum epicarp of fruit
Faraasiyun (White Horehound), فراسیون	Marrubium vulgare	Sumbul-ut-teeb / Jatamansi (common valerian) or Asaroon/Tagar, سنبل الطیب، اسارون	Valeriana Officinalis Linn. Or Asarum europaeum
Fawwah/Majeeth (Indian madder), فوہ/مجیٹھ	Rubia cordifolia root	Kababa / Kabab Chini (Cubeb pepper), کبابہ/کبابہ چینی	Piper cubeba
Filfil abyaz (White pepper), فلفل ابیض	Piper album	Zanjabeel (Ginger), زنجبیل	Zingiber officinale rhizome
Filfilmoya/Pipla Mool (Long pepper), فلفل مویہ / پپلا مول	Piper longum root	Narmushk (Ceylon Ironwood), نارمشک	Mesua ferrea
Foful (Betel nut), فوفل	Areca catechu	Sandal (Sandalwood), صندل	Santalum album wood
Ghariqoon (Agarikon), غاریقون	Polyporus officinalis	Turbud (Turpeth roots), تربد	Ipomoea turpethum Linn
Habb al-Neel/Kala dana, (Ivy-leaved Morning Glory), حب النیل/کالادانہ	Ipomea hederacea	Tukhme Al-Hanzal (Bitter apple seeds), تخم الحنظل	Citrullus colocynthis
Hafad/Rasaut (Barberry), حفض/رسوت	Berberis vulgaris	Foful (betel nut) and Sandal (Sandalwood), فوفل وصندل	Santalum album wood
Irsa (Orris root), ایرسا	Iris germanica root (Rhizoma iridis)	Mazaryun (Mezereum), ماذریون	Daphne mezereum
Jadwar, (Indian Atees) جدوار	Delphinium denudatum Wall.	Zaranbad/Kachoor (White turmeric/Zedoaria) زرنباد	Curcuma zedoaria Rosc.
Jaosheer (Galbanum resin), جاوشیر	Ferula galbaniflua	Laban al-Teen (Milky sap from Figs), لبن التین	Ficus carica Linn.
Jawzboa/Jauz-ut-teeb /Jaiphal (Nutmeg), جوزبو/جَوْزُ الطِّیب	Myristica fragrans Houtt	Sumbul-ut-teeb / Jatamansi (Common valerian), سنبل الطیب	Valeriana officinalis Linn.
Joada (Felty germander), جُعْدَة	Teucrium polium Linn.	Salikha (Chinese cinnamon) bark, شاخ سلیخہ	Cinnamomum cassia bark

Jund Bedastar, جندبیدستر	Castoreum	Filfil/Filfil safed, فلفل	Piper nigrum Linn.
Kaknaj (Chinese lantern fruit), کاکنج	Physalis alkekengi	Bazrulbanj/Ajwain Khurasani (Black Henbane), بزرالنج/ اجوائن خراسانی	Hyoscyamus niger
Kharbaq siah (Black hellebore root), خربق سیاه	Helleborus niger	Kundash (White hellebore) or Ghariqoon (Agarikon), کندش، غاریقون	Veratrum album Linn., Polyporus officinalis
Kharbaq[411] (White hellebore) (White hellebore), خربق	Veratrum album	Mazriyoon (Mezereum), ماذریون	Daphne mezereum
Khayarshamber/Amaltas (purging cassia), خیارشنبر/ املتاس	Cassia fistula pulp	Turbud (turpeth roots) or Rub al-Soos (Liquorice Extract), تربد، رُبّ السوس	Ipomoea turpethum Linn, Glycyrrhiza glabra
Khulanjan (Galangal), خولنجان	Alpinia galanga	Qaranfal (clove), قرنفل	Syzygium aromaticum
Lisan al-asafeer/Inderjao (Kurchi), لسان العصافیر	Holarrhena antidysenterica	Maghz Akhrot (Walnut), مغزاخروٹ	Juglans regia
Marwareed/Lulu (Pearl), مروارید	Mytilus margaritiferus	Sadaf (Oyster), صدف	Ostrea edulis
Mazoo (Aleppo oak), مازو	Quercus infectoria	Jhao fruit/Mayeen Kalan/Tamarisk Galls, جھاؤ کا پھل	Tamarix dioica
Mur (Myrrh), مُر	Commiphora myrrha	Filfil Siyah (Black Pepper), فلفل سیاہ	Piper nigrum Linn.
Nakchikni (Sneeze wort), چھکنی	Dregea volubilis	Filfil (Indian Long Pepper), فلفل	Piper longum
Narmushk/Nagkesar (Ceylon ironwood), نارمشک/ناگیسر	Mesua ferrea	Zanjabeel (Ginger), زنجبیل	Zingiber officinale rhizome
Ood-e-Balsan (Mecca myrrh), عود بلسان	Commiphora gileadensis	Post Salikha (Chinese cinnamon/Cassia, Bark), پوست سلخہ	Cinnamomum cassia
Persiyoshan/Hansraj (Maidenhair fern), پرسیاوشان	Adiantum capillus-veneris Linn	Banafsha (Sweet violet), بنفشہ	Viola odorata
Qardamana/Elachi (Green cardamom), قردمانا	Elettaria cardamomum	Izkhir (Camel grass), اذخر	Cymbopogon schoenanthus

---

[411] If only written as Kharbaq, then this refers to Kharbaq Safed (White Hellebore), which is Veratrum album. It is known to be poisonous and is rarely used.

Qust (Costus root), قسط	Saussurea lappa root	Aqarqarha (Pellitory), عاقرقرحا	Anacyclus pyrethrum
Rewand[412] (Rhubarb), ریوند	Rheum officinale	Gul Surkh (Rose petals) or Sumbul-ut-teeb (Common valerian), گل سرخ، سنبل الطیب	Rosa damascena, Valeriana Officinalis Linn.
Rogan Balsan[413] (Mecca myrrh)	Commiphora gileadensis	Olive oil, روغن زیتون	Olea europaea
Rogan Gul (Rose oil), روغن گل	Rosa damascena	Rogan Banafsha (Sweet violet oil), روغن بنفشه	Viola odorata
Saffron (Zafran - Crocus sativa stigma), (Saffron), زعفران	Saffron - Crocus sativus Linn	Sumbul-ut-teeb / Jatamansi (Common valerian) سنبل الطیب	Valeriana officinalis Linn.
Sakbinaj (Sagapenum), سکبینج	Ferula persica Willd.	Behroza/Qinnah (Chir, Pine), بہروزہ	Pinus longifolia Roxb.
Sarw (Cypress), سرو	Cupressus sempervirens	Anzaroot (Pinersarcolla Resin), انزروت	Astragalus sarcocolla gum
Sazij Hindi/Tez paat (Malabar leaf), ساذج ہندی	Cinnamomum tamala	Sumbul-ut-teeb / Jatamansi (common valerian) سنبل الطیب	Valeriana Officinalis Linn.
Shahatraj/Shahatra (Fumitory), شاہترج/ شاہترہ	Fumaria parviflora Linn.	Sana (Senna) or Halela zard (Yellow myrobalan), سناء، بلیلہ زرد	Cassia angustifolia Vahl., Terminalia chebula yellow
Shahdanaj/Tukham Qinnab (Hemp seeds), (شہدانج (تخم قنب	Cannabis sativa Linn. seeds	Marzanjosh (sweet Marjorum), مرزنجوش	Origanum marjoram
Shaqaqul (Wild parship), شقاقل	Pastinaca secacul Linn	Boozaidaan (Sweet Pellitory), بوزیدان	Tanacetum umbelliferum Boiss.
Sheetraj Hindi (Ceylon Leadwort), شطرج ہندی	Plumbago zeylanica	Fawwah/Majeeth (Indian madder), فوہ/مجیٹھ	Rubia cordifolia root
Sibr/Elva (Aloe vera), ایلو/ صبر	Aloe barbadensis Miller	Rasaut/Hudod (Indian lycium), رسوت/ حضض	Berberis lyceum
Sosan (Orris flower), سوسن	Iris germanica	Nargis (Paperwhite), نرگس	Narcissus tazetta Linn.

---

[412] Different types are used based on origin for example **Indian rhubarb** but more commonly Rewand Chini - Chinese Rhubarb.
[413] i.e., Rogan Ood-e-Balsan - sap obtained from the Balsan tree by making cuts - Balsam Mecca

Sumbul-ut-teeb/Jatamansi (Common valerian), سنبل الطیب	Valeriana Officinalis Linn.	Izkhir (Camel grass), اذخر	Cymbopogon schoenanthus
Suranjan (Yellow colchicum)[414], سورنجان	Colchicum luteum	Barg-e-Hina (Henna leaf) or Muqil azraq (Guggul), برگ حناء، مقل ازرق	Lowsonia inermis Linn, Commiphora mukul Linn.
Taj /Salikha (Chinese cinnamon), تج قلمی/سلیخہ	Cinnamomum cassia bark	Kamun/Zeera safed (Cumin seed), کمون	Cuminum cyminum
Taj Qalmi/Salikha (Chinese cinnamon), تج قلمی/سلیخہ	Cinnamomum cassia bark	Darchini/Darsini (Cinnamon), دارچینی/دارصینی	Cinnamomum zeylanicum
Tambol / Paan (Betel Vine), تانبول	Piper betel Linn.	Qaranfal (Clove), قرنفل	Syzygium aromaticum
Thafsia (Drias Plant), ثافسیا	Thapsia garganica	Baloot (White oak), بالوط	Quercus alba
Ushaq (Gum ammoniac), اشق	Dorema ammoniacum	Darmana (Sea wormwood), درمنہ	Artemisia maritima
Ushna/Charila (Black stone flower), اشنہ	Parmelia perlata	Qirdmana (Cuckoo Flower), قردمانا	Cardamine pratensis
Ustukhuddus (Lavender), اسطوخودوس	Lavandula stoechas	Faraasiyun (White Horehound), فراسیون	Marrubium vulgare
Zaranbad/Kachoor (white turmeric/Zedoaria), زرنباد	Curcuma zedoaria Rosc.	Sheetraj Hindi (Plumbago zeylanica), شطرج ہندی	Plumbago zeylanica
Zarawand Taveel (Bereztem), زراوند طویل	Aristolochia longa Linn	Rasaut/Hudod (Indian lycium), زرنباد	Curcuma zedoaria Rosc.
Zarawand Taveel (Bereztem), زراوندطویل	Aristolochia longa Linn.	Jadwar, جدوار	Delphinium denudatum Wall.
Zard Chob/Haldi (Turmeric), زرد چوب/ہلدی	Curcuma longa	Mameeran (used for the eyes i.e., as a kohl [eye powder]), مامیران	Coptis teeta

Beneficial and adverse effects of drugs

Some drugs, even though they are used because of their beneficial effects on diseases, may also have some adverse effects. In such cases, it may be necessary to modify the drug. This can be done through detoxification (Mudabbar) methods such as roasting, frying, or burning the drug to a charring stage without reducing it to ash or through processes like calcination, sublimation, decantation, separation, removal of froths, washing, cleaning, or dissolution.

---

[414] more commonly this is Suranjan talkh [bitter] i.e. سورنجان تلخ

Another way to modify the effects of a drug is to change the route of administration. For example, if a drug causes vomiting and discomfort when taken orally, it might be administered through an enema instead.

A third approach is to add another drug that can reduce the side effects of the main drug. This additional drug is known as a Musleh (corrective).

Correctives drugs (Muslehat)

A Musleh (corrective) is used to reduce the toxicity of a drug or to increase its potency. It can also be added to extend the expiry date of a drug. There are mainly four single drugs, such as Gum acacia (Gond-e-Babool), Astragalus gummifer (Samag-e-Kateera), Sugar, and Honey, that have corrective properties to reduce the toxic effects of other drugs. Therefore, these drugs are added as excipients with most of the compound formulations.

For instance, if a drug is too acidic and its use may cause ulceration in mucous membranes, then a Musleh can be added to dilute the drug with water and decrease its acidic effects. Mucilages such as Samagh Arabi (Acacia arabica) gum, Kateera (Astragalus gummifer gum), honey, or Amber (Ambra grosea) can also be used to achieve this purpose.

To illustrate how a Musleh works, let us consider the example of Qurs Tinker (Tinker tablets), a well-known Unani formula primarily used for the treatment of digestive disorders. It contains Elva (Aloe vera), Filfil Siyah (Piper nigrum fruit), Ajwain Khurasani (Hyoscyamus niger), and Tinker (borax). Although Aloe vera is very effective in removing gas, it can cause intestinal cramps. Therefore, Ajwain Khorasan is added as a Musleh to reduce the effects of cramping.

Another example is when we want to increase the potency of a drug such as Turbud (Ipomea turpenthum root), which is used as a laxative but is not effective in removing thick Balgham (phlegm). In that case, we can add Sonth (Zingiber officinale – dried ginger) to the formula, which helps Turbud in its potency to remove phlegm.

If we wish to extend the life of a drug, we can add honey, salt, or sugar to the formula. For example, a Majun contains honey as a preservative and becomes the corrective (Musleh) of the short-lived dried powdered herbs.

Treatment with single and compound drugs

If a single (mufradat) drug is used for treatment, it is referred to as 'ilaj bil mufrad'. On the other hand, if more than one drug is used in the form of a decoction, infusion, distillate, powder, electuary, or syrup, then this type of treatment is called 'ilaj bil murakkab' or 'treatment with compound (murakkabat) drugs'.

The benefits of using only single drugs

Unani physicians assert that it is always preferable to use a single drug for treatment. This is because using multiple drugs together can result in adverse effects. However, if a single drug is not sufficient due to any reason or condition, it is recommended to use the minimum number of drugs possible. Long prescriptions are not only objectionable but also abnormal, as mentioned by Ibn Sina in The Canon. Therefore, it is important to remember that experimented and experienced drugs are better than non-experimented drugs, and the use of a few drugs is more beneficial than the use of many drugs.

The use of compound drugs

Conditions that may require a physician to prescribe compound drugs are:

1. **Use of Musleh (corrective) drugs:**
   We have previously discussed the use of adding a Musleh (corrective) drug to create a compound formulation.
2. **Islah-e-dawa (In order to change taste, odour and colour):**
   There are several reasons why some drugs may not be well-tolerated by the body. For example, a drug may have an unpalatable taste, such as Aloe vera (Elva), or a strong odour, such as Amaltas (Cassia fistula). Additionally, the form, shape, and colour of a drug may be unpleasant to look at. To address these issues and make the drug more palatable, efforts are made to improve its taste, odour, and appearance. For instance, sugar and honey can be added to many drugs to make their taste and odour more tolerable.
3. **Izafa-e-quwwath (Increase potency of the drug):**
   When a drug contains constituents that have different properties, it may produce dual effects. However, sometimes, the effect of one action may be weaker than what we require. In such cases, we can add another drug to strengthen the first drug's effect if it is not strong enough. For instance, Chamomile has resolvent (tahlel) and astringent (qabiz) properties, but its astringent power is weaker than its resolvent power. Therefore, we add an astringent to increase the overall astringent effect.
4. **Tazeef-e-amal (Reduce potency of drug):**
   In some cases, a drug may be too potent for the specific disease being treated. In such situations, additional drugs can be added to decrease its potency. For instance, camphor (Kafoor) is often added with Saffron (Zafran - Crocus sativa stigma) to achieve the required potency level.
5. **Ibtab e nafuz (Slowing the penetrative action of a drug):**
   In some cases, drugs may have a rapid effect, which needs to be slowed down by adding an additional medication to ensure that the medicine remains in the body long enough to achieve the desired results. For instance, Saqmonia (Scammonia resins) and Ghariqoon (Polyporus officinalis) are powerful purgatives, but they may be excreted out of the body before they can take effect. To prevent this, we need to add an additional drug to slow down the penetrative power of the primary medicine before it is eliminated from the body. There are two types of these additional drugs:

Directly acting drugs (Ibtay-e-nufuz zati): These medications decrease the penetrative power of the primary drug directly. Examples of such medications include vinegar mixed with water or Sankhya (Purified Arsenic trioxide) with Ghee (clarified butter).

Indirectly acting drugs (Ibtay-e-nufuz arzi): These medications do not directly decrease the penetrative power of the primary drug, but instead, they act on the body organs to make them less penetrative. Alternatively, they regulate an opposite mechanism to cancel out the undesirable effects of the primary drug. For example, adding a diuretic (mudir-i-bawl) to a Muarriq (diaphoretic) can help achieve the desired results.

6. **Surat-e-nufuz (Increasing the penetrative action of a drug):**
   Drugs that have a slow penetration rate can be aided by the addition of other drugs that increase their ability to penetrate the body. These types of drugs are known as Badraqa[415] ('vehicle' drugs). or instance, when applying oil to the skin, we can mix it with drugs that can be dissolved in the oil, such as opium and camphor, which help in quick and easy absorption into the skin. Similarly, we can mix sugar and salts with water since they are soluble.
   Drugs that are slow to penetrate have two forms:
   i. With the addition of a second drug results in an increase in the primary drug's penetrating power.
   ii. Or when the addition of a second drug increases the penetrating power of the drug towards a specific organ or increases its direction towards that organ.

7. **Ilaj-e-amraz-e-murakkabah (Treatment of compound diseases):**
   When more than one disease exists, and a single drug cannot always treat all the diseases, then in such situations, based on each disease, a composite prescription is prepared. For example, when there is a fever and a cold, a compound prescription that treats both is prepared.

8. **Tahafuz-e-dawa (drug preservation):**
   It is common to add a secondary drug to the primary drug to prevent it from getting contaminated, corrupted, or losing its potency. The technique of adding a honey or sugar mixture is often used to preserve seasonal fruits or flowers, such as Gulqand (flower conserve). In addition, salt and vinegar can also be used to prevent drugs from decaying and getting corrupted.

9. **Drug which is small in quantity:**
   The quantity of a drug can be minute on its own. For example, Rai (Mustard seeds) or poppy seeds would be hard to consume on their own due to their small dosage, so we can simply add, for example, a mixture of starch, sugar, and honey water with the herb, thereby making it easy to take as a dose.

10. **Other types of diseases:**

---

[415] drug enhancing absorption of another drug; a drug or substance which helps the main drug in absorption and reaching its target; it may be an inert substance or of therapeutic value in potentiating the effect of the main drug.

Sometimes a second drug is added for reasons than the above-mentioned. For example:
   a. Multiple treatments of a disease: In some cases, a disease may require more than one type of treatment. This is called multiple treatments of a disease. For example, in the case of septic fever, a laxative may need to be added to the fever medication in order to keep the intestine clear during the fever. Alternatively, diaphoretics (Muarriqat) or diuretics (Mudirat-i-Bawl) may be added to the fever medication to help evacuate substances through sweat or urination.
   b. Multiple disorders of a disease: When there is a single disease, but it has multiple disorders, then along with the drug for the actual disease, we need to add drugs to help with the order disorders.
   c. Sometimes we can add two or more drugs in order to create a secondary synergistic action. For example, where vapours are created to release gas which has built up in the stomach through belching.

Antagonistic drugs and antagonism

Antagonistic drugs

There are certain drugs that have opposing effects on the body. For instance, they can either constrict or dilate the vessels, accelerate or decelerate blood flow, or cause constipation or diarrhoea. Such drugs are called antagonistic drugs, as their effects counteract.

For example, Ibn al-Nafis explains that sourness and saltiness are counteractive to each other. When combined, they alter each other's mizaj (temperament).

The role of an antagonist is not necessarily to represent evil but rather to provide a counterbalance to the protagonist. In the same way, an antagonistic herb would block certain pathways or actions, similar to how a story's antagonist blocks the protagonist's goals. This herb may help prevent excessive activity of a process, such as controlling the dilation of blood vessels to maintain balance in the body's system.

Antagonism: Types

Functional antagonism

Refers to the direct counteraction of the effects of a drug. For example, if one drug causes dilation and another causes constriction, their effects may neutralize when mixed. However, if one drug is more potent, its effect will dominate. Sometimes, an antagonist is introduced to mitigate the extreme effects of a drug. For instance, the potent drug Jamal gota (Croton tiglium) can be paired with a Mushil (Purgative) to reduce its severe side effects, such as severe cramps.

Mizaj (temperament) antagonism

Related to a drug's inherent nature or temperament. It has two subtypes:

Absolute antagonism (tanaqiz suri)

This results in an actual change in drug temperament upon combination, producing a distinct compound. This new entity can be:

- Beneficial to the body.
- Detrimental to the body.
- Neutral in effect.

For instance, some acidic substances, when combined with saline ones, can produce vapors that aid in digestion and gas release. Such combinations are medically recommended, while the harmful or neutral ones are generally avoided.

Outcomes of absolute antagonism can be evident, like sediment formation, termed visible antagonism (tanaqiz jili). Alternatively, they might be subtle or unseen, called antagonism (tanaqiz khaffi).

Qualitative/Relative antagonism (tanaqiz mizaji)

Here, the drugs maintain their individual mizaj (temperament) post-combination. However, they might form incompatible mixtures. For instance, introducing an acidic substance to Asal Alsoos (Glycyrrhiza glabra - liquorice roots) makes it cloudy and precipitates its essence. Combinations of insoluble substances, such as chalk and resin, fall under this category.

The mixing and synthesis of drugs

Ibn Sina explains[416] that mixing medicines can sometimes strengthen their function or correct their side effects. Moreover, in the chapter on properties of composition, Ibn Sina notes[417] that certain drug combinations can lead to adverse effects, while others can enhance the effects and function of the drugs.

Examples of when the function of drugs is enhanced

Ibn Sina has mentioned some examples:

1. A drug may have potency potential, but it may need another specific drug added, as its essence may not naturally contain a specific component. When this additional drug is added, its action is enhanced. For instance, Turbud (Ipomea turpethum root) has purgative powers (Quwwath-e-mushil), but these are weak and incapable of

---

[416] In the Canon of medicine volume 2
[417] In the Canon of medicine volume 5

dissolving thicker matter. However, when ginger (Zanjabeel - Zingiber officinalis) is added to Turbud, its purgative actions are enhanced. This allows it to remove sticky matter and expel cold and vitreous humour (Zujaji khilt) through the bowels.
2. Aftimoon (Cuscuta reflexa) is a weak purgative, but if a demulcent (Mulattif) like pepper (Filfil) is added, then it increases the frequency of stools because pepper, due to its dissolving power, can assist Aftimoon in its purgative action.
3. Asrol (Rauwolfia serpentina Root) has a strong astringent power (quwwath-e-qabiza), but it also possesses a deobstruent (Mufattih) property that weakens its astringent power. However, when Hajar-e-Armani (Lapis anninium) is added to Asrol, its astringent power becomes strong and potent.

Examples of ineffectual drug combinations

It is important to note that some drugs can become ineffective due to incorrect mixing combinations. For instance, when Banafsha (Viola Odorata) and Halela (Terminalia chebula) are mixed, their effects become ineffective. This is because Banafsha is a resolvent[418] (mullaiyin) that weakens and moves an active substance, whereas Halela is a purgative that squeezes (Mushil bi'l Asr[419]) and constricts (Takthif). Therefore, if both are consumed at the same time, their expected effects will be cancelled out. Even if Halela is used before Banafsha, the results will be similar. In this case, Banafsha will soften the stomach, and Halela will have a squeezing and moistening action.

An example of an effective drug combination:

The combination of Sibr (Aloe vera), Kateera (which comes from Astragalus gummifer gum), and Mukul (which comes from Commiphora Mukul) can be very effective. Although Aloe vera is known for its purgative and intestine-cleansing properties, it can also cause intestinal irritation and lead to bleeding. However, Kateera and Mukul are astringents, which means they have properties that can help reduce bleeding. When these three ingredients are combined, the irritation caused by Aloe vera is countered by the adhesive qualities of Kateera and the astringent properties of Mukul. This helps constrict the dilated blood vessels, effectively preventing bleeding. By neutralizing the potential adverse effects of Aloe vera, this combination can be very beneficial.

Benefits of drug composition

After a mixture of certain drugs, some strong and beneficial effects can be produced that were not present in the single drug. Ibn Sina explains this phenomenon in the following way:

'It should be noted that some useful drugs, such as antidotes, have functions and properties that depend on their components, while others are due to their nature, which results from mixing. To achieve the required action, an antidote may be fermented for

---

[418] An agent which softens or resolves the inflammatory exudates.
[419] Drug that excretes morbid humours by squeezing from neighbouring organs of body and inducing diarrhoea.

some time so that a new mizaj (temperament) is created, with new potent effects in the constituents, which are more potent than the effect of a simple drugs.'

Drug Types: Their function and characteristics

Aasir عاصر **(Squeezing):** These drugs are highly astringent in nature and are dry in temperament. This helps in eliminating liquid matter from vessels by squeezing such as Amla (Emblica officinalis fruits), Balela (Terminalia blerica fruit), and Post Anar (Punica granatum epicarp of fruit).

Akkal اکال **(Corrosive):** These drugs can aid in the healing process of a wound by removing any unwanted tissue. For example, Choona (Calcium hydroxide - Quick lime), Zangar (Cupric sulphate), and Mardarsung (Litharge[420]).

Dafe Humma دافع حمّیٰ **(Antipyretic):** Antipyretic drugs reduce fever. For example, Karanjwa seeds (Caesalpinia bonducella) and Shahatra (Fumaria parviflora Linn.), Khaksi (Sisymbrium irio seed), Kasoos (Cuscuta reflexa herb), Gilo (Tilifora indica herb), Chiraita (Swertia chiratta herb), Bakayan (Melia azedarach - all parts), Palas Papra (Butea monosperma - seed), Abrak (Talc), Brahmadandi (Tricholepis glaberrima), Jadwar (Delphinium denudatum root), Falsa (Grawia asiatica fruit), Atees (Aconitum heterophyllum root), Phitkri (Alum), Anisoon (Pimpinella anisum seed), Afsanteen (Artemisia absynthium), Aslussoos (Glycerrhiza glabra root), Tabasheer (Bambusa arundinasia), Biranjasif (Achillea millefolium - Yarrow), and Arusa (Adhatoda vasica leaf).

Dafi-i-Taaffun دافع تعفّن **(Antiseptic):** Drugs that can be used either internally or externally to prevent or stop infections. They work by altering the substance of the infection, inhibiting the growth of organisms, altering the temperament of their host, or by using any other method. Examples of Dafi-i-Taaffun (Antiseptic) include Para (Hydrargyrum -Mercury), Raskapur (Calomel), Zangar (Cupric sulphate), Darchikna (compound of mercury and arsenic), Barg Neem (Azadirachta Indica - leaves), Gul Barg Neem (Azadirachta Indica - flowers), Sat Podina (Mentha arvensis extract - Menthol), Sat Podina, Menthol (Mentha arvensis extract), Kafoor (Cinnamomum camphora), Gulab (Rosa damascena), Zahar mohra (Serpentine), Ajwain Desi (Trachyspermum ammi), Hing (Ferula asafoetida), Qaranfal (Caryophyllus aromaticum bud), Mur (Commiphora myrrh gum), Tezpat (Cinnamomum tamala leaf), Loban (Boswellia serrata gum), Javitry (Myristica fragrance fruit coat), Sat Ajwain (Thymol), Roghan, Qaranfal and (Caryophyllus aromaticum oil).

Dafi-i-Tashannuj دافع تشنّج **(Antispasmodic/anticonvulsant):** These drugs relieve muscle and nerve spasms by depressing nervine centres. Examples include Datura metel (leaf) and Atropa belladonna (leaf). Other examples are Berg Datura (Datura metel, leaf), Berg Yabruj (Atropa belladonna - leaf), Ood Saleeb (Paeonia officinalis root), Affiyun (Papaver Somniferum), Hilteet (Ferula foetida gum), Asrol (Rauwolfia serpentina root),

---

[420] one of the natural mineral forms of lead(II) oxide.

Roghan Suddab (Ruta graveolens oil), Jadwar (Delphinium denudatum root), Qaranfal (Caryophyllus aromaticum bud), Karanjwa seeds (Caesalpinia bonducella), Anzarot (Astragalus sarcocolla gum), Sumbul-ut-teeb / Jatamansi (Valeriana officinalis Linn.), Kafoor (Cinnamomum camphora - camphor), and Roghan Podina (Mentha arvensis oil).

Ghassal غسّال **(Abluent):** This refers to a liquid agent that cleanses the parts applied to, owing to its detergent properties. Its detergent power, known as Quwwat-e-Jalia, combined with its viscosity, enables it to flow smoothly over surfaces, efficiently cleaning them in the process. The terms 'abluent' and 'detergent' are interconnected. Examples of Ghassal include Maul Asl (Honey water), Aash-e-Jau (Barley water), and Maul jubn (Whey).

Habis Dam حابس دم **(Haemostyptic):** Drug that stops bleeding either by constricting blood vessels locally or by reducing blood circulation to the affected area. These drugs stop the bleeding in the following ways.

(i) They act as astringent and close the vessels or capillaries. These drugs have a strong astringent power (quwwath-e-qabiza).

(ii) Some drugs are mucilaginous and sticky in nature, so they coat the mouth of vessels and capillaries and stop blood flow.

(iii) Drugs which have a cold temperament constrict the blood vessels and arrest the flow of blood.

(iv) Drugs which are narcotic in nature also decrease the blood flow.

(v) Some drugs divert the blood inside the blood vessels.

Examples are Phitkri (Alum), Safedi Beza (Egg white), Kaharba (Amber Sucomum), Sange Jarahat (Magnesium silicate), Geru (Red Ochre Powder - Alumina silicate and iron oxide), Dam-al-akhwayn (Dracaena cinnabari - Socotra dragon tree), Sadaf sokhta (Ostrea edulis), Mazoo sabz (Quercus infectoria), Post khashkhash (Papaver somniferum seed coat), Muqil (Commiphora mukul gum), Affiyun (Papaver somniferum), Khabsul Hadeed (Ferroso-Ferric Oxide Calx), Tukhme Anjbar (Polygonum Bistorta - seeds), Tukhme Bartang (Plantago major - seed), compounds formulations of Iron, etc.

Haliq/Hallaq حالق **(depilatory drug):** A drug that removes hair by stimulating and irritating nerve endings, for example, Safeda (Plumbi carbonas), Hartal (Arsenic trisulphide), Raakh (Ash), and Choona (Calcium hydroxide - Quick lime).

Hazim/Hadim هاضم **(Digestive):** These drugs aid digestion by either toning up the stomach or the intestine. Examples include lemon, Jawakhar (potassium carbonate), ginger, black salt, cardamom, Suhaga (borax), chicken gizzards, cinnamon, Javitry (Myristica fragrance fruit coat), Zeera Siyah (Carum carvi seed), Zeera Safed (Cuminum cyminum seed), Ajwain (Carum capticum, Trachyspermum ammi seed), Barberry (Zarishk), black pepper, radish, mint, and all gastric tonics (Muqawwi-i-Mida).

Jali جالی **(Detergent):** These drugs help clear the body's pores of sticky fluids, like Abhal (Juniperus communis fruit), Babchi (Psoralea corylifolia Linn seed), Beladur (Semicarpus anacardium fruit), Boora armani, (Arminium bole), Kharbaq (Helleborus niger root), Shora qalmi (Potassium nitrate), Aqarqarha (Anacyclus pyrethrum), Asl (Honey), Nagermoth (Cyperus scariosus root), Kalonji (Nigella sativa seed), and Phitkri (Alum).

Jazib جاذب **(Absorbent/Siccative/Desiccant):** Drugs that have a hot and volatile nature which enables them to move secretions and humours in the body, thus helping to eliminate them. These drugs can cause dryness and some examples of such drugs are Jundbedster (Caster beaver secretion), Ghareeqoon (Polyporus officinalis), Lehsun (Allium Sativum - garlic), Behroza (Pinus longifolia Roxb.), and Rai (Bressica alba, B. nigra seed).

Kasir Riyah کسر ریاح **(Carminative):** Drugs that promote digestion in the stomach and expel gases. They are characterised as hot, dry, and slightly acidic. Here are some common examples: Hing (Ferula asafoetida), Pudina (Mentha arvensis herb), Zanjabeel (Zingiber officinalis rhizome), Namak Siyah (black salt), Muqil (Commiphora Mukul, gum), Suhaga (Borax), Sat Podina, Menthol (Mentha arvensis extract), Kalonji (Nigella sativa seed), Darchini (Cinnamomum zylenicum bark), Baboona (Matricaria chamomile flower), Filfil Siyah (Piper nigrum fruit), Aslussoos (Glycerrhiza glabra root), Khulanjan (Alpinia galanga root), Karafs (Apium graveolence seed), Badiyan (Foeniculum vulgare seed), Ilaichi (Elletaria cardamomum fruit), Lavender (Lavandula stoechas), Zeera (Cuminum cyminum seed), and Mur (Commiphora myrrha gum).

Kawi/Kavi کاوی **(Escharotic agent/Corrosive/Caustic):** These are drugs or substances that destroy or burn the surface of tissues due to their irritating and drying properties. They are primarily used to seal open wounds and fistulas. Examples include: Tezab Gandhak, Mehlool (sulphuric acid), Tezab Namak (Hydrochloric acid), Choona (Lime), Tezab Shora (Nitric acid), Phitkri (Alum), Heera Kasees (Ferrous sulphate), and Tootia (Copper sulphate).

Khatim خاتم **(Cicatrizant):** these drugs are known for their dry nature which aids in drying up wounds and their secretions. This eventually leads to the formation of a scab over the wound. As the wound heals, the scab falls off, leaving new skin. Some examples of Khatim drugs include Tootia (Copper sulphate), Sadaf sokhta (Ostrea edulis), Elva (Aloe vera dried juice of leaf), and Anzarot (Astragalus sarcocolla gum).

Laaze/Ladhi لاذع **(Irritant):** Drugs that can cause a burning sensation or irritation. They increase blood circulation and may also induce pain. These are all Hakkak (Irritant) drugs and are has been described under them. All Muhammirat (Rubefacients), Mubassirat (Eruptives) and Munaffitat (Vesicants) are irritants.

Man-i-Araq/Qati-i-Araq قاطع عرق/منع عرق **(reducing perspiration/sweating):** These refer to processes or drugs that reduce excessive sweating by affecting the sweat glands, nerves, or by sealing body pores. Some examples are: Yabruj (Atropa belladonna root),

Azraqi/Kuchla Mudabbar (Strychnos nux-vomica), Sheelam (Claviceps purpurea - Ergot fungus), Ghareeqoon (Polyporus officinalis), Datura (Datura metel, seed), and ice.

Mani-i-Nawbat مانع نوبت **(Antiperiodic):** A drug that prevents the recurrence of the episode of fever by blocking the action of the diseased substance. Examples are Atees (Aconitum heterophyllum root), Phitkri (alum), Barg-e-Tulsi (Ocimum sanctum Linn leaf), Chirata (Swertia chiratta herb), Dar Hald (Berberis aristata bark), Samm-ul-far (arsenic), and Karanjwa seeds (Caesalpinia bonducella).

Muaddil معدّل **(Alterative):** These drugs normalize body humours when faced with qualitative or quantitative changes. They can function as blood purifiers (Musaffi-i-Dam) or concoctives (Munzijat).

Muarriq معرّق **(Diaphoretic):** Drugs that induce perspiration. Examples include Tea, Shora qalmi (Potassium nitrate), Khaksi (Sisymbrium irio seed), Garlic, Raddish, Beesh (Aconitum nepallus root), Aqarqarha (Anacyclus pyrethrum), Kafoor (Cinnamomum camphora - camphor), and Tukhme Karafs (Apium graveolens seed).

Muattis معطس **(Errhine):** Drugs that induce sneezing by irritating the nasal passage, diverting matter towards the nose for excretion. Examples include Nakchikni (Dregea Volubilis - Sneeze wort), Tobacco, Berg Shabit (Anethum sowa – dill leaf), and Jund Bedastar (Castorium).

Mubakhkhir مبخّر **(Flatulent):** The drug that produces abnormal gases and substances in the intestine by disturbing the digestion, which disrupts the temperament of the body and results in a slight temperature rise, such as Shallots (Allium ascalonicum seed) and Onions (Scilla indica bulb).

Mubarrid مبرّد **(Refrigerant):** Drug which reduces body temperature and cools the body. This category includes Qabiz/Qabid-i-'Uruq (vasoconstrictor), Habis Dam (Haemostyptic), and Mukhaddir (anaesthetic).

Mubassir/Mubaththir مبثّر **(Eruptive):** Drugs that produce eruptions on the skin due to their heat and excessive irritation. Examples are Onion, Zarareeh (Canthradin), Roghan Jamalgota (Croton tiglium oil), Azraqi/Kuchla Mudabbar (Strychnos nux-vomica), Garlic (Allium Sativum), and cloves (Caryophyllus aromaticum bud).

Mudir-i-Bawl/bol مدرّ بول **(Diuretic):** These drugs increase kidney activity by irritation or filtration (mechanism discussed earlier). Example: Tukhme Kharpaza (Cucumis melo seed), Tukhme Khayaren (Cucumis sativa seed), Tukhme Kasni (Cichorium intybus seed), Persiyoshan/Hansraj (Adiantum capillus-veneris Linn), Badiyan (Foeniculum vulgare – fennel seed), Kharkhasak (Tribulus terrestris fruit), Tukhme Kasoos[421] (Cuscuta epithymum Linn, seeds), Tukhme Khurfa (Portulaca oleracea - purslane seeds), Anisoon

---

[421] Also known as Aftimoon hindi which are the seeds from the pods of Aftimoon.

(Pimpinella anisum seed), Ispand (Peganum harmela seed), Tukhme Kaddu (Pumpkin seed), and black tea.

Mudirr-i-Hayd/Haiz مدرّ حيض **(Emmenagogue):** Drugs that can induce or increase menstrual bleeding. For more information on their mechanisms of action, refer to earlier text. For example, Abhal (Juniperus communis fruit), Ispand (Peganum harmela seed), Habbe Balsan (Commiphora opobalsamum, seed), Rewand Chini (Chinese Rhubard - Rheum emodi), Akleelul Mulk (Trigonella uncata), Tukhme Kasoos (Cuscuta epithymum Linn, seeds), Kharkhasak (Tribulus terrestris fruit), Persiyoshan/Hansraj (Adiantum capillus-veneris Linn), Jadwar (Delphinium denudatum root), Aqarqarha (Anacyclus pyrethrum), Ghareequn (Polyporus officinalis), Karafs (Apium graveolence seed), Hab-ul-Qilt (Dolichos biflorus Linn, seed), Gul-e-Tesu (Butea monosperma – flower), Mia Saila/Silaaras (liquidambar orientalis - Storax), Elva (Aloe vera dried leaf juice), and Dar Chini (Cinnamomum zeylanicum bark).

Mudirr-i-Luab Dehen مدرّ لعاب دہن **(Sialagogue):** Drugs that can help increase saliva production by stimulating the salivary glands. Some examples include Rewand (Rheum officinale), Aqarqarha (Anacyclus pyrethrum), Sonth (Zingiber officinale – dried ginger), Tamarhindi (Tamarindus indica fruit), lemon, vinegar and all sour foods and herbs.

Mudammil مُدَمِّل **(Cicatrizant/vulnerary agent):** These refer to types of drugs that aid in the healing process of wounds and scars. These drugs possess drying properties that promote wound healing. Examples of these drugs include Dam-al-akhwayn (Dracaena cinnabari - Socotra dragon tree), Sange Jarahat (Magnesium silicate), Behroza (Pinus longifolia Roxb.), Raal (Shorea robusta – Yellow resin, Kameela (Mallotus philippinensis) Gile multani (Silicate of aluminia, magnesia oxides of iron), and Aab Barge Bartang (juice from the leaves of Plantago major).

Mufattit-i-hasat مفتّت حصات **(Lithotriptic):** Drugs that break down kidney and bladder calculi. Examples are Hajrul yahood (Lapis judaicus), Shora qalmi (Potassium nitrate), Aqrab Sokhta[422] (Burnt and processed Scorpion), Hab-ul-Qilt (Dolichos biflorus Linn seed), Jawakhar (Potassium Carbonate/potash), and Mudirat-i-Bawl (diuretics).

Mufattih مفتّح **(Deobstruent):** Drugs that clear blockages from luminal[423] organs and dilate vessels. They either dilate the vessels (Mufattih-i-'Uruq[424]) or dissolve viscous substances (Ghaleez Mavaad) making them thin and liquid, using a Jali (detergent) and resolvent (Muhallil). Examples include Lavender (Lavandula stoechas), Afsanteen (Artemisia absynthium), Anisoon (Pimpinella anisum seed - aniseed), and others.

Moreover, Laaze (Irritant), Muhammir (Rubefacient), Muhallile (Resolvant), Kawi (caustic), and Mubassir (eruptive) also classify as Mufattihat (Deobstruents). Some

---

[422] The process by which drugs are burnt to the charring stage but not reduced to ash. Drugs which undergo this process are suffixed with the term Muharraq or Sokhta'. For example, Crab - Sartan Muharraq and Scorpion - Aqrab Sokhta.
[423] the inside space of a tubular structure, such as an artery or intestine.
[424] مفتّح عروق

Mudirat-i-Bawl (diuretics) and Muarriqat (diaphoretics) also share this deobstruent function.

Mufattih-i-Thuqba Inabiyya مفتّح ثقبه عنبيه **(Mydriatic drug):** Drugs that dilate the pupils of the eyes include Safeda (Plumbi carbonas), Jungle piyaz (Urginea scilla - Sea Onion), Heera Kasees (Ferrous sulphate) and Suhaga/Tinker (borax).

Mufarrih مفرّح **(Mood elevator):** Drugs that can act as exhilarants and mood elevators. These drugs can help relieve symptoms like tachycardia, palpitations, and thirst. They are considered to have a cooling effect. Some examples of these drugs include Cardamom, Abresham (which comes from the silk-cotton tree), Badranjboya (made from the leaves of Catnip), Balangu (which comes from the seeds of Lallemantia royleana), Javitry (which is made from the fruit coat of Myristica fragrance), Gule Gurhal (Hibiscus rosa sinensis, flower), Gul Gaozaban (Borago officinalis, flower), Gule surkh (Rosa damascena flower), Lemon, Pomegranate, Sandal safed (Santalum album wood), Arq Gulab (Rosa damascena aqua), Kewra (Pandanus odoratisimus) and Arq e Bedmusk (distillate of flowers of salix caprea).

Mughazzi/Mughadhdhi مغذّى **(Nutritive):** Drugs that provide nutrition to nourish the body. Examples are Almonds, pumpkin seed, figs, honey, raisins, Nishasta (starch), Ghee, Butter, and eggs.

Mughalliz-i-Mani مغلظ منى **(Semen inspissant/thicker):** Agents that increase semen viscosity due to their astringent nature. This category includes Singhara (Trapa Bispinosa - Water Chestnut), Shaqaqul Misri (Pastinaca secacul Linn – Wild Parsnip), Safed musli (Chlorophytum arundinaceum, root), Musli Siyah (Curculigo orchioides, root), Satawar (Asparagus racemosus root), and others.

Muharrik-i-A'ṣab محرّك اعصاب **(Nervine stimulant):** Drug that stimulates nerves. Examples are Azraqi/Kuchla Mudabbar (Strychnos nux-vomica), Yabruj (Atropa belladonna root), Naushader (Ammonium chloride), Sheelam (Claviceps purpurea - Ergot fungus), Musk (Moschus moschiferus), Sumbul-ut-teeb (Valeriana Officinalis Linn.), Bhang (Cannabis sativa leaf), Sammulfar (Purified Arsenic trioxide), Zarareeh (Canthradin), Coffee, and Heeng (Ferula foetida latex).

Muharrik-i-Dimagh محرّك دماغ **(Brain Stimulant):** Drug that enhances brain functions by stimulating it. Examples are tea, alcohol, and cannabis.

Muharrik-i-Dawran-i-Khun محرّك دوران خون **(Circulatory Stimulant):** A drug that stimulates blood circulation through various mechanisms. Examples are Alcohol, Azraqi/Kuchla Mudabbar (Strychnos nux-vomica), Kafoor (Cinnamomum camphora - camphor), Tea, and Sumbul-ut-teeb (Valeriana officinalis Linn.).

Muhammir محمّر **(Rubefacient):** Local application of certain drugs can cause capillary dilatation and increased blood circulation, resulting in skin redness. Examples include, Zarareeh (Canthradin), Roghan Behroza (Pinus longifolia oil), Roghan Jamalgota

(Croton tiglium oil), Roghan Suddab (Ruta graveolens oil), Rai (Bressica alba seed), Lemon oil, Yabruj (Atropa belladonna root), Rai (Bressica alba seed), Garlic and cloves (Caryophyllus aromaticum bud).

Mujaffif مجفّف **(Siccative/drying):** A dryness-producing drug that causes dryness by decreasing exudation resulting from constrictions of local blood vessels, thus aiding in wound healing. Examples are Habbul Aas (Myrtus communis fruit), Persiaoshan (Adiantum capillus herb), Qust (Sassuria lappa root), Mako (Solanum nigrum fruit), Post Anar (Punica granatum epicarp of fruit), Sadaf sokhta (Ostrea edulis), Gile Armani (Arminium bole), Marjan (Corallium rubrum), Sange Jarahat (magnesium silicate), Tootia (Copper sulphate), Berg hina (Lawsonia alba leaf), Ushq (Dorcus ammonicum gum), Tabasheer (Bambusa arundinasia), Habbe balsan (Commiphora opobalsamum, fruit), and Sumbul-ut-teeb (Valeriana Officinalis Linn.).

Mujammid مجمّد **(Coagulant/Condensing agent):** An agent that induces or aids coagulation; drugs with cold and astringent properties affect humours and constituents of blood or other liquids. Examples include Phitkri (Alum), Geru (Red Ochre Powder - Alumina silicate and iron oxide), Sange Jarahat (magnesium silicate), Samagh Arabi (Acacia arabica gum), Kateera (Astragallus gummifera gum), Kaharba (Amber Sucomum), Sadaf sokhta (Ostrea edulis), Ajwain Khurasani (Hyoscyamus niger), Marvareed (Pearl), and ice.

Mukhaddir مخدر **(Narcotic/Anaesthetic):** These drugs affect the sensory nerve and reduce sensation by causing loss of sensation in an organ. They can act as both local and general anaesthetics. Examples of such drugs include Beesh (Aconitum nepallus root), Post Khashkhash (Papaver somniferum seed coat), Bhang (Cannabis sativa leaf), Yabruj (Atropa belladonna root), Roghan Qaranfal (Caryophyllus aromaticum – clove oil), and Tukhme Kahu (Lactuca sativa Linn seed).

Mukhrij-i-Janin wa Mashima مُخرج جنين و مشيمه **(Abortifacient):** These drugs induce uterine contractions, leading to fetal or placental expulsion, and can also act as emmenagogues. Examples include Post Amaltas (Cassia fistula fruit epicarp), Abhal (Juniperus communis fruit), Zaravand (Aristolochia longa, A. rotunda root), Persiaoshan (Adiantum capillus herb), Sarakhs (Dryopteris filix-mas), Jund Bedastar (Castorium), Hanzal (Citrullus colocynthis fruit). And all strong purgatives, diuretics and emmenagogues.

Mukhrij-i-Didan-i-Am'a مُخرج ديدان امعاء **(Vermifuge):** the drugs that expel intestinal worms without killing them include Roghan Bedanjir (Ricinus communis, oil), Saqmoonia (Convolvulus scamony root latex), Kameela (Mallotus philippinensis), Palas Papra (Butea frondosa seed), Rasaut (Berberis aristata extract), and Beikh Jalapa (Exogonium purga, Ipomoea purga root).

Mukhashshin مُخشّن **(Roughening agent):** Some drugs are known as roughening agents because they cause inflammation and accumulation of fluids on the skin surface. This effect can be achieved through the use of certain substances such as Rai (Brassica alba seed) and Beladur (Semicarpus anacardium), or by using drugs with astringent properties such as Escharotics (Kawi) and Rubefacients (Muhammir).

Mulayyin-i-Waram ملیّن ورم **(Resolvant):** Drugs that resolve inflammation and reduce swelling. Examples include Beikh Kasni (Cichorium intybus root), Afsanteen (Artemisia absynthium), Tukhme Katan/Alsi (Linum usitatissimum seed), Barge mako (Solanum nigrum, leaf), Tulsi (Ocimum sanctum Linn), Dar Hald (Berberis aristata bark), Aanba Haldi (Curcuma amada root), Jaosheer (Ferula galbaniflua secretion), Darmana (Artemisia maritima herb), Izkhir (Cymbopogon schoenanthus), Jadwar (Delphinium denudatum root), Dooqu (Pencedanum grande seed), Asarun (Valeriana wallichii root), and Berg Aak (Calotropis procera leaf).

Mulattif ملــطّــف **(Attenuant):** Drugs that disintegrate morbid material into smaller particles, thin out viscous substances, and liquefy Akhlat (humours) through their mild heat. Examples include Suddab (Ruta graveolens), Abresham (Bombax mori), Chamomile (Babuna - Matricaria chamomilla), Beikh Kasni (Cichorium intybus root), Jadwar (Delphinium denudatum root), Ood saleeb (Paeonia officinalis root), Biranjasif (Achillea millefolium - Yarrow), Kabab Chini (Piper cubeba), Satar Farsi (Zataria multiflora), Inab-us-Salab (Solanum nigrum), Zaravand (Aristolochia longa, A. rotunda root), Persiyoshan/Hansraj (Adiantum capillus-veneris Linn), Ghaafis (Agrimonia eupatoria), Zufa (Hyssopus officinalis, flower), Izkhir (Cymbopogon schoenanthus), Kasoos (Cuscuta epithymum Linn, seeds), Tea, and Vinegar.

Mulayyin-i-Ama ملیّن امعاء **(Laxative):** Drugs that mildly increase peristaltic movements of the intestines or make them slippery, or dilute the stool so that it can be excreted more easily. Examples are dried plums, Psyllium husk (Aspaghol), Roghan Alsi (Linum usitatissimum seed oil), Figs, Tamar Hindi (Tamarindus indica fruit pulp), Almond oil, Raisins (Maveez), and Hing (Ferula asafoetida).

Mulayyin-i-Waram ملیّن ورم **(Swelling-softening drug):** These drugs relieve congestion, dilute, and increase the absorption of inflammatory swelling. Examples are Tukhme Khatmi (Althea officinalis seed), Ajwain Khurasani (Hyoscyamus niger), Chamomile (Babuna - Matricaria chamomilla), Tukhme Katan (Linum usitatissimum – Flaxseed), Akleelul Mulk (Trigonella uncata), Muqil (Commiphora Mukul, gum), and Mur (Myrrh - Commiphora myrrha).

Murkhi مــرخــی **(Laxity-producing drug):** When applied externally, laxity-producing drugs soften skin by loosening it. Examples include flaxseed oil (Tukhme Katan/Alsi), almond oil, beeswax, olive oil, and fats.

Mumallis ممّلس **(Emollient):** Greasing drugs that lubricate when applied to the skin surface or mucus membrane. For example, Behi dana (Quince seed - Cydonia oblonga Miller), Sapistan (Cordia latifolia fruit), Tukhme Katan/Alsi (Linum usitatissimum seed), Samagh Arabi (Acacia arabica gum), Kateera (Astragalus gummifer gum), Tukhame Rehan (Ocimum sanctum – Basil seeds), Bel Giri (Bael Fruit - Aegle marmelos), Psyllium husk, Almond oil, and Rose oil.

Mumsik-i-Mani ممسک منی **(Semen retentive agent):** Drugs that delay ejaculation. They are dry in nature and prolong the period of intercourse. Examples are, Aqarqarha (Anacyclus pyrethrum), Clove (Caryophyllus aromaticum bud), Behi dana (Quince seed - Cydonia oblonga Miller), Tukhme Imli (Tamarindus indica, seeds), Affiyun (Papaver Somniferum), Kuchla (Strychnos nux-vomica) and Cannabis sativa leaf.

Munzijat/Mundijat منضجات **(Concoctives):** Drugs which modify and prepare morbid humours for evacuation from the body.

Mundij-i-Balgham منضج بلغم **(Phlegm concoctive):** Drugs which modify and prepare phlegm for evacuation from the body. Examples are Gul Gaozaban (Borago officinalis, flower), Tukhme Katan (Linum usitatissimum seed), Beikh Kasni (Cichorium intybus root), Persiaoshan (Adiantum venustum herb), Tukhme Khatmi (Althea officinalis seed), Aslussoos (Glycerrhiza glabra root), Biranjasif (Achillea millefolium - Yarrow), Tukhme Khubazi (Malva sylvestris, seeds), Shukai (Onopordum acanthium), Figs, and Raisins.

Mundij-i-Safra منضج صفراء **(Yellow Bile concoctive):** Drug which modifies and prepares yellow bile for evacuation from the body. Examples are Gul Banafsha (Viola odorata, flower), Beikh Kasni (Cichorium intybus root), Tukhme Kasni (Cichorium intybus, seed), Unnab (Zizyphus sativa fruit), Tukhme Kahu (Lactuca sativa Linn, seed), Pumpkin seed, Tukhme Khurfa (Portulaca oleracea - purslane seeds), dried plums, Imli (Tamarindus indica), Taranjabeen (Alhagi pseudalhagi), Sharbat Nilofar (Nymphaea lotus, syrup), Sharbat Banafsha (Viola odorata, syrup), Tabasheer (Bambusa arundinasia), Sikanjbin (Oxymel), Gulqand (flower conserve), and Watermelon water.

Mundij-i-Sawda منضج سوداء **(Black bile concoctive):** Drug which modifies and prepares black bile for evacuation from the body. Examples are Lavender, figs, fennel, Beikh Kasni (Cichorium intybus root), Persiaoshan (Adiantum capillus herb), Tukhme Khubazi (Malva sylvestris, seeds), Tukhme Khatmi (Althea officinalis seed), Sapistan (Cordia latifolia fruit), and Sumbul-ut-teeb (Valeriana officinalis Linn.).

Munaffith-i-Balgham منفّث بلغم **(Expectorant):** Drugs which facilitate expectoration. Examples are Baqla (Vicia faba), Khatmi (Althea officinalis), Aslussoos (Glycerrhiza glabra root), Aroosa (Adhatoda vasica), Zufa (Hyssopus officinalis), Katan (Linum usitatissimum – Flaxseed), Sapistan (Cordia latifolia fruit), Abresham (Bombax mori), Unnab (Zizyphus sativa fruit), honey, Kuchla (Strychnos nux-vomica), Gaozaban (Borago officinalis), and Gau danti (gypsum).

Munaffit منفّط **(Vesicant):** Drugs which produce blisters on the surface of the skin when applied locally. Examples are Beladur (Semicarpus anacardium), Sheer Mudar/Aak (Calotropis procera, latex) and Zarareeh (Canthradin).

Munawwim منوّم **(Hypnotic agent):** Drugs which induce sleep. They either act on the brain as a sedative or analgesic. Examples are Afiun (Papaver somniferum seeds, Kahu

(Lactuca sativa Linn), latex, seed, seed coat), Post khashkhash (Papaver somniferum seed coat), Chob Chini (Smilax china root), and Kasoos (Cuscuta reflexa seed).

Muqawwiyat-i-Asnan-o-Lissah مقویات اسنان و لثه **(Teeth and gum strengthening drugs):** Drugs that are used for toning and binding gums while also strengthening teeth. These drugs have different properties, including astringents, irritants, and antiseptics. For instance, Phitkari (Alum), Kabab Chini (Piper cubeba), Filfil Siyah (Piper nigrum fruit), Tootia Biryan (Copper sulphate), Gulnar (Punica granatum - flower), cardamom seeds, Qaranfal (Syzygium aromaticum bud), and Kafe Dariya (Sepia officinalis - cuttlefish bone) are some examples of such drugs.

Muqawwi-i-Aaza Raisa مقوّی اعضاء رئیسه **(Tonic for vital organs):** Drugs which strengthen vital organs of the body for their optimal functions. They act on the brain, heart and liver. Generally, they act on a particular organ, but mostly, all vital organs are also improved. For example, Amla (Emblica officinalis fruits), Jadwar (Delphinium denudatum root), Saffron (Zafran - Crocus sativa stigma), Musk (Moschus moschiferus), Marvareed (Pearl), Post Turanj (Citrus modica fruit epicarp), Gul surkh (Rosa damascena flower), Zahar mohra (Serpentine) and Gau danti (gypsum[425]).

Muqawwi-i-Bah مقوّی باہ **(Aphrodisiac):** Drugs used for toning up sexual organs; strengthens sexual organs and improves their function. They act in many ways, such as stimulating nerves, increasing semen viscosity, or normalising increased sensation. Examples are Dried dates (Khurma), Tudari (Cheiranthus cheiri Linn.), Behman (Centaurea behen root), Sataver (Asparagus racemosus root), Sadaf (Ostrea edulis), Pistachio, Pine nuts (Chilghoza), Shilajit (Bitumen Mineral), Saffron (Zafran), Carrots, Mango, Onion, Amber (Amberis grasea), Pineapple, Behi (Pyrus cydonia, Cydonia quincy fruit), Chickpea (Cicer arietinum seed) and Hen eggs.

Muqawwi-i-Basar مقوّی بصر **(Eye tonic):** Drugs used for toning up and improving eyesight. For example, Badiyan (Foeniculum vulgare seed - fennel), Sang-e-Basri[426] (zinc carbonate), Sang-e-Surma[427] (Antimony Sulphide - Surma Stone), Haleela (Terminelia chebula fruit), Amla (Phyllanthus emblica) and Mameera (Coptis teeta, root).

Muqawwi-i-Kabid/Muqawwi-i-Jigar مقوّی کبد / مقوّی جگر **(Hepatotonic/Liver tonic):** Hepatotonic drugs improve liver function by toning up liver cells. Examples include Afsanteen (Artemisia absinthium), Sangdana[428] (Chicken gizzards), Kasni (Cichorium intybus), Kasoos (Cuscuta epithymum Linn, seeds), Bartang (Bartang (Plantago major - seed), Mastagi (Pistacia lantiscus gum), Elva (Aloe vera dried juice of leaf), Zarishk (Berberis vulgaris - barberry), Rosa damascene flowers, Haleela (Terminelia chebula fruit), Dar Chini (Cinnamomum cassia bark), Rewand Chini (Chinese Rhubard - Rheum emodi), Gul Ghaafis (Agrimonia eupatoria, flower), Nagkesar (Mesua ferrea), Naushader

---

[425] Plaster of Paris.
[426] is also known as Hajar al Kohl because of its stone-like appearance and its use in eye ailments.
[427] also known as Kohl.
[428] sang = stone and dana = grain.

(Ammonium chloride), Behi (Pyrus cydonia, Cydonia quincy fruit), Saffron (Zafran - Crocus sativa stigma), Mint, Apple, Raisins, Formulations like Kushta Faulad[429], and Habbe Khabsul Hadeed[430].

Muqawwi-i-Dam/ Muqawwi-i-Khoon مقوّی دام/ مقوّی خون **(Blood tonic):** Drugs that increase haemoglobin content and stabilise other cells in the blood. Examples are Habbe Khabsul Hadeed, Kushta Faulad, fish liver oil, Raisins, Sweet pomegranate, Sour pomegranate, and Sharbat Faulad (Iron, syrup).

Muqawwi-i-Dimagh مقوّی دماغ **(Brain tonic):** Drugs used for improving the brain's faculties. For example, Amla (Emblica officinalis fruits), Lavender, Haleela Siyah (Terminelia chebula unripe fruit), Marvareed (Pearl), Chamomile (Babuna - Matricaria chamomilla), Tukhme Khashkhash (Papaver somniferum seed), Gaozaban (Borago officinalis), Brahmi (Hydrocotyle asiatica), Kabab-e-Khanda (Zanthoxylum rhetsa), Ginger, Almonds, and Pumpkin seed.

Muqawwi-i-Tihal مقوّی طحال **(Spleen Tonic):** Drugs that strengthen the spleen. For example, Kushta Faulad (Iron Calx), Barg Jhao (Tamarix dioica, leaf), and Farash (Tamarix gallica).

Muqawwi-i-Qalb مقوّی قلب **(Heart tonic):** Drugs used for toning up the heart, improving its functions. For example, Abresham (Bombax mori), Amla (Emblica officinalis), Badranjboya (Duperalis- Nepeta cataria), Jadwar (Delphinium denudatum root), Apple, Guava, Pineapple, Pomegranate, Gule Surkh (Rosa damascena flower), Gule Gurhal (Hibiscus rosa sinensis, flower), Musk (Moschus moschiferus), Amber (Amberis grasea secretion), Saffron, Sumbul-ut-teeb (Valeriana officinalis Linn.), Zahar mohra (Serpentine), Cardamon, Tukhame Rehan (Ocimum sanctum – Basil seeds), and Yaqoot (Ruby).

Muqawwi-i-Mida wa Ama مقوّی معده و امعاء **(Gastric and intestine tonic):** These drugs strengthen the stomach and intestines by enhancing digestion. Additionally, they bolster liver function in various ways. Examples include: Amla (Emblica officinalis), Bael Fruit (Bel Giri - Aegle marmelos), Barberry (Zarishk - Berberis vulgaris), Black Pepper, Black Salt, Cardamon, Chicken Gizzard, Cloves (Syzygium aromaticum), Fennel, Ginger, Jaiphal (Myristica fragrans), Javitry (Fruit coat of Myristica fragrans), Lemon and Lemon Peel, Mastagi (Pistacia Lentiscus gum), Mint, Papaya (Papeeta - fruit), Suhaga (borax), Sumac (Rhus coriaria), Taj Qalmi (Cinnamomum cassia bark), Kuchla Mudabbar (Strychnos nux-vomica), and Gul surkh (Rosa damascena flowers).

Muqi مقی **(Emetic):** Drugs that induce vomiting by stimulating the emetic centre. They are considered optimal for the excretion of balghami (phlegmatic) and safravi (yellow bile) wastes, particularly from the liver and stomach, and they also mobilize the humours

---

[429] Unani formulation Iron tablets.
[430] Unani formulation containing Ferroso-Ferric Oxide Calx.

in distant viscera. Examples include warm water, spinach water, liquorice, and radish seeds.

Musakkin-i-Alam/Musakkin al-Waja مسكّن الم / مسكّن الوجع (**Analgesic**): These drugs alleviate pain and can be applied externally or taken internally. They work by affecting the nerves and reducing their ability to transmit pain signals. Some examples of analgesics include Tukhme Kahu (Lactuca sativa Linn seed), Post Khashkhash (Papaver somniferum seed coat), Ajwain Khurasani (Hyoscyamus niger), Flax seed oil (Tukhme Katan/Alsi), Suranjan (Colchicum luteum root), Anisoon (Pimpinella anisum seed), Affiyun (Papaver somniferum), Qaranfal (Caryophyllus aromaticum bud), Bhang (Cannabis sativa leaf), and Qust (Sassuria lappa root).

Musakkin Aasab wa Dimagh مسكّن اعصاب و دماغ (**Brain and nerve relaxant**): These drugs are known to have a relaxing effect on the brain and nerves, helping to alleviate irritability and hyperactivity. Some examples of such drugs are Asrol (Rauwolfia serpentina root), Post Khashkhash (Papaver somniferum seed coat), Affiyun (Papaver Somniferum), and Yabruj (Atropa belladonna root). Additionally, anaesthetics (Mukhaddirat) and sedatives (Musakkinat) can also be used for the same purpose.

Musakkin-i-Tanaffus مسكّن تنفس (**Broncho-relaxant**): Drugs that alleviate respiratory irritation. They have a sedative effect on the respiratory centre, reducing coughing and other spasmodic conditions. Examples of such drugs include Tukhme Kahu (Lactuca sativa Linn seed), Post Khashkhash (Papaver somniferum seed coat), Affiyun (Papaver Somniferum), along with standard Unani formulations like Kushta Qarnulail[431] and Kushta Abrak.

Musakkin-i-Hararat مسكّن حرارت (**Febrifuge**): A febrifuge is a drug that helps to lower abnormal body heat and cool the body. Some examples of febrifuges include cold water, Aab Anar Tursh (sour pomegranate juice), Aab Berge-kasni sabz (juice of Cichorium intybus leaves), Aab Berg-e-Khurfa sabz (juice of Portulaca oleracea leaves), Aab Turanj (juice of Citrus medica), Aab Zulal Tamar Hindi (water infused with Tamarindus indica fruits), Aab Zulal Aaloobukhara (water infused with Prunus domestica fruits), Aab Kashneez sabz (juice of Coriandrum sativum leaves), Aab Leemun (juice of Citrus lemonum), Sheera Tukhme Kahu (ground Lactuca sativa seeds with water), Sirka (Acetic acid), Arq Gulab (Rose water), and more.

Musakkin-i-Qalb مسكّن قلب (**Heart-calming agent**): Heart-calming agents are a type of medication that help reduce cardiac activity and relieve palpitations. These agents include Yaqoot Mehlool (powdered and purified Ruby), Musk (secreted by Moschus moschiferus), Saffron (also known as Zafran and derived from the stigma of Crocus sativa), Crocus sativa (saffron), and the formulation Kushta Tila[432].

---

[431] Contains powdered and prepared Stags Horn.
[432] Contains gold.

Musakhkhin مسخّن **(Calorific drug)** : These are drugs that produce heat within the body. They are used to balance the humors (akhlat) or to treat cold temperaments. Examples include tea, coffee, honey, pepper, Azraqi/Kuchla Mudabbar (Strychnos nux-vomica), Musk (Moschus moschiferus), amber, and alcohol.

Musaffi-i-Dam مصفّي دم **(Blood purifier):** Drugs that remove toxins from blood through urine, stool, and sweat. Mechanism of action previously described. Examples include are Unnab (Zizyphus sativa fruit), Mundi (Sphaeranthus indicus Linn), Nigand Babri (Vitex negundo Linn), Brahmadandi (Tricholepis glaberrima), Sarphuka (Tephrosia purpurea), Neel kanthi (Ajuga bracteosa), Gul Neem (Azadirachta Indica - flowers), Sandal safed (Santalum album wood), Sandal surkh (Pterocarpus santalinus wood), Haleela Siyah (Terminelia chebula unripe fruit), Ushba maghribi (Sarsaparilla europaea herb), Babchi (Psoralea corylifolia seed), and Chhal Mogra (gynocardia odorata).

Musammin Baden مسمّن بدن **(Fattening):** These agents help in increasing the body weight by acting on different parts of the body to raise the Basal Metabolic Rate (BMR), such as dried dates, coconut, pine seeds, pistachio, all dry fruits, beetroot (Beta vulgaris), sesame seeds, Toodri (Lepidium iberis seed), Milk, and Behman (Centaurea behen root).

Mushil مسهل **(Purgative):** These drugs increase the frequency and consistency of stool. They act in several ways, either by squeezing or by increasing peristaltic movements. When specifically removing balgham, sawda, safra they are called Mushil-i-Balgham, Mushil-i-Sawda, Mushil-i-Safra respectively.

In terms of force of action, the following are its types:

- **Mulayyin** ملیّن **(laxatives/softeners):** Drugs which relieve constipation smoothly and act to loosen stool and prevent or treat constipation – these are weak purgatives. Examples include Shir khest (Cotoneaster nummularia), raisin, Muqil (Commiphora mukul gum), tamarind, dried plums, figs, Taranjabeen (Alhagi pseudalhagi), and olive oil.
- **Mamooli Mushilh** معمولی مسهل **(Basic or common purgative):** These drugs induce one or two loose stools. Examples include Ersa (Iris ensata root), Senna (Cassia senna leaf - Cassia angustifolia), Elva (Aloe vera dried leaf juice), Rewand (Rheum officinale), Kameela (Mallotus philippinensis), and Suranjan (Colchicum leutiun root).
- **Qawiyya Mushilh** قویه مسهل **(Strong purgative):** These drugs induce more frequent loose stools, and stools may be watery. Examples include Jamalgota (Croton tiglium fruit), Saqmoonia (Convolvulus scamony root latex), Habb al-Neel (Ipomea hederacea), Shehm Hanzal (Citrullus colocynthis fruit), Turbud (Ipomea turpenthum root), Kharbaq siah (Helleborus niger), Roghan Jamalgota (Croton tiglium fruit oil), and Rasaut (Berberis aristate extract).

Types of Mushilath (purgatives) according to Akhlat (humours):

- **Mushil-i-Balgham** مسهل بلغم **(purgative of phlegm – Phlegmagogue):** Drugs which cause evacuation of balgham (phlegm humour) through purgation. Examples include Senna (Cassia senna leaf - Cassia angustifolia), Suranjan (Colchicum luteum root), Turbud (Ipomea turpenthum root), Tukhme Al-Hanzal (Citrullus colocynthis seeds), Qust (Sassurea lappa root), Dhamasa/Shakai (Fagonia cretica), Ghareequn (Polyporus officinalis), and Muqil (Commiphora mukul gum).
- **Mushil-i-Sawda** مسهل سوداء **(purgative of black bile – Melanogogue):** Drugs which cause evacuation of sawda (black bile humour) through purgation. Examples include Jamalgota (Croton tiglium fruit), Shehm Hanzal (Citrullus colocynthis fruit), Aftimoon vilayati (Cuscuta reflexa), Turbud (Ipomoea turpenthum root), Haleela Siyah (Terminelia chebula unripe fruit), Kharbaq siah (Helleborus niger), and Penwaad (Cassia tora Linn).
- **Mushil-i-Safra** مسهل صفراء **(purgative of yellow bile – Cholagogue):** Drugs which cause evacuation of safra (yellow bile humour) through purgation. Examples include Senna (Cassia senna leaf - Cassia angustifolia), Elva (Aloe vera dried leaf juice), Taranjabeen (Alhagi pseudalhagi), Shir khest (Cotoneaster nummularia), and Shahatra (Fumaria parviflora Linn. herb),

Mushtahi/Mushahh مشتهی / مشهی **(Appetizer):** Drugs that promote appetite by increasing gastric secretions, such as lemon, cardamom, vinegar, fennel, and other carminative drugs.

Musleh مصلح **(Corrective):** These drugs counteract the toxic effects of other drugs, rendering them safe for consumption.

Muwallid-i-Khoon[433] مولّد خون **(Haematogenic/blood producing):** Drugs that improve the production of blood. They increase the red blood count in the blood. Examples are Kushta Faulad (Iron Calx), Khabsul Hadeed (Ferroso-Ferric Oxide Calx), Egg yolk, grapes, pomegranate, mango, and dried dates.

Muwallid-i-Laban مولّد لبن **(Galactopoietic):** These drugs can increase milk secretion or production by correcting nutrients and digestion. Examples are Satever (Asparagus racemosus root), Toodri (Lepidium iberis seed), Pambadana (Gossypium herbaceum seed), Kalonji (Nigella sativa seed), Zeera safed (Cyminum cuminum seed), Shaqaqul Misri (Pastinaca secacul Linn), and Milk.

Muwallid-i-Mani مولّد منی **(Spermatogenic):** Some drugs can help increase semen production by improving health and digestion. Some examples of these drugs include Satever (Asparagus racemosus root), Singhara (Trapa bispinosa or water chestnut), Khurfa (Portulaca oleracea or purslane), Asgand (Withania somnifera), and Behman (Centaurea behen). Additionally, certain foods such as walnut, chickpea, Tudari

---

[433] Khoon (خون) in Urdu is Dam (دم) blood in Arabic and is used interchangeably.

(Cheiranthus cheiri Linn.), hazelnut, pine nut, pistachio, half-boiled egg, sesame seeds, chicken meat, and other tonics can also help increase semen production.

Qabiz/Qabid قابض **(Astringent):** All the drugs described as Habis Dam (Haemostyptic), Radey (Repellent/Divert), Aasir (Squeezing), and Qabiz ama (Intestinal astringent) in this section have astringent properties. They cause the contraction of body tissues and lumen by constricting ducts and openings with their coldness and astringent power (quwwath-e-qabz).

Qabiz Ama قابض امعاء **(Intestinal astringent/constipation-inducing):** Some drugs can cause constipation (qabz) by reducing the secretion and peristaltic movement of the intestine. They can also constrict the blood vessels that supply the intestines. A few drugs can reduce irritation, soreness and hypersensitivity of the intestines by decreasing the secretions. Examples of such drugs include Kehruba (Vateria indica gum), Tabasheer (Bambusa arundinasia), Bel Giri (Bael Fruit - Aegle marmelos), Tukhme Anjbar, (Polygonum bistorta - seeds), Habbul Aas (Myrtus communis fruit), Zarishk (Berberis vulgaris - barberry), Mastagi (Pistacia lantiscus gum), Post Khashkhash (Papaver somniferum seed coat), Tukhame Rehan (Ocimum sanctum seeds), Kushta Faulad (Iron Calx), Khabsul Hadeed (Ferroso-Ferric Oxide Calx), Sange Jarahat (magnesium silicate), Zahar mohra (Serpentine), Geru (Red Ochre Powder - Alumina silicate and iron oxide), Phitkri (Alum), Mazoo (Quercus infectoria), Gile Makhtoom (Makhtoom clay), Post Turanj (Citrus medica – Citron peel), Sumac (Rhus coriaria), and Dudhi (Euphorbia hirta).

Qatil-e-Deedan Ama (Anthelmintic) قاتل ديدان امعاء: Drugs designed to target and eliminate intestinal worms.

These drugs act on different kinds of worms.

(A) Hayyat حيّات (Ancylostoma duodenale - hookworm): Darmana (Artemisia maritima herb), Beikh Bakayan (Melia azedarach - bark), Fufal/Supari (Areca catechu nut), and Bed Anjeer/ Eranda (Ricinus communis - fruit).

(B) Habbul qara حب القرع (Tape worm): Beikh Bakayan (Melia azedarach - bark), Post Toot Siah (Morus nigra bark), Arusa (Adhatoda vasica leaf), Kaknaj (Physalis alkekengi - fruit), Kameela (Mallotus philippinensis), Ushba maghrabi (Sarsaparilla europaea herb), Maghaz Narjeel Kohna (Cocos nucifera - fruit very old), Ajwain (Carum capticum seed), Baobarang (Embelia Ribes), and Post Beikh Anar (Punica granatum root bark).

(C) Dahkili/Sighar داخلی/صــغــار (Thread worm): Internal use: Darmana (Artemisia maritima herb), Fufal/Supari (Areca catechu nut), Mushktramsheey (Ziziphora feruior herb). As an enema: Roghan Tarpeen (Terpene oil), Roghan Bedanjeer (Castor oil), Rogan Zaitoon (Olive oil), Sirka (vinegar), Aab Namak (Salt water), Joshanda Mushk Taramsheya (Mentha Pulegium - Pennyroyal herb - decoction).

(D) Aam Qatil Deedan Ama عام قاتل ديدان امعاء (General anthelmintic): Hing (Ferula asafoetida), Chirata (Swertia chiratta herb), Kalonji (Nigella sativa seed), Zufa (Hyssopus officinalis, flower), Senna (Cassia senna leaf - Cassia angustifolia), Gilo (Tinospora indica herb), Bozidan (Pyrethrum indicum root), Berg Anjeer/Eranda (Ricinus communis leaf), Mur (Commiphora myrrh gum), Ispand (Peganum harmela seed), Babchi (Psoralea corylifolia seed), Kat (Acacia catechu), Rewand (Rheum officinale), and Zanjabeel (Zingiber officinalis rhizome).

Qashir قاشر (**Sloughing agent**): Drugs that assist in the separation of dead tissue from a healed wound. For example, Zaravand (Aristolochia longa, A. rotunda root), Kunjad Siyah (black sesame seeds - Sesamum indicum Linn), Qust (Sassuria lappa root), and Khulanjan (Alpinia galanga root).

Qati-i-Bah قاطع باه (**Anaphrodisiac**): Drugs designed to decrease or suppress sexual desire, typically by reducing vaso-congestion circulation in the genitalia and surrounding tissues. These medications often have anaesthetic (Mukhaddir) and bitter (Tursh) properties. Examples are Shokran (Conium maculatum seed), Yabruj (Atropa belladonna root), Kafoor (Cinnamomum camphora - camphor), Sandal (Santalum album wood), Tabasheer (Bambusa arundinasia), Kahu (Lactuca sativa Linn seed), Lemon, Datura (Datura metel, seed), Irsa (Iris ensata root), Aaloobukhara (Prunus domestica fruit), and Imli (Tamarindus indica fruit).

Radey رادع (**Repellent/Divert**): These drugs redirect matter from one part of the body to another. They are typically applied topically as liniments and have strong astringent properties (quwwath-e-qabiza) and cooling properties (quwwath-e-barida). This constricts the pores and reduces heat absorption (hararat-e-jaziba), which prevents further accumulation of disease-causing substances (madda-e-marz). Examples of such drugs include Kashneez (Coriandrum sativum seed) and Fufal/Supari (Areca catechu nut), Gile armani (Arminium bole), Gile multani (Silicate of aluminia, agnesia oxides of iron), Geru (Red Ochre Powder - Alumina silicate and iron oxide), Gule surkh (Rosa damascena flower), Safedi beza (Egg white yolk), Khatmi (Althea officinalis), Sandal safed (Santalum album wood), Sandal surkh (Pterocarpus santalinus wood), Zarishk (Berberis vulgaris - barberry), Aqaqia (Acacia arabica extract) Mako (Solanum nigrum fruit), Roghan gul (Rosa damascena oil), Rasaut (Berberis aristata extract), Sirka (Acetic acid), and Roghan Zetoon (Olea europia oil).

Sammi سمّى (**Toxic/Poisonous**): These are drugs known to cause harmful and toxic effects, which, in severe cases, can be lethal. Some examples include Sammulfar (Purified Arsenic trioxide) and Hartal (Arsenic trisulphide), Darchikna (compound of mercury and arsenic), Azraqi/Kuchla Mudabbar (Strychnos nux-vomica), Affiyun (Papaver somniferum), Sendur (Borax), Raskapur (Calomel), Zangar (Cupric sulphate), Datura (Datura metel, seed), Shingarf (Compound of Mercury and Sulphur), Beesh (Aconitum nepallus root), Jamalgota (Croton tiglium fruit), Yabruj (Atropa belladonna root), Saqmoonia (Convolvulus scamony root latex), Para (Hydrargyrum -Mercury), and Shokran (Conium meculator seed).

Note: The drugs mentioned above are meant for educational purposes only. Although most of these herbs are generally safe, and some are even used in cooking, a few, particularly those in the Sammi (Toxic) category, can be extremely hazardous. It is crucial to avoid using these herbs without the guidance and prescription of a licensed specialist in this specific domain. Therefore, we strongly recommend you consult your licensed physician or Unani practitioner before using any herb.

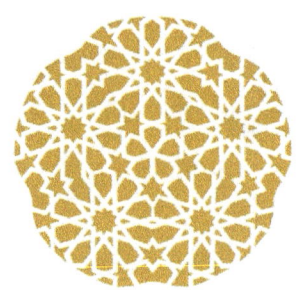

SECTION 5

PRINCIPLES OF TREATMENT

'There are no incurable diseases — only the lack of will. There are no worthless herbs — only the lack of knowledge.'

– Ibn Sina.

Methods Of Treatment

There are three types of general treatment: Regimental Therapy, Diet-o-Therapy, Pharmacotherapy and Surgical treatment.

Regimental therapy (Ilaj-bil Tadbeer) and Diet-o-Therapy (Ilaj-bil Ghiza)

Regimental therapy refers to the changes and modifications in the six essential factors (Asbab Sitta Daruriyya) that have been previously described, and in this section, we will discuss regimental therapy and diet by applying the same foundational concepts explored in the previous section on drugs. Unani medicine follows the principle of mizaj (temperament) and utilizes the opposites concept to restore balance. This principle is fundamental to all treatment approaches, including pharmacology, dietary adjustments, and lifestyle interventions. For instance, diseases caused by cold morbid humour are treated by a hot temperament diet and regimental treatment methods. On the other hand, conditions resulting from a morbid hot humour are managed with a cold temperament diet and corresponding therapeutic practices. There are also some specific rules regarding diet, which are as follows:

Diet plays a dual role in relation to the faculties (quwa) of the body—it is both a sustainer and a potential to harm. It sustains by providing essential nourishment, without which the body's faculties cannot function. Conversely, it can be harmful when it can exacerbate the active substances (Madda) associated with diseases, thereby aggravating and strengthening them. Consequently, strict dietary rules and regulations are essential to ensure that carelessness does not worsen any existing conditions.

Besides, the real healer is not a physician but the Tabi'at (medicatrix naturae[434]). Therefore, if the diet is against the medicatrix naturae, it will be harmful because the Tabi'at, which is the corrector of the body, will focus completely on digesting the food rather than curing the disease and thus will complicate the treatment. Therefore, due to these facts, caution is needed when prescribing dietary changes.

Types of dietary treatment:

1. Tark-e-Ghiza (Stopped diet/nil diet intake):

A physician may advise patients to stop their diet completely to redirect the body's natural healing power (Tabi'at) towards eliminating abnormal substances (munzij) from the

---

[434] Ultimately, the Creator is the Healer.

body. However, this approach is only appropriate for severe conditions where the body is strong enough to cope with the lack of food. If the body is weakened due to malnourishment, even during a crisis, this diet is not recommended and should be discontinued if already initiated.

2. Taqleel-e-Ghiza (Reduced diet intake):

In a reduced diet, patients are given a lower amount of food than their regular intake to preserve their body's faculties and prevent exhaustion. The amount of food provided is based on the patient's strength and is decreased based on the abnormal matter causing the illness. The idea behind this approach is that by reducing the amount of food, the body can focus on resolving the substance causing the disease instead of digesting a large amount of food. The priority is given to the more important of the two things, which could either be the body's faculty or disease matter. If the patient's strength is weak, they are given food to strengthen it. However, if the disease is very strong, food is stopped altogether.

Types of reduced diet:

1. Reduction in kammiyat (quantity) of the diet.
2. Reduction in kaifiyat (quality) of the diet.
3. Reduction in the diet's Kamiya (quantity) and kufiya (quality).

The distinction between quantity and quality lies in the fact that while food may be sufficient in terms of quantity, it may not be sufficient in terms of quality. For instance, melons and watermelons in salads and fruits may fill the stomach, but they may not provide enough nutrients. This type of food is given when the appetite is false, i.e., when you eat even though you are not truly hungry and the body's vessels are full of normal substances. This type of medicine is used to reduce appetite by filling the stomach. Since these foods contain fewer nutrients, the amount of morbid matter (mavaad) in the body does not increase, and the stored matter concocts and dissolves. Alternatively, these types of foods are used during weight loss.

In contrast, some foods are sufficient in terms of quality but not in quantity. For example, a half-boiled egg is given when the aim is to strengthen the faculty, and it is so weak that it cannot digest large amounts of food. The need to reduce food intake usually occurs when the patient suffers from an acute disease (Amrad Hadda) but is not required in cases of chronic diseases (Amrad Muzmina). This is because the crisis of acute disease occurs early, and it is expected that most of the faculty will not be weakened.

Chronic diseases have a long duration and crisis. Therefore, if the faculty is not maintained through diet for this long period, then it will deplete before the peaking of the disease, and the Madda will not be able to concoct as the Madda of chronic diseases concocts late.

Acute diseases have a shorter duration with few complications, but according to the strength of the faculty, diet is increased. But as the complications of diseases increase with time, diet is reduced so as not to put a load on the facility to fight the disease.

In addition to the quantity and quality of the diet, there are three other characteristics of diet:

a. Saree-un-nufuz (Rapidly absorbing diet). This type of diet, after digestion, is easily absorbed by the body, e.g., honey and alcohol. This is administered in cases of excessive debility and during illness as the body can readily utilize them.
b. Batee-un-nufuz (Slowly absorbing diets). This type of diet takes much time to absorb due to its complex and lengthy metabolic process, which is difficult to absorb after metabolism, e.g., Spinach, Radish, and Carrot.
c. Blood produced from the diet which is either
    I.   Ghiza-e-Raqeeq (Liquid diet) produces less viscous blood after metabolism e.g., juice, soups, and wheat porridge.
    II. or Ghiza-e-Ghaleez (Solid diet) produce more viscous blood after metabolism, e.g., solid/semisolid preparations of meat and vegetables.

A rapidly diffusing diet is required when the vital force is weakening, the body does not have the faculty to digest a diet that is slow to digest, and the disease is time-specific. In this case, to generate energy and heat quickly, such as tea, coffee, honey, or alcohol should be given, and weakness and energy loss should be remedied as much as possible.

On the other hand, it is necessary to avoid rapidly diffusing diet when the patient has taken the slow-to-digest drugs; thus, they have not been fully digested. Similarly, a concentrated diet should be avoided when there is a risk of developing an obstruction.

A concentrated, high-calorie diet is beneficial for people who do hard physical work, and a low-calorie diet is good for people whose sweat pores are quickly condensed or when an unusual thickness develops in their blood. As in cholera, the blood becomes concentrated, and a low-calorie is required.

Levels of food in terms of tenuity and concentration

There are three levels of diet:

1. **Light and soft diet:** such as pomegranate water, citrus water, orange water, barley water, tea, coffee, honey, sabudana[435], dilute water of yellow lentils, curd water.

---

[435] 'tapioca pearls' - small, desiccated, translucent white balls of tapioca, extracted from the roots of the cassava plant, sabudana or Indian sago.

2. **Medium diet:** such as khichdi[436], thick barley water, egg yolks, digestible vegetables such as apple gourd, pumpkin, broth, gravy and cow's milk.
3. **Concentrated diet:** meat, pulses, rice and fruits such as mango, banana, etc.

Fruits are often harmful in fevers because the digestion becomes weak during fever, due to which the fruit decays and produces poisonous substances, but in Safra (bilious) fevers, apple juice, pear water, Laooq[437] (linctus), dried plums, etc., are given.

Pharmacotherapy

Pharmacotherapy is carried out under the following three rules:

1. Law on quality of drug
2. Law on the quantity of drug
3. Law on timings of drug

In addition to the above three basic laws, there are a few other laws which have to be observed in pharmacotherapy.

a. By what means should the drug be delivered to the body so that it can reach the organs and show its effect? For example, through mouth, membranes or by inoculation.

b. In what form should the drug be used, for example, Habbub (pills), Joshanda (decoction), Khesanda (Infusion), Laooq (linctus), Majun (electuary), Arqat (distillates)[438].

c. Medication should be taken individually or in combination. In cases where a single drug is sufficient, a combination of drugs is not required, and in cases where a combination of drugs is required, a single drug is not sufficient.

d. It is important to use medicines when they are fresh because some drugs lose their effectiveness when they get old. For instance, Gul Banafshah (Viola odorata flower), Gul-e-Nilofer (Nymphaea alba flower)[439], Maghz Akhrot (Juglans regia – walnut), Maghz Pista (Pistacia vera – pistachio) and other such medicines have a shorter shelf life. On the other hand, some medicines become more potent with age. For example, Itrifal is more effective when it is pressed into grains and allowed to age for a certain period.

---

[436] a dish of rice and moong daal.
[437] Also, spelt La'uq is a semisolid preparation used in diseases of the lungs and pharynx. The half-grounded drugs are soaked in water overnight and boiled the next day till the quantity of water is reduced to half. The decoction is then strained and mixed along with some other powdered drugs in a sugar base.
[438] Note all these terms have been defined in the previous chapter on drugs.
[439] In the Unani system of medicine, plant-origin drugs are most commonly used. The parts used are root, stem, fruits, flowers, leaves, seed, gum and peel. You will commonly see these words in front of names of plants: Flowers (Gul) and leaves (Barg), Seeds (Tukhm) and fruits (Phal), Roots (Asl), Branches (Shaakh) and barks (Chaal), Shrubs (Bootiyan), Gums (Gond).

e. When selecting a medicine, it is important to consider its essence. For instance, if multiple medicines have the same effectiveness in treating a particular condition, choose the one that has a more suitable essence. For example, if you need a digestive medicine, and there are multiple options available, choose the one that is fragrant and sweet, as it is more likely to be effective.

Law on quality of drugs

Quality of drug refers to the nature of the action of the drug, i.e., adopting the law of the quality of drug can give correct guidance when the Tabi'at (medicatrix naturae) knows the type and nature of the disease. Therefore, a drug is chosen which is opposite to the quality of the actual disease, because the disease is treated heteropathically[440].

Heteropathy (Ilaj bil Didd) [441]

This means that, for example, in the case where blood vessels become dilated due to a disease, which can result in haemorrhage (Jarayan al-dam), it is recommended to use drugs that constrict the blood vessels. This helps in retaining the blood. Such drugs are called haemostyptic (Habis-i-Dam).

Conversely, when a disease causes vessel narrowing, it can lead to weakness due to a lack of nutrients. In such cases, vasodilators (Mufattih-i-Uruq) should be used to dilate the vessels.

When the body is sick, the intestine's expulsive faculty (Quwwat Dafia) and the rotatory movement (Harakat Dawariyya) decrease. This leads to a reduction in the secretion of fluid from the mucous membrane. To treat this, drugs that can help accelerate the expulsive faculty and peristalsis while increasing fluid secretion are used. This is usually seen in the case of constipation. Such types of drugs are called Mushilath (purgatives) and Mulayyinaat (laxatives).

On the other hand, when peristalsis increases and the secretion of fluids becomes excessive, drugs that reduce the secretion of fluids are used. These drugs can help decrease peristalsis and are called Qabidat (astringent) and neutralizers of the Musakkinat (heat) of humours.

When the body temperature rises, as in the case of remittent fever, antipyretic drugs, also known as refrigerants, are used. On the other hand, when the body temperature decreases, as in the case of cold or syncope (fainting), hot medicines are used.

---

[440] That mode of treating diseases, by which a morbid condition is removed by inducing an opposite condition; allopathy
[441] Essentially this is the main concept of treatment in Unani – treating with opposites.

Exceptions

There are some diseases where the principle of Ilaj bil Didd (heteropathy) cannot be applied. For example, in disorders of stools where faeces are being passed, Mushilat (purgatives) are used. In vomiting, Muqiyyat (emetics) are used, which can be helpful in both types of diseases. The cure for these diseases is to expel the rotten substances that cause vomiting and stools. In other words, in the case of fullness, the excess Madda (matter) is treated by excretion, which is a form of heteropathy. Similarly, Safra (bilious) fever is a hot temperament ailment but is treated with Saqmoonia (Convolvulus scammonia root latex), which is a hot drug, and it is a Mushil-i-Safra (cholagogue), i.e., it helps to excrete putrescent bile through faeces.

Like for like treatment (Ilaj bil-Misl)

Reciprocal therapy applies to diseases and medicines whose nature is not known. It is a fact that we don't know the nature of many diseases. Similarly, the type of action of many medicines is also unknown, although certain medicines have been proven to cure certain diseases. Some hot drugs are useful for hot diseases, while cold drugs are useful for cold diseases. Physicians call these types of drugs Zulkhassa, meaning their mode of action is unknown.

Furthermore, some drugs mix with the matter in the body and alter its temperament and structural parts. However, it cannot be said that they break down, for example, the cold matter due to the cold temperament. For instance, Sammulfar (purified arsenic trioxide) was used to treat syphilis.

The law of quantity of drug

The law that has been enacted for the quantity of medicine can lead only when the physician knows:

(1) The nature of the organ, (2) the quantity of the disease, and (3) other factors to consider when prescribing.

The nature of the organ

This means that four things should be known about the organs.

1. The temperament of the organ
2. The structure of the organ
3. The position and location of the organ
4. The faculty and function of the organ

The temperament of the organ

To understand the diseased temperament of an organ, it is essential to know its normal temperament. By understanding how far the organ's temperament has deviated from normal, estimating the appropriate amount of medicine required to restore it to its normal state is possible.

The structure of the organ

It also consists of four parts

1. The shape of the organ
2. Virtual pores of the organ
3. The cavity of the organ
4. The surface of the organ

Certain organs possess a porous structure which enables easy entry and exit of substances through them. Such organs can eliminate waste with the aid of a small quantity of drugs. Conversely, non-porous organs necessitate more potent medication to function efficiently.

The location of the organ:

This is based on two things

1. The association of organs
2. The position and location of the organs

Physicians can benefit greatly from understanding the association of organs. Knowing the involvement of organs helps doctors choose the best course of action for the patient's recovery. For instance, Mudirat (Diuretics), Mushilath (purgatives), Muqiyyat (emetics), and Muarriqat (Diaphoretics) are used based on this principle. The primary advantage of this knowledge is that it makes it easier for Madda to divert and excrete, leading to better treatment outcomes.

Knowing the location of the diseased organ is beneficial for three reasons:

Firstly, the proximity of the application site to the affected organ can significantly influence the required dosage of the drug. A smaller amount of the drug may suffice if the target organ is near the application site. Conversely, if the organ is distant, its effectiveness may diminish as it travels, necessitating stronger drugs. The drug's potency is determined by its weight and degree of action. Medicines like Majun (electuary, a semi-solid preparation), Jawarish (digestive paste), La'uq [442] (Linctus), Safuf (powdered medicine), and Huqna (enema) are used based on this principle.

Secondly, understanding the location of the diseased organ aids the physician in choosing appropriate substances for the medicine to ensure its effects reach the specific organ. For

---

[442] Plural of Laooq

instance, if the disease affects the urinary system, diuretics might be added to the medication to facilitate its transmission to the urinary organs.

Thirdly, knowing the specific location of the disease helps determine the most effective delivery method for the medication. For example, if an ulcer is in the inferior intestine, the drug might be administered through mucous membranes (sublingual or buccal) to ensure direct absorption. Conversely, medications for ulcers in the upper part of the intestine are typically delivered orally.

The faculty and function of an organ:

There are two benefits in knowing the faculty of an organ:

1. Consideration of the supporting organs: If the disease affects the supporting organs such as the heart, the brain and the liver, then potent drugs should be used with great caution so as to not harm the organs.
2. Consideration of the sharpness and dullness of the sensation of the organs: If the disease has arisen in the sensory organs, then the drug should be used with great caution.

The intensity of a disease

To use the drug according to its degree of intensity. This is an important principle because, in diseases where, for example, heat is intense, potent refrigerants are used. But if the temperature is mild, then slightly cold drugs are sufficient.

Factors to consider when prescribing

The following factors are relevant when determining the appropriate dosage of a drug:

1. Gender
2. Age
3. Habit
4. Time
5. Country and race
6. Profession
7. Faculty/Power
8. Temperament
9. Physique
10. Climate and weather
11. Previous measures
12. Time of disease
13. Crisis of the disease
14. Mode of drug administration
15. Patient's thoughts
16. A full or empty stomach

17. Current diseases
18. Specific nature
19. The active principle of drugs
20. Deposition of the drug in the body

Gender

In general, women are prescribed lower doses of medicine than men due to their relatively lower physical strength. During treatment, the menstrual cycle of women needs to be taken into account since certain medications can either prolong or shorten the duration of menstruation. Moreover, pregnancy is a critical factor that needs to be considered during medication.

Age

When it comes to medication, it is typically recommended to administer smaller and lighter doses to children compared to adults. Medical literature generally records the dosage required for adults, often referred to as a full dose. However, this amount is adjusted and reduced for children and senior citizens.

For instance, if the adult dose of a medication is 12 grams, the following dosage adjustments are recommended:

- For children under 2 years: 0.5g

- For children aged 2-3 years: 1.5g

- For children aged 3-4 years: 2g

- For children aged 4-6 years: 3g

- For children aged 6-10 years: 4g

- For children aged 10-13 years: 5g

- For teenagers aged 13-16 years: 6g

- For teenagers aged 16-18 years: 8g

- For young adults aged 18-21 years: 10g

- For adults aged 21-60 years: the full dose

- For adults over 60 years: the dose is reduced according to age, and the specific health conditions of the individual, with particular caution employed for potent and toxic medications.

Habit

When a person becomes dependent on a drug, the prescribed dose of the medicine may not have the desired effect. This is because the body builds up resistance to toxic drugs like opium, cannabis, alcohol, and others, causing their desired effects to gradually decrease. Hence, the patient's usage habits should be assessed to determine the appropriate dose of medicine.

It is worth noting that the effectiveness of certain medications can vary depending on the time of day they are taken. Drugs such as Mufarreh (exhilarants), Muharrikat (stimulants), and Muqawwiyat (tonics) are more likely to have a stronger effect in the morning and evening, when the patient's natural energy levels may be lower. Therefore, larger doses of these drugs may be more beneficial to optimise their therapeutic impact during these periods.

Country and race

Different countries have different temperaments, just like the quality of food. As a result, people living in colder regions can tolerate hot medicines better than cold medicines. On the other hand, people living in warmer areas can tolerate cold medications better than hot medicines. It is important to be cautious while using hot drugs in hot countries and cold medicines in cold countries.

Profession

Individuals who work in occupations that cause sweating or loss of body fluids, such as blacksmiths, carpenters, and bath attendants, should avoid being treated with hot, dry drugs or potent purgatives. Conversely, people whose work produces cold in the body, such as sailors or fishermen, may be treated with hot medicines.

Faculty

Stronger people can tolerate potent drugs in larger doses, but weaker people cannot tolerate large doses, and small amounts of drugs are enough for them.

Temperament

It is important to remember that different patients have different temperaments: Damawi (sanguine), Balghami (phlegmatic), Saudawi (melancholic), or Safra (bilious). Sensitivity levels also vary; some patients exhibit mild sensitivity, while others may have sharp sensitivity. Therefore, when determining the appropriate medicine dosage, it is crucial to consider the patient's specific temperament and sensitivity level.

Physique

Obese and muscular individuals may require higher doses of medications, such as purgatives and toxic drugs, compared to those who are thin and lean.

Climate and weather

It's important to take climate into account when choosing a treatment for an illness. As Ibn Sina said, certain diseases are more prevalent in hot and humid climates, while a change in climate can cure many ailments. When it is hot, the Muhallil drugs (resolvent) work better and require a smaller dosage. However, their effect is reduced when it is cold, and a relatively larger dose may be necessary. Some hot drugs should be avoided during summer or used only in small doses if required. Similarly, cold drugs are not recommended during cold weather but can be used in small doses if needed.

Previous treatment

It is important to gather information from the patient regarding their previous medication history and any measures they have taken. This is especially important in the case of spasmodic (Tashannuj) drugs. For instance, if the patient has previously taken spasmodic drugs, then a larger dosage of antispasmodic (Dafe Tashannuj) drugs will be required for them to be effective.

Phase of disease

The phase of the disease refers to the stage of the illness. For instance, if swelling initially increases, a repellent drug (Radi'[443]) will be used. If the swelling is regressing, Mulayyin (resolvents) are used. However, if the swelling is between the two, then both types of drugs will be used in combination. Similarly, for all diseases, the phase of the disease will be considered.

Crisis

While prescribing the dosage and potency, the crisis period should also be considered. So, if defecation or diarrhoea is needed, Mushilat (purgatives) are strictly avoided during crises. And if they are urgently required, only mild forms are given.

Mode of drug administration

The method of administering a drug can affect the required dosage of that drug. Generally, oral medications require smaller doses than those administered through an enema. However, there are exceptions, such as the drug Kuchla (Strychnos nux-vomica), which requires smaller doses when given as an enema. Drugs also require smaller doses when applied topically or injected into muscles or veins.

The patient's thoughts and beliefs

The beliefs and thoughts of a patient can have an impact on the dosage of a drug prescribed. If a patient strongly believes that a particular medication is very effective, even

---

[443] رادع Drug which diverts matter from one part of body/organ to another part.

a small amount can have a significant effect. Conversely, if a patient has a negative belief about a drug and considers it ineffective, a higher dose of the medicine may be needed to achieve the desired results. Therefore, false beliefs and thoughts can play a critical role in medication effectiveness.

A full or empty stomach

An empty or full stomach also affects the dose of the drug. A small quantity of drugs on an empty stomach has a significant effect, whereas some drugs lose their effect when taken on a full stomach. Therefore, it is usually better to take most drugs on an empty stomach.

Current diseases

Large amounts of certain drugs are tolerable in the presence of certain diseases. For example, in syphilis, the tolerance of compounds of Para (purified mercury) and Sammulfar (purified arsenic trioxide) compounds increases, whereas in kidney diseases, small amounts of purified mercury and purified arsenic are also intolerable.

Specific nature

Some individuals may respond differently to certain medications or diets than expected. In some cases, large quantities of a drug or specific dietary regimen may not affect certain individuals. It is important to remember that this knowledge is typically only gained through experience and observation.

The active substance of medicine

Compound medication can be administered in a higher dose with multiple ingredients; however, if the active ingredients are extracted from the mixture, they can only be used in small amounts.

Deposition of the drug in the body

Once the body absorbs and metabolises a drug, it is excreted through urine, faeces, or sweat. However, if toxic drugs are used in non-toxic quantities, they can accumulate in the body and may cause symptoms after some time. Therefore, it is important to use toxic drugs with breaks, such as Kuchla (Strychnos nux-vomica seed), Sammulfar (purified arsenic trioxide), afyoon (opium), etc. This helps to ensure that the amount of the drug is absorbed gradually and does not produce poisonous effects.

Law on drug timings

Physicians say that the timing of drug administration depends on the disease stage. For instance, when dealing with the early stages of acute swelling (Waram Harr), repellent drugs (Radi'at) are used. However, during later stages, treatment shifts to resolvents and relaxants to further alleviate symptoms. Resolvents such as Aanba Haldi (Curcuma amada root), Dar Hald (Berberis aristata bark), Rai (Brassica alba seed), Alsi (Linum usitatissimum seed), Barg Kasni (Cichorium intybus leaves), Barg Mako (Solanum nigrum leaves), saffron, aloe vera, chamomilla, along with vinegar and honey are commonly employed. Relaxants like flaxseed and olive oil also help ease the condition.

Beyond this basic principle, several other considerations are taken into account:

1. Some medicines are specially used on an empty stomach; for example, the best time to use an anthelmintic (Qatil Deedan Ama) drug such as Tukhm Bakain (Melia azedrach seeds) Kamela (Mallotus phillipinensis), Senna (Cassia senna leaf), Gilo (Tinospora indica herb), Neem (Melia azadirachta) etc. is on an empty stomach.
2. Toxic drugs such as compound preparations that include opium, Strychnos nux-vomica and compounds of Burada Faulad (processed iron powder) are usually taken after food.
3. Slow-acting purgatives (Mushilat) such as Senna makki (Cassia Angustifolia - Arabian Senna), aloe vera, and aloe vera compound formulations like Habb-e-Shabyar, as well as laxatives (Mullein Ama) like Haleela (Terminalia chebula fruit), are typically administered at night before going to sleep. This allows them to work through the night and be expelled in the morning.

Additional guidelines include:

- It is common to take a Emmenagogue (Mudir Haiz) before the start of menstruation.
- Protective drugs that help against stomach acid are potent and saline. They are usually taken shortly before or after a meal.
- It is best to avoid giving the medicine when the patient needs to wake up to take it. However, it may be better for the patient not to sleep in some diseases. Sleep is not considered a factor in these cases, such as in litharghus (phlegmatic meningitis).
- Diaphoretics (muarriqat) work best when the air in the patient's room and their skin is warm. They are not effective when the environment is cold, or the skin is cool. Therefore, before administering diaphoretics, the patient should be kept in a warm room and instructed to cover themselves with a sheet or blanket, depending on the weather. This will help them to experience the full benefits of the medication. Keeping the patient in the open air before giving them diaphoretics is not advisable.
- Diuretics are more effective when the skin and room environment are cool. The kidneys and the skin have opposite functions, so when the kidneys are working harder, the skin's sweating function decreases. Conversely, the kidneys' function decreases when the skin is sweating more.

Principles of treatment and other considerations

Use of potent therapies

According to Ibn Sina, if a patient is suffering from a dangerous disease, and there is a risk that the natural healing ability of the patient will be depleted if the required treatment is delayed or reduced, then it is necessary to start a more potent therapy. However, in diseases where there is no such risk, a mild treatment should be used initially. If this does not work, gradually move towards a stronger, more potent therapy.

It is a fundamental principle that the more potent a drug is, the stronger it works against the body's natural healing ability. Therefore, such drugs or therapies should be introduced into the body only when necessary. Powerful treatments, such as the use of toxic drugs, potent purgatives and vomiting, should be avoided as much as possible during extreme weather conditions.

Drug resistance

It is well-documented that the efficacy of a drug can diminish after prolonged use, which must be considered during treatment. Ibn Sina noted that despite this phenomenon, adherence to the correct treatment protocol is crucial. It is not advisable to continue using the same treatment or drug when it fails to show benefits. Instead, it is necessary to switch medications if the expected therapeutic effects are not observed. This is because the body can become accustomed to and resistant to a drug, rendering it ineffective. For instance, individuals who develop an addiction to opium may find that the standard dose no longer provides relief from pain as their tolerance builds.

Pain relief is a priority in treatment

Ibn Sina summarised that pain can be associated with a disease in different ways.

The first is when disease and pain co-exist but are present in separate organs and don't precede each other. For example, acute conjunctivitis and headache.

The second is when a disease presents with pain, and the cause of the pain is the disease itself. For example, colic and syncope (fainting), where syncope is due to colic.

The third is when pain is a symptom of a particular disease. For example, acute or traumatic inflammation or syncope.

In all these cases, pain should be relieved cautiously using Mukhaddirat (anaesthetics) because the pain-resolving faculty can diminish the Tabi'at (medicatrix naturae) and weaken immunity. The local arteries dilate due to pain, causing rapid absorption and effusion of the Madda at the site of abnormality. This can either lead to the progression of the disease or give rise to another one. Therefore, the Tabi'at diverts from the actual illness, resulting in prevailing disease.

Restrictions on the use of potent anaesthetics

Ibn Sina advised against using strong anaesthetics as they can impair bodily functions and slow down the mind. However, when faced with severe and unbearable pain that may lead to collapse or fainting, opium and its derivatives or other active components may be considered based on the severity of the pain.

Managing hyperaesthesia

Ibn Sina says that when the sensitivity of any organ, i.e., hyperaesthesia[444], becomes a problem, such things that thicken the blood and refrigerants are used—for example, lettuce (Lactuca sativa) seeds or leaves.

Psychotherapy

It is widely accepted that negative emotions like worry, grief, sadness, rage, and fury can have harmful effects on the physical body. They can cause disorders, illnesses, and even fatal diseases like TB. Conversely, positive emotions such as happiness and pleasure can help alleviate psychiatric issues. In some cases, they may even provide a permanent cure, although pharmacotherapy may be necessary in others.

Change in location and environment

Ibn Sina suggests that relocating to a different city and altering one's environment can be a part of psychotherapy. This change can positively impact the patient's health in two ways: firstly, if the patient moves to a good and pleasant environment from an unpleasant one, then their illness may improve. Secondly, the change in scenery can provide new and interesting sights, creating pleasure, which can be an effective treatment that positively affects the body's functions, such as nutrition, growth, and development. Ibn Sina referred to this treatment as a way to improve the condition without requiring medication.

Change in order

Ibn Sina suggested that certain medical conditions could be effectively addressed by changing one's posture and behaviour. For instance, people suffering from Strabismus (squint) were advised to focus on a shiny and bright object placed on the opposite side of the squint. Additionally, patients with facial palsy (Laqwa) were encouraged to observe their own facial movements in a mirror and attempt self-correction, which was a precursor to mirror feedback therapy.

---

[444] extreme sensitivity to touch, pain, pressure, and thermal sensations.

Furthermore, adopting good and positive company and replacing harmful habits with beneficial ones can be a way to treat mental and emotional disorders. This understanding highlights the importance of environmental and behavioural factors in mental health.

Apparent conflicts in treatment

Ibn Sina, in his exposition of the laws of treatment, highlights that physicians must exercise caution in situations where conflicting treatments are indicated for the same disease. For example, some conditions may necessitate cooling, while the underlying cause might require heat. In instances like a fever due to blood vessel obstruction, the fever itself calls for cold treatment, but the obstruction causing the fever needs heat. Similarly, colic might require heat for the discomfort and reduction of the offending matter (Madda), but its underlying cause might require coldness and anaesthesia (Takhdir).

Illustrative Examples:

Cough with Fever

Thirst during fever usually demands cold interventions like ice water and cold drugs, which, however, can exacerbate a cough. Conversely, warm water and hot drugs that soothe the cough may intensify the fever. The recommended treatment involves drinking warm water to alleviate the cough, using fresh, well water to quench thirst, and selecting drugs like Behi (Cydonia oblonga, C. quince seeds), Unnab (Zizifus sativa fruit), and Sapistan (Cordia latifolia fruit) prepared as a Joshanda (decoction) and Unnab as a Sheera[445], which are effective against cough but not detrimental during fever.

Cough with Naif al-dam (haemorrhage)

It can be difficult for doctors to treat patients with cough-related haemorrhage, mainly if the bleeding is caused by internal organs such as the lungs or stomach or due to an abortion. The primary objective is to stabilise the patient and prevent coughing, which could lead to increased blood loss.

Doctors may prescribe warm medications instead of cold to treat coughs, which can worsen coughing. Poppy seeds, opium, and their derivatives are commonly used to treat both coughs and bleeding. However, these drugs can cause severe constipation, especially if the patient is also suffering from haemorrhoids (Bawasir), which can worsen the obstruction and lead to complications. To prevent constipation, patients can take opium and its derivatives with almond oil mixed in milk before going to bed.

Physicians must carefully consider their approach when faced with complex medical cases and conflicting requirements. They must decide whether to leave the diseases to the

---

[445] mainly seeds ground in water and used with or without straining it is called sheera. Its consistency is more or less like milk. See the previous section on drugs.

body's natural healing process (Tabi'at) without any treatment or to treat them and prioritize which component needs to be addressed first. Young doctors with limited experience may find this challenging, while experienced physicians rely on their knowledge and expertise to make the best decisions.

Treatment in cases where the diagnoses is difficult

Determining the appropriate treatment can be challenging when a disease cannot be diagnosed. According to Ibn Sina, it is best to allow the body's natural healing process (Tabi'at) to take over in such situations. Acting hastily due to ignorance should be avoided. Either the body's natural healing process will overcome and eliminate the disease, or the disease will become more severe, presenting with clear signs and symptoms that can be diagnosed.

For example, treating an undiagnosed fever can be difficult. In such cases, it is recommended to provide a light and easily digestible diet. Although it is harmful to leave the disease to the Tabi'at without any drug or treatment, it is more dangerous to give the wrong treatment due to ignorance.

Physicians may prescribe mild-acting and broad-spectrum drugs without a clear diagnosis based on their medical knowledge. These drugs should not cause harm if they do not benefit the patient.

General acting drugs

Example: Digestive disorders

Nuskha khalale shikam[446] (prescription for digestive disorders):

HUWA SHIFA (HE is the curer)[447]

Gul Banafshah (Viola odorata flower)	7 grams
Maveez Munaqqa (dried Vitis vinifera)	9 pieces
Beikh Kasni (Cichorium intybus root)	7 grams
Badiyan (Foeniculum vulgare seed)	5 grams
Gaozaban (Borago officinalis, flower)	5 grams

---

[446] This is a famous formula for abdominal organ illnesses with great benefit even for the very old and stubborn conditions in which a humour is actually in excess is not clear. It is essentially a munzij (concoctive) – that clears corrupted matter through excretion. Additional herbs may be included for fevers, etc.
[447] Meaning The Creator is the ultimate curer and not the physician as she/he merely facilities.

To prepare Nuskha khalale shikam, soak overnight in one glass of hot water. In the morning, drain the water and drink it on an empty stomach with 5g teaspoon of khamira banafsha for ten days.

If the patient is suffering from an unknown type of septic fever, such as Balghami or Safrawi fever, this formula can be used with Khaksi (Sisymbrium irio) water or honey. For cold, flu, cough or shortness of breath that cannot be diagnosed, add Tukhme Khatmi (Althea officinalis seed), Tukhme Khubbazi (Malva sylvestris seed), and Aslussoos muqashshar (Glycyrrhiza glabra root-liquorice root peeled) as required.

If the digestive system needs to be cleared or softened, add Mushil (purgative) or a Mulayan (laxative) after ten days of using the above formula.

Example: Fever

If a patient is experiencing an undiagnosed fever, mild laxatives such as Itrifal Mulayyan or Sharbat Ward can be used frequently to relieve the symptoms, provided there is no bowel disease in which laxatives are contraindicated. It is important to note that the use of potent and irritating purgatives (Mushilat) is not recommended for several conditions, such as enteric fever (Humma Mi'wiyya), dysentery or haemorrhoids. However, mild laxatives are not prohibited if required.

Example: Inflammation

When there is inflammation in the body, but it is unclear whether it is in the liver, stomach, intestines, or kidneys. The type of hot swelling or composition of its corrupted matter is unknown. In such a case, Aab-e-Murawwaqain (i.e., juice of Kasni leaf (Cichorium intybus) 50g and Mako leaf (Solanum nigrum) 50g - obtained through Tarwiq [the process of cleansing a liquid drug]) is used with Nuskha khalale shikam (see above).

Example: Kidney and urine

Mudirat (Diuretics) are very beneficial for most kidney and urine diseases, such as Tukhme Kharpaza (Cucumis melo seed - Muskmelon seeds), Kharkhasak (Tribulus terrestris fruit), Tukhme Khayaren (Cucumis sativus seed- cucumber seeds) and Ma-ush-shaeer (Barley water)[448] in the diet.

Example: Heart

Muqawwiyat Qalb (Heart tonics/ Cardiotonics) and Mufarrehat (Exhilarants), which are useful in many heart diseases, are compound formulations which are readily commercially available such as Khamira gaozaban ambari jawahar wala, Dawa Ul Misk Motadil Jawahar

---

[448] See previous section on drugs.

Wali, khamira abresham hakim arshad wala, Khamira Marwareed, Jawahir Mohra, Habbe Jawahar, Qurs Malti Basant, etc.

Example: Uterus

In many uterus-related diseases, Mudir Haiz (Emmenagogue) is normally used.

Example: Septic fever

In the treatment of septic fever, Talyin (soften), Ta'riq (diaphoresis)[449] and Qay (vomiting) are effective treatments. It is a beneficial treatment adopted when the type of septic fever cannot be diagnosed. However, using Tabreed (Cooling), i.e., cold treatments, would be an exceptional case, as it will harm the individual.

The principle of treatment for abnormal temperaments (su-e-mizaj)

There are two types of Su-e-Mizaj (abnormal temperament/dyscrasia)[450]

1. Su-e-Mizaj Sada (abnormal temperament)
2. Su-e-Mizaj Maddi[451] (abnormal temperament with a substance(s))

Su-e-Mizaj Sada (abnormal temperament)

Su-e-Mizaj Sada refers to a simple increase in heat or cold in the organs without any association with morbid matter (Madda) that requires its removal from the body by ripening and elimination. It is also known as abnormal simple temperament without morbid matter. For instance, walking in the sun can cause headaches that can be cured by staying in a cool place. However, prolonged sun exposure or cold exposure can significantly alter an abnormal simple temperament by oxidizing the body's humours and disrupting their functions.

In the same way, living in an extremely cold and unbearable environment coagulates the humours, alters them, and increases coldness in their temperament. This decreases their flow, which disrupts their functions.

According to Ibn Sina, whenever an abnormal temperament exists without morbid matter (Madda), treating it with contrasting measures is sufficient. For example, treat the organ with cold measures if the organ is suffering from heat. Similarly, if the organ is

---

[449] Expulsion of humours by sweating is beneficial in certain fevers, ascites, obesity and joint pain. It is done by using some specific drugs which induce sweating, or it can be done by hot chamber, Hammam.
[450] Also known as a dyscrasias/dys-temperament/in-temperament.
[451] This is an abnormal temperament but also there is matter or substance also involved.

suffering from coldness, provide heat to treat it. However, no eliminatory measures should be taken, such as purging (Ishal) and diaphoresis (Ta'riq).

Su-e-Mizaj Maddi (abnormal temperament with a substance(s))

When there is an abnormal substance in the body and an abnormal temperament (Su-e-Mizaj Maddi), it becomes necessary to mature and remove this substance. An abnormal substance results from an imbalance in the body, which leads to the accumulation of waste or excess of particular humour.

There are two types of substances in a disease:

1. Some substances can be easily expelled through elimination. For example, blood can be easily evacuated through Fasd (Venesection). Similarly, substances in the stomach and intestine can be easily expelled through vomiting and diarrhoea.

2. Some substances penetrate the cavities of the organs, veins, and fibres so that they can't be excreted by simply purging through emesis or diarrhoea only. In such conditions, necessary changes need to be introduced in the substance before their elimination. Such changes are called Nudj (concoction), and the drugs that enable such changes are called Mundij (concoctive).

Ibn Sina says, if some of Su-e-Mizaj remains with the substance, i.e., the disease has not entirely been eradicated, then additional therapies or treatment will be required.

Different levels of Su-e-Mizaj (abnormal temperament) and their treatment

There are three levels of Su-e-Mizaj (abnormal temperament) and their treatment:

1. If there is no risk of developing Su-e-Mizaj, preventive measures alone are sufficient. These measures aim to prevent the onset of any abnormal temperament. They may include maintaining a balanced diet, regular physical activity, managing stress, and avoiding known imbalance triggers, such as extreme weather conditions.
2. If Su-e-Mizaj is still in its early stages of development, then measures will be taken to prevent the progression of the disease. For example, suppose acute inflammation is in the initial stage. In that case, medicines that reduce the heat absorption of an organ (ravaadiaat) are used along with purgation to remove any excess or Madda and to decrease progressive inflammation.
3. If Su-e-Mizaj is fully developed, it is now called Su'-i-Mizaj Mustawi (a steady abnormal temperament). In such cases, Ilaj bil Didd (heteropathy) is applied. For example, infective fever caused by organisms found in stagnant water that can lead to an enlarged spleen can be treated with Gilo (Tinospora indica) and habbe Karanjwa (Caesalpinia bonducella pills). To control the heat in the body, cold air, cold water, and ice can be used. Also, the treatment requires managing

the Kayfiyat Arba'a (the four physical properties)[452], namely a regimen of moistening (tartib) and drying (Tajfif) is required.

For the treatment of Su-e-Mizaj, internal and external coldness is delivered to the body, and this process is called tabreed (cooling); the measures to increase the fluid in the body are called tartiib (moistening), and sometimes measures are taken to Tahlil (dissolve) the body fluids which is called Tajfif (drying).

But all of this is done under specific requirements because, in some cases, the body temperature rises above normal, whereas in some diseases, it decreases. Hence, the first situation requires cooling, and the second requires heat (Taskhin). For this purpose, cold water, ice, etc., are used in severe fever, but during shock, when the hands and feet become cold, then at that time, compound formulas such as Dawa al-Misk are used, and external medications are applied. In the same way, in the case of cachexic oedema/anasarca and diarrhoea, where the body loses fluid, fresh water is used, and the blood flow to the organs is increased.

Negligence during warming and cooling should be avoided. In hot and severe diseases such as meningitis (Sarsam), high fever, and hot Madda-like bile excitation, refrigerants are given externally and internally, which decreases the temperature rapidly to normal or below normal levels. In such situations, Ibn Sina says that refrigerants can give rise to other problems along with the weakening of vital power. In extreme cases, a refrigerant can worsen the patient, and some patients even get so cold that their temperature cannot be raised.

Sometimes due to excess tabreed (cooling), hot diseases and hot humours do not concoct i.e., their transformation and metabolism stops. It is because due to high Tabreed, the body faculty depletes and so when the faculty is weakened by the disease, the excess cold produces abnormal cold substantial temperament which is the contrary to the temperament that can be treated by refrigerants.

Sometimes, when the body is excessively cooled, it can prevent the proper transformation and metabolism of hot diseases and humours. This happens because too much cooling depletes the body's natural faculties. As a result, when a disease weakens the body's faculties, the excess cold produces a morbid cold temperament with substance (Su-e-Mizaj Barid Maddi).

---

[452] The four natural properties or qualities associated with matter - hot, cold, moist and dry.

Evacuation (Istifragh)

Evacuation/elimination refers to the expulsion of such substances from the body that may be harmful to the body. Since substances and wastes help spread disease, it is necessary to expel them.

Types of elimination

1. **Purging (Ishal):** The expulsion of the active substances through the intestine is called Ishal. Often, expulsion through diarrhoea is very useful in diseases due to active substances. It is especially beneficial in most gastrointestinal and liver diseases and can prove especially beneficial in diseases of joints, which is due to Madda (matter/substance that has accumulated).
2. **Emesis/vomiting (Qay):** The ejection of Mavaad through the mouth is called emesis. It is extremely useful for kidney, bladder, stomach and chest diseases.
3. **Diaphoresis (Ta'riq):** Expulsion of Mavaad through sweating. This process is useful in different fevers, oedema, obesity, and joint pain.
4. **Diuresis (Idrar[453]):** The removal of Mavaad (matter) through urination is called diuresis. It is useful in kidney, bladder, urethra, and liver diseases, as well as arthritis (al-mafasil) and hemiplegia (Falij). Diuretics also include medicines for menstruation, semen and lactation. Emmenagogues are used in diseases of the uterus (Rahim) and Damawi (sanguine) ailments, and galactagogues are used during low milk secretion and mastitis.
5. **Expectoration (Tanaffus):** Expulsion of phlegm through the throat.
6. **Venesection (Fasd):** Evacuation of blood by incising veins. It is useful in Damawi ailments and pain.
7. **Cupping (Hijama):** Cupping instruments, which are typically made of plastic nowadays, are used to absorb and divert Mavaad. In cases where blood evacuation is necessary, cupping with scarification (hijama ma'l shart) is useful for treating Damawi ailments and pain. When applied to the lower part of the shin and soles, cupping instruments prevent Mavaad and Bukharat[454] (vapours) to reach the brain, so it is useful in the treatment of brain ailments.
8. **Hirudo therapy/leeching (Taliq Alaq):** It refers to the use of leeches and is a substitute for Fasd.

---

[453] Idrar is the process of increasing the flow of any liquid from the body, e.g., urine, menstrual blood, saliva, milk, etc.
[454] The gaseous substances usually form due to extra matter retention, leading to an abnormal state. Their impact may be on organs to cause disease.

Conditions of Evacuation/Elimination

During any elimination, the following ten things should be considered:

1. **Congestion (Imtila):** Imtila is a condition where bodily fluids, particularly blood, accumulate in different body parts. Istifragh is contraindicated in this situation as it can cause the emptying of humours.
2. **Faculty/power of the patient:** Elimination should not be carried out on weak patients unless there are no other options. In such cases, elimination can be done, but the weakened faculty of the patient must be treated later.
3. **Temperament (Mizaj):** A mizaj that is excessively hot, dry, cold or in a state of anaemia elimination can decrease the fluids in the body, as useful fluids are expelled during the elimination, resulting in weakness.
4. **Physique:** Elimination is contraindicated if the patient is under weight or excessively over weight. It is because useful fluids are lost during the elimination in underweight patients, and fluid loss in overweight patients causes the reduction of vessels in flesh and fats and depletion of pneuma and innate heat.
5. **Excluded conditions:** If the patient is prone to diarrhoea or has an ulcer in the intestine, elimination should be avoided.
6. **Age:** Elimination is generally contraindicated in the elderly and children due to lower faculty in these age groups.
7. **Time of elimination:** Avoid elimination during extreme hot or cold weather conditions. This is because in extremely hot weather, the body is already weakened due to a lack of fluids, and elimination can further increase fluid loss. Similarly, elimination may be ineffective in extremely cold weather as the body's humours become less active.
8. **Climate and environment:** Elimination is not recommended in extremely hot or cold environments.
9. **Occupation:** In professions where bodily substances metabolize rapidly, such as blacksmiths, elimination is not recommended as they don't have enough substances that can be evacuated.
10. **Habits:** If a person is not accustomed to elimination, they should not be given potent elimination drugs as they may be more used to excreting waste through other means.

Aims and objectives of elimination

Five things should always be considered in every elimination:

1. That madda (substances/matter) which has corrupted in quantity or quality (its kafiyat i.e., hot/cold/dry/moist) should be evacuated.
2. Elimination should be limited according to the patient's tolerance.
3. Elimination should be done as to the type of Madda. For example, when a patient is experiencing nausea, emesis should be performed and if the patient has stomach cramps, purgation should be carried out. But it is not necessary to

follow this in case of complications, as in using emesis which could have the possibility of being harmful to the brain; in such situations, purgation is preferred over emesis.
4. Always evacuate the Madda through its natural route as this route is better for the Tabi'at (medicatrix naturae). If there is any obstruction or inflammation, the route can be modified but only towards the lesser organs. The Madda should never be directed towards the supporting organs as it will result in greater damage. Also, there should be a connection or relation between both the organs; from which the Madda is directed so that they can aid each other in the removal of waste.
5. Before evacuating any substance, it is necessary to concoct it. Nudj (concoction) means to make the Madda ready for expulsion. Therefore, if a Madda is concentrated and sticky, it cannot be expelled unless it has been diluted. However, if it is diluted and thin then it would need to be concentrated so it can be more easily removed.

Instructions for elimination

1. If the matter that is being excreted during a bowel movement is flowing normally and the individual is able to endure the process, there is no reason to be concerned about large amounts of discharge in fact in some cases, the need for elimination is so intense that it may even cause fainting.
2. Physicians often find it easier to remove body wastes that do not accumulate in large quantities in batches instead of evacuating them all at once. For instance, in ascites, where there is a large amount of fluid in the peritoneal cavity, it is not excreted all at once or in a single day. Similarly, if the fluid accumulates in a single place, such as the accumulation of pus in the pleural cavity, elimination is not performed in one go, but in batches, as evacuating it all at once may worsen the condition.
3. In cases where individuals have a high amount of morbid matter (Mavaad) in their bodies and are not physically strong, elimination should be performed gradually. This approach is also recommended when the morbid matter is viscous, mixed with blood, impossible to remove, or has penetrated the cavities of organs, such as in cases of sciatica, arthritis (Waja al-Mafasil), carcinoma (Saratan), chronic flow, and chronic boils.
4. Leaving the potential excretory matter inside the body is not as painful as expelling it out forcefully and to the extent where the physical faculty is exhausted. The Tabi'at (medicatrix naturae) often dissolves the remaining matter itself.
5. Note that morbid matter (Mavaad) in joints is harder to remove than from vessels.
6. After undergoing elimination treatments like taking purgatives (Mushilat), it is not advisable to start a heavy diet. This is because the body's natural healing process (Tabi'at) will digest indigestible foods quickly. However, if necessary, the diet can be gradually increased over time.

Concoction[455] (Nudj)

Nudj[456] (concoction) is obligatory in the treatment of chronic diseases. In acute diseases, it is better to concoct the substance, but if there is a risk of damage to the supporting and vital organs by the Madda (active matter) while waiting for its concoction, then the concoction process should be stopped immediately.

Concoction refers to the process by which the morbid material is made ready to be expelled or evacuated from the body. For this purpose, concentrated humour is converted into dilute and dilute humour is changed into concentrated humour. Thus, Safra (bilious) Madda is changed to a concentrated form, and melancholic (cold and dry) Madda is turned to a dilute form.

Benefits of concoction

The importance of concoction is that it modifies the Mavaad (morbid matter) to allow it to be expelled from the body. For instance, pleurisy (inflammation of the lungs and ribs) requires concoction because the Madda (active matter) cannot be expelled through the mouth until it has undergone concoction.

The need for the concoction

1. Chronic diseases and illnesses that last more than forty days require treatment with a concoction. In some cases of acute diseases, a concoction may also be necessary, particularly if the illness has persisted for more than seven days.
2. In treating phlegmatic and melancholic ailments, it is necessary to administer concoctives before purgatives (Mushilat). It is recommended, but not necessary, to do so for Safra (bilious humour) ailments. For Damawi (blood humour) ailments, it is not required; however, if blood humour has been corrupted by one of the other humours, then that corrupted humour must be concocted from blood. It is important to know which humour type oxidation has produced the abnormal sauda (black bile humour) while treating with concoctives.

Duration for concoction

The duration for concocting each type of humour is as follows:

- Sufra (yellow bile humour) usually takes three days to concoct, while some atypical sufra may take up to five days.
- Diluted balgham (phlegm humour) takes five days to concoct, while concentrated balgham takes twelve days.
- Sauda (black bile humour) requires fifteen to forty days of concoction time.

---

[455] Some sections of this material has has been adapted from Usool-e-tibb by Hakeem Hamdani.
[456] نضج is sometimes written as nuzj (I have retained the original Arabic pronunciation).

- The regulation of Damawi (blood humour) is carried out by Damawi moderators and not through the concoctives.

Signs of concoction

To determine whether the Madda (matter) in the body has matured, one can observe the colour of the urine. When Safra Madda is present, the Madda is considered concocted if the urine turns yellowish. If Sauda Madda is present, the urine should turn blackish to show that the Madda has matured. During the concoction process, if a Balghami and Saudawi substance is present, the urine becomes more concentrated.

The pulse is also an indicator of the maturity of the substance. If the pulse is initially hard (Nabd Sulb), it will become soft (Nabd Layyin) after maturation. On the other hand, if the pulse is initially soft, it will become hard after maturation.

In the same way, if the pulse is initially full (Nabd mumtali), it will become empty (Nabd khali) after the substance matures. However, in cases of melancholic ailments, the pulse is soft during the concoction of the substance (madda).

The principles of Concoctives (Munzijat)

1. Munzijat (Concoctives) are different for each type of humour.
2. The prescription for a concoctive must include drugs specific to the disease being treated. For instance, lavender (Ustokhuddoos) is necessary for head-related conditions like sleep issues, and drugs for arthritis must include Colchicum luteum root (Suranjan).
3. If Madda is present in the joints and nerves, as seen in conditions like hemiplegia, facial palsy, arthritis, or gout, the concoctives should be given for an extended period, and Mushilat (purgatives) may need to be repeated until the Madda is removed.
4. Cold-related head diseases such as hemiplegia and facial palsy require specific filtration along with the Munzijat. After initial purgative therapies have reduced the excess pathological matter, it is recommended to introduce formulations such as Habbe Ayarij and Habbe Shabyar to support further detoxification and enhance neurological recovery. Habbe Ayarij is particularly useful for improving cerebral circulation and aiding in nerve function, while Habbe Shabyar supports overall nerve health and helps manage paralysis.

The concoctives (Munzijat) of each humour, known as Munzijat, are listed below:

Yellow bile humour concoctive (munzij sufra)

1. To prepare the drink, soak 5 Unnab (Zizyphus sativa fruit), 7 grams of Gul Banafsha (Viola odorata flower), 7 grams of gul-e-nilofer (Nymphaea alba flower), 7 grams of Shahtra (Fumaria officinalis herb), 7 grams of Tukhm kasni (chicory seeds), 7 grams of Beikh kasni (Cichorium intybus root), and 7 grams of Gul surkh (Rosa damascena flower) in hot water overnight. In the morning, strain the mixture and mix it with 25 ml of sharbat (syrup) Nilofer syrup or 25 ml of Sikanjbeen[457] (vinegar and honey water) and give it to drink.
2. Or take 7 grams of Gul Banafsha (Viola odorata flower), 7 grams of Gul Surkh (Rosa damascena flower), 7 grams of Nilofer (Nymphaea alba flower), 7 grams of Enabussalab/Mako (Solanum nigrum), 7 grams of Tukhme Khatmi (Althea officinalis seed), 7 grams of Shahtra (Fumaria officinalis herb), 7 grams of Tukhm Kasni (chicory seeds), 5 Unnab (Zizyphus sativa fruit) seeds, and 5 Aloo Bukhara (Prunus domestica fruit - plums). Soak these herbs in hot water overnight. In the morning, strain the mixture and mix it with 50 grams of gulqand-e-aftabi[458] (rose petal jam)[459] or 50 grams Turanjabeen (Tamarix indica) or 50 grams Khamira banafsha and give it to drink.

Phlegm humour concoctive (munzij balgham)

1. To prepare a drink, add 9 seedless raisins (maviiz-e-munaqqaa), 5 grams of fennel seed (Badiyan), 7 grams of peeled liquorice root (Aslussoos muqashshar), 7 grams of Hansraj / Persiyoshan (Adiantum capillus), and 7 grams of figs to boiled water. Mix the ingredients with Gulqand (rose petal jam) and then drink.
2. Or boil 7 grams each of Beikh Badiyan (fennel root), Beikh karafs (Carum roxburghianum root), Beikh izkher (Cymbopogon jwarancusa roots), and Beikh kasni (Cichorium intybus root) along with 7 grams of lavender (Ustokhuddoos - Lavandula stoechas), 9 seedless raisins and 2 figs in water. Strain the mixture and add 25 grams of pure honey before drinking it.

Black bile humour concoctive (munzij sauda)

Soak 5 Unnab (Zizyphus sativa fruit), 7 grams Gaozaban (Borago officinalis flower), 7 grams Shahtra (Fumaria officinalis herb), 7 grams Badranjboya (Melissa parviflora herb), 7 grams lavender (Lavandula stoechas), 9 grams Sapistan (Cordia latifolia fruit), and 7 grams of peeled liquorice root in hot water overnight. In the morning, strain the mixture

---

[457] See the chapter on drugs.
[458] Qulqand: Different kinds of flowers, dry or wet, are mixed with sugar or honey and called gulqand-e-shakri and gulqand-e-asli, respectively. When the gulqand is kept under sunlight, it is called gulqand-e-aftabi; when kept under moonlight, it is called gulqand-e-mehtabi.
[459] Contains barberry, pomegranate seeds, melon seeds, dried rose petals, coriander, poppy seeds, black pepper seeds and sugar - equal weight.

and add 25 grams of rose petal jam (gulkand) or 25 grams of Turanjabeen (Tamarix indica). Mix well and serve as a drink.

Types of mushhilat (purgatives)

A. Purgatives, in terms of severity and mildness, these are as follows:

1. Mild purgative (Mushil-e-khafeef): They increase bowel movement and secretion of moisture and expel thick stools with mild abdominal cramps. Such as Elva (Aloe vera dried juice of leaf), Revand (Rheum palmatum root), Suranjan (Colchicum leutiun root), Senna (Cassia senna leaf), etc.
2. Strong purgative (Mushil-e-Qavi): These result in the discharge of frequent loose motion that may be watery. They include Beikh Jalapa (Exogonium purga, Ipomoea purga root), Jamalgota (Croton tiglium fruit Kherbaq), Rasaut (Berberis aristata extract), Saqmoonia (Convolvulus scammonia root latex), etc.

B. Purgatives, in terms their effects

1. Purgative by softening (Mushil bil Talyin): These drugs help the morbid matter by softening it and reducing water absorption from the intestine, for example, Sheerkhisht (Fraxinus ornus secretion).
2. Purgative by lubrication (Mushil-bil-izlaq): Purgative drugs that lubricate the intestinal tract scatter morbid matter and facilitate the smooth passage of the matter, such as Aloo Bukhara (Prunus domestica fruit - plums), Sapistan (Cordia latifolia fruit), Tukhme Khatmi (Althea officinalis seed) etc.
3. Purgative by cleansing (Mushil-bil-jail): These drugs break down the matter into smaller particles and clear the mucosa of the intestine, such as Boora Armani (Arminium bole), etc.
4. Purgative by the power of evacuation (Mushil-bil-Quwwat Mushila): Those which are purgatives according to their essence (Surat Naw'iyya) and not from the qualities (Temperament). Ghareeqoon (Polyporus officinalis), Saqmoonia (Convolvulus scammonia), etc. Tukhm Hanzal (Citrullus colocynthis seed) and Elva (Aloe vera) have special properties for purifying the brain and nerves, Ghareeqoon (Polyporus officinalis) for expelling phlegm from the lungs and chest, and Suranjan Shirin (Colchicum leutiun root) for joints.
5. Purgative by squeezing (Mushil-bil-aasir): These drugs increase the astringent power of intestines and squeeze the morbid matter out, such as Haleela[460] (Terminalia chebula), Sharbat ward mukarrar, etc.

It is best to take strong purgative medicines with cold water, as the cool temperature can help moderate the intensity of the purgative's effects.

---

[460] Note if the herb is noted as Haleela only, this refers to Haleela zard (Terminalia chebula half-ripe fruit), which is yellow.

C. Purgatives, in terms of their mode of action: Various kinds of purgatives are based on their actions and properties.

1. Some drugs, such as Turbud (Ipomoea turpenthum root), possess dissolving power and morbid matter-diluting abilities in addition to being purgative.
2. Some drugs, such as Haleela (Terminalia chebula), squeeze (stimulate) the intestine and cause defecation and are known as Mushil-bil-aasir.
3. Certain medications act as purgatives and have a resolvent (Mulayyin) effect. An example is Turanjabeen (Tamarix indica).
4. Certain medications can cause the intestinal contents to expand, resulting in their expulsion through defecation. For example, psyllium husk, dried plums (Aloo Bukhara) etc.
5. Some Zulkhasa drugs (those whose mode of action is unknown) are cholagogues, like Saqmoonia (Convolvulus scamony root latex).
6. Some drugs, such as borax salts (Boraqiya Namakiya), cause defecation by breaking down the active substance.
7. Certain drugs can dissolve Mavaad (matter) and eliminate it from the body. One such drug is Turanjabeen (Tamarix indica).
8. Potent purgatives have a toxic action and cause defecation by overriding the body's natural processes. These effects can be countered with anti-toxins.
9. Some purgatives have different tastes and properties that affect their effectiveness. Bitterness and rapid action help dissolve active Mavaad, while lubricating (muzliq) drugs help to swell the substance.

When administering medications, it is important not to combine lubricating drugs and squeezing drugs, as they can have the same effect. It is recommended to give the lubricating drugs first to soften the Mavaad, and then give the squeezing drugs to expel the softened substance. This method should be followed when prescribing all other drugs as well.

Purgation (Ishal)

The uses of purgatives

1. Purgatives are used to eliminate matter-related diseases, such as inflammations caused by matter (madda).
2. Taking a purgative can help reduce body temperature by inducing bowel movements. This, in turn, can help alleviate fever.
3. Purgatives are effective for severe constipation and colic but should not be used for chronic constipation.
4. Purgatives can be used to remove fluids, such as ascites (fluid accumulation in the abdomen).
5. Purgatives can be used to eliminate Balgham (phlegm humour), safra (yellow bile humour) and sauda (black bile humour) from the body.
6. Purgatives can be used to lower blood pressure.

Softening (Talyeen)

Softeners (Mulayyin) and Purgatives (Mushilat):

Softeners (Mulayyin) are designed to expel matter from the stomach and related organs through the intestine, while purgatives (Mushilat) are intended to squeeze and expel matter from the vessels of the stomach, intestine, and nearby organs.

The function of Softeners:

Softeners increases the peristalsis by stimulating the stomach and intestine muscles, which results in softening.

Softeners drugs:

Figs, raisins, Aloo bukhara (Prunus domestica fruit - plums), Sheerkhisht (Fraxinus ornus exudate), Turanjabeen (Tamarix indica), Tamar Hindi (Tamarindus indica fruit pulp), Maghaz faloos Khayarshamber (Cassia fistula pulp), Haleela (Terminalia chebula), Almond Oil, Olive Oil etc.

Uses of Softeners:

They are usually used for severe or chronic constipation.

Contraindications of purgatives:

Administering a purgative to individuals with an extremely hot or cold and dry temperament can be relatively harmful. It can cause harm when there is swelling in the membranes or heaviness or dryness in the intestines. However, the use of a softener is not contraindicated and can be safely used.

Pregnant women should avoid taking purgatives, especially before their fourth month and after their seventh month of pregnancy. It is also contraindicated during menstruation and should be avoided by infants and those who are weak.

If purgatives are required after the age of forty-five. In that case, sticky, viscous type of drugs such as Sheerkhisht (Fraxinus ornus), Tukhme Khatmi (Althea officinalis seed), and Tamar Hindi (Tamarindus indica fruit) should be given.

When to take purgatives:

It is not advisable to take purgatives during extreme heat or cold. Moreover, it should be avoided if there is a risk of Madda (matter) being corrupted or if the risk of stimulation is high due to using purgatives.

The ideal seasons for purgation are spring and autumn. However, it should be avoided during windstorms and rain. Purgatives should be taken early in the morning during summer and spring and two hours after sunrise during winter and autumn.

Additional instructions related to purgatives:

1. If the patient suffers from a fever or a fever-related illness, it is advisable to avoid giving purgatives for at least a week. However, if the condition of the patient is severe and there is a risk to their life, then purgatives can be given on the fifth or sixth day.
2. When treating individuals with dry temperaments, it is recommended to avoid potent purgatives and instead use soft and viscous drugs such as Cassia fistula pulp, Fraxinus ornus, Tamarindus indica fruit, etc.
3. A person who is not accustomed to using purgatives should not be given potent purgatives.
4. Do not administer purgatives to those with indigestion, viscous humours, inflammation, wounds, or membrane obstructions.
5. Purgation is prohibited during severe winters and summers, and emesis is prohibited during Fasd (Venesection) and Kaiyy (cauterization).
6. During the day of purgation, as well as three days before and after, the patient must avoid activities that may lead to dehydration. Such activities include fatigue, sexual intercourse, and any strenuous physical exertion if the patient has a strong nervous illness. In addition, the patient's diet should consist of soft, easily digestible foods.
7. Before giving a purgative to someone with a sensitive stomach, feed them a soft diet like barley water to protect their stomach from yellow bile.
8. It is recommended to wait at least four hours before drinking water after taking purgatives to avoid interfering with the action of the purgatives.
9. The person taking purgatives should keep himself and his stomach warm.
10. If there is a build-up of dry heaviness in the intestines, such as in the case of colic. In that case, it is recommended not to use purgatives until the dry heaviness has been expelled through a Huqna (enema) or Mullein Ama (Laxative) suppository or some other lubricating drug.

Measures to be taken during purgation

The purgative should be taken early in the morning on an empty stomach. If the patient has a hot temperament and a weak stomach, they should be given a pomegranate or a light meal like soup or porridge before the purgative. If the patient feels nauseous due to the unpleasant odour of the purgative, they can try taking it while holding their nose closed. If the taste of the purgative is unpleasant, they can chew on cinnamon or Aqirqarha (Anacylus pyrethrum root) or numb their tongue by putting ice on it. If there is a risk of vomiting while taking the purgative, hold the patient's arms and legs and let them smell fragrances like Sandal (Santalum album wood - sandalwood), Arq Gulab (Rosa damascena aqua – rose water), etc. After taking the Mushilat, chew and suck on pomegranate, mint and Behi (Cydonia oblonga, C. quincy fruit).

Fifteen minutes after administering purgatives, a paste made by mixing Arq Gulab (rose water) and Sandal Safed (sandalwood) is wrapped and placed on the stomach.

If the purgative is in pill form, it can be soaked in honey or sugar, covered with a silver leaf foil, or taken as capsules.

After taking purgatives, it is best to avoid movement for some time to prevent the drug from being expelled through vomiting. Walking is fine after a while, but any intense activity should be avoided. On the other hand, sleeping can help speed up the purgative process. Eating or bathing right after taking a purgative can nullify its effects. A light massage is okay, but avoid intense massages. If there is tenderness after taking the purgative, you can apply butter or rose oil or wash the area where there is tenderness with boiled Khatmi (Althea officinalis).

Managing issues with purgatives

If a person is taking purgatives but is not able to defecate, some measures can be taken to avoid any issues. If the purgatives are causing a delay in bowel movements, you can give them honey water or a mixture of 50 ml of Sharbat Ward Mukarrar and 120 ml of Sharbat Dinar to drink.

If the purgatives are too strong, and the person experiencing this is young and has not passed stool yet, you can give them cold water or Sikanjbeen (vinegar and honey) to sip on slowly. If the person cannot defecate due to their Mizaj being cold or cold weather. In that case, they can be given an equal mixture of Arq Badyan (fennel water) and Arq-e-Gulab (rosewater) to sip or 120 ml of honey water.

If the person still cannot defecate even after trying the above measures and is experiencing symptoms such as pain, headache, dizziness, cramps, syncope, etc., you can mix around 500ml of warm water, 2 grams of salt, and 60 ml of Sikanjbeen and give it to them to drink to induce vomiting. If the purgatives have already reached the intestines, you can give them soap with salt as a Huqna (enema) to prevent the matter from reaching the vital organs. However, avoiding more than two purgations in a day is important to avoid further issues.

Ailments related to purgatives:

If a person experiences cramps after taking purgatives, they can benefit from taking small sips of warm water and walking.

If they feel thirsty, give them lukewarm water, Arq Gulab or Arq Badyan to drink.

If the purgative is too hot, give cold water, sour yoghurt buttermilk or sour pomegranate juice to drink. Similarly, formulas like Jawarish amla, Jawarish anarain, Jawarish bahi, and other astringent medicines should be given. Massage of palms, foot bath, and a bath are also beneficial. And the patient should go to sleep.

If a person has dysentery, give them 7 grams of Khatmi (Althea officinalis) mucilage and 3 grams of Behi (Cydonia oblonga, C. quincy seed) mucilage.

If they get a fever after taking purgatives, a prescription of nuskha tabrid (cold formulas) should be given, which is mentioned below.

Diet after purgation:

It is recommended to follow a specific diet after undergoing purgation. On the day of purgation, it is advised not to consume any food in the morning. In the evening, it is recommended to have moong dal (mung beans) Khichdi[461], yoghurt, rice, broth, etc. If magnesia or other salty purgatives are used, it is recommended that milk and rice be consumed. For purgatives that help in removing phlegm, broth is a good option.

In the case of purgatives containing Jamal Gota, it is recommended to have cold water, milk lassi, and pills that contain turbid, zanjabeel, etc., mixed in cold water.

Similarly, for Mushilat (purgatives) of sheer Zaqqum (Euphorbia antiquorum, milk), it is suggested to consume these with cold water. For Revand Chini (Rheum palmatum root), colocynth seeds, Elva (Aloe vera dried juice of leaf), and Jalapa (Ipomoea purga root), lukewarm water should be consumed after taking these purgatives.

Cooling after purgation:

After a purgation, cooling prescriptions are often given. These prescriptions are called Tabreed. Ancient physicians used to prescribe psyllium husk (Asphaghol - Plantago ovata) for hot temperaments, Tukhme Rehan (Ocymum sanctum) for moderate temperaments, and Tukhme Teratezak (Lepidium sativum Linn) for cold temperaments.

Modern physicians prescribe other cooling drugs after purgation. For instance, Khamira Goazaban wrapped in silver leaf can be eaten, and a mixture of 3 grams of Behi (Cydonia oblonga) and 5 Unnab (Zizyphus sativa fruit) juice in 120 ml of Gaozaban (Borago officinalis) water, mixed with 25 ml of Gul Banafsha (Viola odorata flower) syrup and sprinkled with 7 grams of Tukhme Rehan (Ocymum sanctum) can be consumed.

Some physicians prescribe 5 ml of Sheera Badiyan (fennel seed ground in water), Sheera Unnab (5 pieces of Zizyphus sativa in water), and 25 grams of Gul Banafsha (Viola odorata) syrup as two parts and one-part Murabba Halela (a jam of Haleela - Terminalia chebula) for cold mizaj (temperaments).

What to do after purgation:

After purgation, the patient needs to rest and avoid activities such as yoga, sexual intercourse, and physical exercise for a few days. Mental exertion should also be limited. Additionally, the patient's diet should not include heavy foods for two or three days and

---

[461] rice and lentils dish

should instead consist of easily digestible items such as moong dal (mung beans) Khichdi, chapatti (flatbread), soup, and vegetables.

Purgative prescriptions

Yellow bile purgative - Cholagogue (Mushil-i-Safra):

Habb-e-Mubarak is a pill that is specifically used to expel safra (bile): Grind and sieve 90 grams maghaz Khayarshamber/ Amtalas (Cassia fistula pulp), 18 grams post halela zard[462] (Terminalia chebula - yellow), 18 grams halela kabuli (Terminalia chebula mature), 18 grams halela siyah (Terminalia chebula - black), 18 grams Senna makki (Cassia angustifolia – Abrabian Senna), 18 grams Zarishk (Berberis aristata fruit), Gul Banafsha (Viola odorata flower), 9 grams Kateera (Astragallus gummifera gum) and 5 grams Saqmoonia (Convolvulus scamony root latex), mix it with 25 ml sweet almond oil and some honey to make pills, and wrap them in silver leaf. Prescribe 7-9 Grams.

Joshanda (decoction) Purgative for safra:

These are commonly used to expel safra (yellow bile):

Cover and boil 12 grams Post Turanj (Citrus medica fruit epicarp[463]), 5 pieces halela zard, 15 Aloo bukhara (plums), 20 pieces Sapistan (Cordia latifolia fruit), 9 Shahtra (Fumaria officinalis), Senna makki (Cassia angustifolia – Abrabian Senna), 9 Unnab (Zizyphus sativa fruit), 7 grams Tukhm kasni (chicory seeds), and 7 grams Tukhme Kasoos (Cuscuta reflexa seed) in water and bring to boil then strain and add 25 grams Sheerkhisht (Fraxinus ornus exudate), 50 grams maghaz faloos Khayarshamber (Cassia fistula pulp) and 25 grams Turanjabeen (Tamarix indica), then mix this with 7 ml almond oil and give to drink.

Phlegm Purgative - Phlegmagogue (Mushil-i-Balgham):

Mushil-i-Balgham (Balgham Purgative) pill; 3 grams of Ayarij fiqra, 3 grams Turbud[464] (Ipomoea turpethum), and 3 grams Habb-ul-Neel (pills), powder and knead with water and make one gram size pills. Give 9 grams to 12 grams with lukewarm water in the morning.

Joshanda (decoction) purgative for Balgham:

This decoction removes Balghami (phlegmatic) Mavaad (matter) through stools and is also beneficial for chronic cough.

---

[462] Terminalia chebula Retz - In Unani medicine, three types of berry fruits have been mentioned. These are small-size Halela siyah (black colour), medium-Halela card (yellow colour) and the large size and relatively mature Halela kabuli.
[463] outermost layer
[464] Also written as Turbud Safed/Nisoth

Boil 15 raisins, 15 Unnab (Zizyphus sativa fruit), 15 Sapistan (Cordia latifolia fruit), 9 grams Zoofa khusk (Hyssopus officinalis flowers - dried), 9 grams Gul Banafsha (Viola odorata flowers), 9 grams Hansraj / Persiyoshan (Adiantum capillus), 9 grams Badiyan (Foeniculum vulgare – fennel seed), 9 grams Aslussoos muqashshar (Glycyrrhiza glabra root - liquorice root peeled) and 7 dry figs in one litre water, when this is reduced to half, add 36 grams Maghaz faloos Khayarshamber (Cassia fistula pulp), 36 grams Turanjabeen (Tamarix indica secretion) and 36 grams gulqand (rose petal jam), after cleaning and sieving add 3 ml almond oil and give it to drink.

Black bile purgative - Melanogogue (Mushil-i-Sawda):

Mushil-i- Sawda (Sawdawi Purgative) pill:

Grind and sieve 3 grams of Ayarij fiqra, 4 grams Lajward (Lapislazuli), 4 grams Ghareeqoon (Polyporus officinalis), 4 grams mash safeed (urad dal - white mung bean), 4 grams grams Gugal safeed/ Muqil (Commiphora mukul), 4 grams treated Turbud (Ipomoea turpethum), 4 grams Kateera (Astragallus gummifera gum) and 4 grams halela zard (Terminalia chebula - yellow), then grease with 3 ml sweet almond oil and prepare gram size tablets. Wrap 7 to 9 grams in 3 silver leaves. Classically this is given during the middle of the night with warm water.

50 grams Sheerkhisht (Fraxinus ornus exudate), 50 grams gulqand aftabi (rose petal jam) and 60 grams Maghaz faloos Khayarshamber (Cassia fistula pulp) dissolved in 140-gram sabz Badiyan (Foeniculum vulgare – fennel leaf) and 230 grams sabz kazni (Cichorium intybus green leaf) chicory is added in water and strained. Then mixed with 4 ml almond oil to be taken in the morning.

Diet: Give chickpea water as food in the afternoon.

Purgative powder (Sufuf Mushil):

Commonly used in the removal of Balgham (phlegm humour) and sauda (black bile humour).

Grind and sieve 4 grams Turbud (Ipomoea turpethum), 4 grams halela zard (Terminalia chebula - yellow), 0.5 grams Senna makki (Cassia angustifolia - Arabian Senna), 0.5 grams Zanjabil (Zingiber officinalis rhizome), 1 gram soft Ghareeqoon (Polyporus officinalis), 1 grams Revand chini (Rheum palmatum root), 1 grams Bisfaij (Polypodium vulgare Linn root), 1 grams Ustokhuddoos (Lavandula stoechas - lavender), 1 grams Afteemoon (Cuscuta reflexa), 1 gram buds of rose flowers, 1 grams Kateera (Astragallus gummifera gum) and 70 grams Misri (rock sugar). Powder the herbs and grease with some 7 ml almond oil. Give 7 to 9 grams with warm water.

Ayarij pills as a purgative: Expels all three humours (balgham, safra, sauda) from an ill body.

Grind finely and sieve the following herbs: 5 grams ayarij fikra, 9 grams peeled Turbud (Ipomoea turpenthum root), 1 gram Habb-ul-Neel (pills), 1 gram Anisoon (Pimpinella anisum seed), 1 gram Ghareeqoon (Polyporus officinalis), 1 gram Tukhm Hanzal (Citrullus colocynthis seed), 0.5 grams Simagh Arabi (Acacia arabica), 0.5 grams Kateera (Astragallus gummifera gum), 0.5 gram Gul surkh (Rosa damascena flower), 0.5 grams black salt, 0.5 gram Mastagi (Pistacia lentiscus gum), 5 grams Azaraqi (Strychnos nux-vomica Linn seed). Add Ghareeqoon (Polyporus officinalis), grease it with 9 ml almond oil then make peanut-sized tablets using Aab-e-Muqil (Commiphora mukul water). Give half tablets at night and the rest in the morning on an empty stomach.

Afteemoon (Cuscuta reflexa) pills as a purgative: causes defecation and protects the stomach and vital organs from sauda (black bile humour).

4 grams Saqmoonia (Convolvulus scamony root latex), 7 grams ayarij fiqra, 7 grams Indrain/Hanzal guudaa (Citrullus colocynthis fruit – its pulp), 7 grams Ghareeqoon (Polyporus officinalis), 7 grams Afteemoon (Cuscuta reflexa), 7 grams guggal (Commiphora mukul), 7 grams hajar-e-armani (Lapis armenus stone) and 7 grams Turbud (Ipomoea turpethum) - Grind and sieve these and mix with water and make gram size tablets, prescribe 7 to 9 Grams.

Salateen pills (Habb-us-Salateen) as a purgative: Expels viscous humours from the depths of the body and kills intestinal worms.

9 grams cleaned Jamalgota (Croton tiglium oil), 5 grams Turbud (Ipomoea turpethum), 5 grams Darmana (Artemisia maritima herb), 5 grams Revand Chini (Rheum palmatum root). Mix and grind these herbs and then grease with almond oil and make small black pepper-sized tablets; give 3-5 tablets.

Note: If these pills cause a lot of diarrhoea or loose stools, mix Arq Gulab (Rosa damascena aqua) with cold buttermilk to drink.

Majun Senna as a purgative: Gently helps in defecation, removes fever, stomach and joint issues, and eliminates the excessive matter of each humour. To prepare Majun Senna, you need to include 180 grams of Senna makki (Cassia angustifolia - Arabian Senna), 60 grams of Afteemoon (Cuscuta reflexa), 60 grams of Bisfaij (Polypodium vulgare Linn), 60 grams of Turbud (Ipomoea turpenthum root), and 60 grams of Gul Banafsha (Viola odorata flower). Grind and sift all these herbs and use them as a majun (semi solid paste).

Enema (Huqna)

Enema is a medical procedure in which a liquid medicine or nutriment is injected into the anus through a device. It benefits patients who cannot defecate and when purgation has failed. It can also be useful in constipation, colic, inflammation, and the intestine, kidney, and bladder pain.

The idea of an enema was derived from watching a seagull by Galen. The seagull ate fish near a beach, and when it got stomach pain, it took seawater in its beak and put it in its anus. After a while, the water, along with faeces, came out of the anus, which is why the enema is also known as 'Amal-e-Ta'ir[465].

There are many types of syringes for enema available, but two types of syringes are more commonly used:

1. Rubber syringe: It has a plastic spout about 7 to 10 cm long at one end and a rubber or plastic band at the other end. The middle part of the syringe is round and swollen. To use it, the spout end is lubricated with Vaseline, glycerine, or castor oil and inserted into the anus. The other end is kept in the instrument with the medicine, and the middle part of the syringe is pressed, which expels the air and then fills with water. Similarly, the water or medicine passes to the anus and into the rectum and from there to the colon by repeatedly pressing.

2. Douche syringe: The difference between this and a rubber syringe is that there is a glass or tin can douche with a hole in the bottom from where a 150 to 180-cm-long rubber tube is fitted. The other end of the tube is fitted with an ivory or plastic spout. To use it, the douche can is filled with an enema drug or water and hung on a wall 60 or 90 cm high near the patient's bed. The spout is lubricated by Vaseline or castor oil and inserted into the patient's anus. The water from the douche can pass through the rubber tube into the intestine through the anus.

Enema Procedure:

1. Place a rubber sheet on the patient's bed.
2. Place the patient on the left side and ask them to pull their legs towards the stomach or move them yourself.
3. Lubricate the spout with Vaseline and slowly insert it into the anus.

It is better to rotate it a little while inserting it to prevent injury to the walls of the anus.

Insert at least 5 cm of the spout inside the anus. If the patient's retentive faculty is weak, then press the edges of the anus to prevent expulsion of enema drug or water. When a certain amount of water enters the intestine, remove the empty tube from the anus after a minute or two. At that time, instruct the patient to keep the enema water inside for at least eight to ten minutes and then allow the patient to expel the water. If necessary, the enema can be repeated after 3-4 hours, but if the patient is weak, postpone the procedure to the following day.

---

[465] Tahir – is bird – so act of a bird.

Enema guidelines: :

Please keep in mind the following guidelines for administering an enema:

1. Always perform the enema when the temperature is moderate, neither too hot nor too cold.
2. Use lukewarm water and appropriate oils for enemas before administering the enema.
3. Advise the patient to avoid sneezing, coughing, or hiccups.
4. Administer the enema slowly to prevent premature contraction of the intestines, which could result in the expulsion of the enema water.
5. Use lukewarm water and a drug of moderate consistency for the enema. The volume of water or drug in the enema should be 250-300 ml. This amount can be adjusted for children and other reasons.

Steps during an enema: :

Here are the steps to follow when administering an enema for different conditions:

1. Lay the patient flat for brain-related disorders and place a pillow under their head and neck.
2. For stomach and intestinal pain such as colic, have the patient lie on their knees with their abdomen raised and a pillow under their head and chest.
3. For dysentery, have the patient lie flat with a pillow under their back.
4. The patient should lie flat with a pillow under their head for kidney disease.

Prescriptions for enema

Enema for severe constipation and colic:

Dissolve toilet soap in lukewarm water, add castor oil, and administer as an enema.

Other enemas for constipation:

Mix Arq Gulab soap (which contains Rosa damascena aqua) with lukewarm water to administer the enema.

Other enemas for concoction, constipation and stomach worms:

Mix turpentine oil and olive oil in lukewarm water for the enema.

Nutritive enema:

In cases where a person cannot ingest food through the mouth, such as during unconsciousness or throat disease, it is possible to provide nutrition through an enema. To prepare for this, one can mix either meat/chicken broth (Yakhni), arrowroot (Maranta arundinacea), or eggs mixed with milk and administer 150 to 200 grams every 6 hours through an enema. It is important to use a rubber catheter for the enema and to apply oil on it before inserting it gently up to 12 to 15 cm into the anus. The person should be lying down comfortably during the process.

Laxative enema (Huqna layyina):

Huqna layyina (Laxative enema) is beneficial for individuals with meningitis (Sarsam) and fevers. To make this enema:

1. Combine 12 grams of each of the following: Unnab (Zizyphus sativa fruit), Sapistan (Cordia latifolia fruit), Gul Banafsha (Viola odorata flower), Tukhme Khatmi (Althea officinalis), peeled and slightly brushed Ikleelulmalik (Trigonella foenum-graecum bud), and wheat bran.
2. Add 5 figs and 1.5 litres of water, bring to a boil and let it simmer down to ½ litre.
3. Strain the mixture and add 60 grams of sugar.
4. Add slightly warm 18 grams of Gul Banafsha (Viola odorata flower) oil, almond oil, and 35 grams of sesame oil.
5. Give the enema twice.
6. Add 25 grams of Maghaz faloos Khayarshamber (Cassia fistula pulp) and 12 grams of Senna makki (Cassia angustifolia - Arabian Senna) to make this enema more potent.

Other enemas:

Beneficial in Sarsam Safrawi[466] (bilious meningitis).

Mix 60 grams of barley water, 30 grams of psyllium husk, 30 grams of sweet almond oil, and 30 grams of sweet pumpkin oil together. Shake thoroughly before administering as an enema.

Enemas for dysentery:

Mix a decoction as required of rice with fresh milk, cook until thick, and add gum Arabic. Administer as an enema.

Suppository (shiyaf)

There are two types of suppositories: drug suppositories and cloth suppositories. Suppositories are used for various purposes such as defecation, anti-purification, antiseptic, and to affect adjacent organs like the uterus and bladder. However, suppositories are limited to the rectum, so their effects do not extend beyond that area.

A purgative suppository is used if purgation does not show the desired effect. However, in the case of obstruction of the intestine due to causative colic, suppository purgatives

---

[466] The inflammation of the brain's meninges due to Safra's predominance (yellow bile).

are not given until the obstruction is removed. If the suppository gets expelled from the rectum without causing any effect, another suppository should be given.

Drug suppositories are conical in shape, 2.5 cm long, and weigh only 1-2 grams, which gets absorbed in the rectum. On the other hand, Cloth suppositories are 5 cm long and inserted so that some parts are kept outside, making them easy to remove.

Emesis (Qay)

Humans don't completely digest all the food they eat. The undigested food either gets excreted or remains in the stomach. If the food keeps collecting in the stomach, it can cause damage and sometimes lead to vomiting. According to Hippocrates, vomiting should be done twice a month to maintain good health. Besides cleaning the fluids from the stomach, vomiting is also beneficial in treating kidney, bladder and liver diseases and paralysis.

Vomiting involves the stomach, oesophagus, throat, muscles, and head muscles. The centre of vomiting is located in the medulla oblongata. This is why some people vomit when they see or smell bad things. Occasionally, vomiting can also be caused by the build-up of Balgham (phlegm humour) and Safra (yellow bile humour) or other fluids in the stomach or due to excitation of sensory nerves of the stomach, intestines, liver, kidneys, heart, uterus, or gastrointestinal tract.

Benefits of emesis:

Vomiting clears the stomach, increases appetite, relieves some types of headaches, and improves vision. It creates agility by removing body fatigue. Vomiting is also useful in treating kidney and bladder diseases, jaundice, oedema, gastric ulcer, paralysis, and tremors. Vomiting is sometimes inevitable, such as when something is stuck in the throat or oesophagus, poisoning, spoilage of food, or accumulation of phlegm in the airways, and thus is beneficial in treating shortness of breath, cough, diphtheria, and sore throat.

Overuse of emesis:

Excessive vomiting can cause damage and weaken the stomach, leading to a build-up of waste matter. It can also harm the teeth by increasing the release of waste products, particularly if the matter is sour. In addition, excessive vomiting can be harmful to eyesight and hearing as it may carry waste products to the ears and eyes and sometimes cause tiny vessels to rupture.

Emesis contraindication:

Emesis is prohibited in certain diseases or conditions, including:

1. Hernia

2. Throat swelling

3. Anal discharge

4. Uterine prolapse

5. Weak stomach and intestine

6. Miscarriage/Abortion

7. Haemoptysis or phthisis (sill)

8. Obesity

9. Emaciation

10. Eye and ear diseases

11. Constriction of chest and neck

Emesis requirement:

Performing two consecutive emesis each month can help safeguard health. If the matter has not been completely expelled the first time, it may be expelled the second time. Additionally, waste that has fallen into the stomach during the first emesis may also be cleared. However, it is important not to fix a specific date for emesis so that the medicatrix naturae (Tabi'at) does not become accustomed to emesis during specific days.

Emesis timings:

Summer and spring are the best seasons for emesis if there is no emergency. The afternoon is the best time for emesis as heat also helps with vomiting. However, 8 or 9 a.m. is suitable if the patient prefers early morning. Those with a moist mizaj (temperament) should avoid emesis in the early morning. If emesis is required in chronic diseases with potent drugs, perform it early in the morning.

Emesis guidelines:

A day before emesis, eat soft food like khichdi, and exercise a little to excite the humours.

Before emesis, bandage the abdomen and eyes to prevent eye and intestine damage. Then, give an emetic. If vomiting occurs voluntarily, that is preferable. Otherwise, try to vomit by putting a finger or pigeon feather in the throat. Remember to clean the pigeon's feathers and soak them with rose oil. If this does not cause vomiting, then take a hot bath. This will cause excitation of the matter and then vomiting. Massage of the stomach and the soles of the hands and feet can also help in emesis. The client should be sat upright with the head tilted forward during emesis and gently press their stomach.

Appropriate measures after emesis:

1. After emesis, the patient should rinse their mouth with vinegar mixed with warm water and wash their face with cold water.
2. If the person feels thirsty after emesis, give chicory water or pomegranate syrup mixed in water to drink slowly.
3. Food should not be given soon after emesis. However, it can be taken if the person is feeling very hungry. After emesis, delicate and easily digestible food, such as chicken soup, is best.
4. If emesis is performed because of ingestion of a poisonous substance, then after vomiting, give ghee mixed in milk and then the person should vomit again or give 2 grams Daryai Nariyal (Lodoicea maldivica - sea coconut) boiled in 750 ml milk.

Emesis issues and their treatment:

If someone is experiencing issues with vomiting, several treatments can be tried:

- If an emetic does not work and the person feels anxious, a mixture of 2 grams of salt, 25 ml of almond oil, and half a litre of warm water can be given. This can either cause vomiting or relieve anxiety.
- Massaging the area with warm rose oil or a cloth soaked in warm water may help if the person feels tightness or pain around the rib cage.
- If there is a burning sensation or inflammation in the stomach, a mixture of 12 grams of almonds, 3 grams of lettuce seeds, and 3 grams of cucumber seeds can be ground and dissolved in 250 litres of cow's milk. Add 25 grams of sugar candy (misri) and give the mixture to drink. Chicken soup is also a good option.
- If the person experiences hiccups after vomiting, sips of warm water may help. For severe hiccups, give them barley water to drink.
- If there is excessive vomiting, a mixture of ground cardamom and white mastic gum, mixed with 6 grams of Jawarish Ood Tursh formula, can be given. Sikanjbeen (vinegar and honey-oxymel) in Arq Gulab (Rosa damascena aqua) with ice is also a good option.
- If blood is expelled with vomit, add 3 grams of Sheera Zarshak (Barberries syrup), 3 grams of Sheera beekh Anjabar (Polyganum viviparum root syrup), and 3 grams of Sheera Tukhme Karafs (celery seed syrup) to some water. Strain and add 1 gram of Gile Armani (Arminium bole) and 25 grams of pomegranate syrup to the strained water and give it to drink.
- If there is a risk of blood clotting in the oesophagus and stomach, adding ice to honey water and giving it to drink can help.
- If vomiting is followed by convulsions, tension, tremors, or confusion, the person's hands can be tied from the armpits to the wrists and their legs from the thighs to the ankles. Massaging the stomach with jasmine oil or henna may also help.

Some emetic prescriptions:

1. Mix 12 grams of table salt with warm water and give it to drink.
2. Mix 2 grams of rye powder with warm water and give it to drink.
3. Mix 2 grams of Tukhme Khayaren (cucumber seeds) and karpuza (cantaloupe roots) powder with 125 ml of water and give it to drink.
4. Dissolve 0.01 grams of Tootia (copper sulphate) in 125 ml of water and give it to drink.
5. Soak 6 grams of ground Tukhme Turb (radish seeds), 3 grams of Tukhme Shabit (dill seeds), 3 grams of Tukhme Gandana (shallot seeds), and 3 grams of table salt in water overnight. Strain it in the morning, add 25 grams of honey and give it to drink.
6. Mix 35 ml of Sikanjbeen (with Vinegar and Honey - oxymel) with 70 ml of Aab barg Turb (radish juice) and give it to drink.
7. Boil 3 grams of white Rai Safeed (mustard seeds) and 6 grams of table salt in one litre of water. Then dissolve it in 25 ml of Sikanjbeen and give it to drink.

Emetic Drinks:

1. For treating epilepsy caused by phlegm in the stomach (Sar Meda Balghami), mix 60ml of soy water, 60ml of Aab barg Turb (juice of Raphanus sativa), and 25ml of Sikanjbeen. Give this mixture to the patient to drink.
2. To induce vomiting in asthmatics, boil and strain 12 grams of half-sliced soya beans and 12 grams of half-sliced Tukhme Turb (Rafanus sativus seed). Add 25 grams of pure honey and 2 grams of salt to the mixture. Give this drink to the patient.
3. For inducing vomiting in a patient, clean the feather of a hen, coat it with honey, and sprinkle Rai (Brassica alba seed) powder. Then, tickle the patient's throat until they vomit.

Fasd (Venesection)

Fasd is the procedure of evacuating blood from the body by incising. This is done as a preventative measure to avoid the risk of developing Damawi ailments caused by the corruption of blood. It is also necessary if there is suspicion of blood clotting, contusions, apoplexy, or other accidental incidents.

However, Fasd is contraindicated in cases of chronic constipation, colic, pregnancy, menstruation, hot Mizaj, weak and anaemic individuals, obese people with loose body fats, severe cold and heat weather, fever, patients under the age of fourteen and over sixty without any urgent need, after eating or having sex, and during illness or crises. It is strictly prohibited for those suffering from colic, diarrhoea, sprue (a chronic disease affecting the digestive system), weak stomach and liver, and chronic fevers.

The best time to perform Fasd is in the middle of the lunar month and during late morning times. Fasd in the spring is useful for Damawi ailments.

When deciding on the width of an incision, it is essential to consider the patient's health status. A narrow incision is recommended as a preventive measure for healthy patients. Also, opening a wide incision is unsuitable for weak and lean patients.

In cases where patients need to redirect morbid humours, a narrow incision should also be made. For instance, in conditions such as haemoptysis, epistaxis, and menorrhagia, if there is a need for Fasd to redirect morbid humours, a large quantity of blood should not be evacuated through a single wide incision. Rather, a narrow incision should be opened, and small quantities of blood should be expelled in steps, gradually reducing the amount of blood expelled each time.

However, for patients with thick, corrupted sauda (melancholic) substances in their bodies, a wider incision should be made. In mental health patients, the incision should also be wider.

Although venesection can be carried out on either veins or arteries, arteries are generally not cut during venesection to prevent severe bleeding that could lead to an aneurysm. However, cutting an artery during venesection can be advantageous if the procedure can be safely performed, particularly in cases where arterial venesection is necessary. The most effective approach is to cut the artery closest to the organ experiencing abnormal symptoms. If an excess build-up of blood causes the symptoms, a safe venesection of the nearest artery can significantly benefit the organ.

Rules of Fasd:

1. To prepare for Fasd, you need to locate the correct blood vessels. Once found, tie a bandage around the vessel so that it swells and becomes easier to see. However, do not proceed with Fasd until the swelling has gone down. To reduce the swelling, gently massage the vessel and open it up for Fasd. Waiting until the swelling has reduced before starting the procedure is important.
2. If an artery is accidentally cut during Fasd, immediately open the bandage and try to stop the arterial bleeding. Apply an astringent (qabiz) and haemostatic (habis) powder that has already been prepared, and tie the bandage tightly to stop the bleeding.
3. If someone faints due to a weak heart or excessive bleeding, you should immediately use a feather to induce vomiting, as previously explained. Additionally, splash fresh, cold water or rose water (Rosa damascena aqua) on the person's face, let them smell perfume or camphor (Cinnamomum camphora dried extract), or tie their arms and legs.
4. If the client experiences hiccups, yawning, or nausea after opening the venesection point and their pulse is weak, immediately close it. If there is a risk of nausea, they should try emesis with Sikanjbeen and warm water before having Fasd.
5. If the consistency of the blood is thick and the colour is dark, continue until it becomes clearer.

6. After the procedure, apply a cloth soaked in Rosa damascena aqua (Arq Gulab) on the wound and bandage it or apply antiseptic ointment before bandaging.

Principles of Fasd:

1. It is recommended that the client should not go to bed immediately after Fasd and instead wait for at least six hours.
2. For a few days after Fasd, the client should consume easily digestible food, and the food quantity should be reduced.
   If a fever or other diseases occur due to the excitement of the active substance after fasting. In that case, the Fasd area should be reopened, or other appropriate measures should be taken.

Important veins for fasd

VEIN	LOCATION	DISEASES IN WHICH FASD IS BENEFICIAL
Warid-i-Basaliq (Basilic vein)	Runs along the medial side of the forearm and upper arm, joining the brachial veins near the armpit (axilla). It is located on the ventral aspect of the arm.	Pleurisy, stomach ache, liver pain, liver swelling, spleen swelling, piles, anal swelling, uterus swelling, endometritis. It is useful for cleansing the whole body.
Warid-i-Qifal/sararo (Cephalic vein)	Runs along the lateral side of the forearm and arm. It is prominent near the elbow joint, on the dorsal aspect of the wrist, and continues up to join the axillary vein near the shoulder. It is also called sararo[467] because this point cleans the head and face.	It is useful in head and neck diseases, for example, acute meningitis, earache, conjunctivitis, Ludwig's angina, swelling, etc.
Warid-i-Akhal/Haft Andam[468] (Median cubital vein)	It lies in front of the elbow joint and connects the basilic and cephalic veins. As it drains blood from all over body so it is also called Nahr-ul-Badan	It is useful in head and neck diseases such as melancholy, headache, pleuritis and abdomen diseases.

---

[467] Farsi for head.
[468] the great vein that runs through the arm.

Warid-i-Habl al-Dhira (Accessory cephalic vein)	A branch of the cephalic vein lies on the dorsal aspect of the forearm and joins the cephalic vein near the elbow joint.	It is useful in head and neck diseases.
Warid-i-Ibti (Axillary vein)	The axillary vein is formed by the continuation of the basilic vein and the brachial veins. It lies in the axilla (armpit) and continues towards the subclavian vein.	It is helpful in chest pain, heart pain, and pleurodynia.
Warid-i-Usaylim (Salvatella vein/ third dorsal metacarpal vein)	The salvatella vein, is a superficial vein located on the back of the hand, running from the little finger.	It is helpful in treating liver diseases, spleen swelling, and heart diseases. It improves liver function, alleviates spleen enlargement, and reduces symptoms of heart-related conditions by enhancing blood flow and reducing congestion.
Warid-i-Safin[469]/ Mahfooz rag (Saphenous vein)	Saphenous vein runs along the medial aspect of the leg, is prominent on the ventral aspect of the ankle and divides into branches on the posterior aspect of the leg.	Useful in back pain, kidney swelling, menstrual retention, testes swelling, joint pain and shin swelling.
Warid-i-'Irq al-Nasa (Small saphenous vein)	This vein runs along the back of the leg, from the foot's outer side up to the popliteal vein near the knee. This vein is often twisted and knotted. To perform Fasd, the practitioner identifies the appropriate location along the vein, which can be on the outer side of the heel or in the area above or below the space between the hip and the heel.	Beneficial for sciatica, varicose vein, gout, and giddiness.

Hijama (Cupping therapy)

Hijama, also known as cupping therapy, is a type of regimenal therapy used to divert and remove morbid matter from the blood. In the past, animal horns were used for this therapy, but today, metal or plastic cups and a small suction pump are used to create a vacuum and suction on the body's surface. There are two common types of cupping:

---

[469] Safin means 'the thing which is always safe and preserved' as its easy approach to the vein during Fasd, as no artery is running parallel or along with this vein, which can lead to confusion or inconvenience, thus performing Fasd in this vein is quite safe.

cupping with scarification (Hijama Ma Shart/ Hijama bil shart - wet cupping) and cupping without scarification (Hijama Bila Shart - dry cupping).

Cupping with scarification involves making a slight incision with a scalpel in the required place and then applying a cup to draw the blood out to achieve local evacuation of morbid matter. Cupping without scarification involves placing a cup on the required part of the body and creating a vacuum without incision to divert morbid matter.

In addition to these two methods, fire cupping is another method. In this method, a glass cup is warmed and placed upside down on the required part of the body. This method can also be done with or without an incision.

Rules and Conditions for Cupping:

Cupping should be avoided by people under the age of ten and over sixty. It is not permissible at the beginning and end of the lunar month because of the lack of strong moonlight, which causes moisture and internal body humours to become static. As a result, waste material cannot be expelled easily.

If the intention is to divert the active matter from the supporting organ to the lower organs, it should be done before the presentation of swelling. If an organ has excess matter, Fasd should be performed first, followed by cupping. This is because general matters will be released first via Fasd.

Cupping should be done 1 and 1/2 hours after sunrise in summers and 3 hours after sunrise in winters. Before cupping, patients should be given orange juice, pomegranate, apple juice, or similar juices to avoid passing Safra (bile) and related matter into the stomach.

Patients with concentrated blood should take a warm bath before cupping to dilute the blood and make it easier to expel. It is recommended not to give food to patients immediately after cupping as it may affect the purpose of cupping. However, people with a Safra (yellow bile) temperament can drink milk or pomegranate water after cupping.

Hot, salty, and spicy foods and baths should be avoided after cupping. Obese people should avoid cupping as much as possible.

Cupping Location points and benefits: :

LOCATION	BENEFITS
Top of the head and occiput	Vertigo, prevents premature greying of hairs.
Under the chin	Teeth and throat troubles and head and jaws cleanse.
Nape of neck	It is useful in dysentery, putrid fever, diphtheria.
Calf muscles	Useful for kidney pain, swelling, uterus, provokes menstrual flow.
Lateral side of hip and over the buttocks	Sciatica, gout, piles, inguinal hernia. Draws the humour from the whole body, benefit intestines.
Above anus (around the coccyx)	Useful when gases are formed in the stomach (tabkheer) and rise towards the upper limbs.
Hands and feet	Useful in headache, meningitis, high fever, rising 'vapours' (saoud Bukharat) etc.
Base of spine (between the pelvic bones)	Useful in swelling of the uterus, swelling of anus and swelling of testes, polymenorrhagia (Istihada).
Interscapular region	Haemorrhagic diseases of the chest and sanguineous asthma, haemoptysis[470], shoulder pain, throat pain.
Over the umbilicus	Severe colic, flatulent distension of the abdomen, dysmenorrhoea.
Below breasts	Useful in treating conditions such as heavy menstrual bleeding (Kathrat-i-Hayd) and Lochia (Postpartum Bleeding).
Lower back region (near the kidneys)	Inflammatory masses in upper part of thigh, bladder and uterus, pustules, gout, piles, pruritus of back (renal congestion) and elephantiasis.
Anterior aspect of thigh	Orchitis, boils of thigh and leg.
Posterior aspect of thigh	Inflammatory swellings and boils of buttock.
Over malleoli	Amenorrhoea, gout, sciatica.
In popliteal space	Aneurysm, long standing abscess, septic ulcers of leg and foot.

---

[470] Blood coming from the respiratory tract.

Leech therapy[471] (Irsaal-e-alaq)

According to Ibn Sina and Indian physicians, leeches benefit skin diseases and are better than cupping in removing blood from deeper tissues. Leech therapy treats conditions like scabies, lymphadenopathy, psoriasis, sinusitis, old ulcers, and carcinomas.

Properties of useful leeches:

Not every leech found in ponds is useful for medical purposes. The best leech for medical purposes grows in water, has a lot of algal growth, and contains small frogs. A liverish red leech, which is as small as a rat's tail and has a small head, is useful. However, leeches with shiny stripes like birds on their bodies are not useful, and those that grow in mud and dirty water should also be avoided.

Method of leech application:

To apply a leech, place it in water to observe its speed. Catch the fast ones, clean them with a cloth, and place them on the required part of the body. Before applying the leech, wash the affected area with salt water and rub it until it turns red using your hand or a soft cloth. Then, attach the leech to this part. If the leech does not stick for some reason, rub fuller's earth (Multani mitti) on the affected area to make the leech stick immediately.

Methods of leech detachment:

Leeches drain the local blood, swell, detach and fall off by themselves. If they don't separate on their own, sprinkle a little salt or ash on them and separate them.

After separating the leech, it is useful to suck a little blood from that place through a cup so that the blood collected at the site of the leech bite is expelled and no complication occurs. And if the blood does not clot on its own after removing the leech, sprinkle some haemostatic drugs on it, such as Dammul akhven (Dracaena ombet), Gile armani (Arminium bole), Sang Jarahat (Soap stone), etc.

Diaphoresis/sweating (Ta'riq)

Sweat glands in the skin produce sweat. It helps cool down the body when the temperature rises above normal. The brain generates this impulse and stimulates the sweat glands. Excessive heat affects the temperature centre in the brain and can cause localised and generalised effects. If the body temperature rises, the entire body will sweat, raising the blood temperature and increasing perspiration.

---

[471] Or hirudo therapy.

Aims:

1. Thermolysis (Taqlil-i-Hararat[472]):

Reducing body heat is essential during fevers. Sweating helps lower body temperature and excretes waste from the blood, thereby reducing heat. For this reason, diaphoretics (Muarriqat) are also known as heat reducers (Muqallilat).

2. Blood purification (Tanqiyya-e-khoon/ Tanqiyya-e-dam):

Diaphoresis is used in the following diseases to cleanse the blood from waste material:

a. Expulsion of fluids from the body in Anasarca[473] and Ascites[474].
b. In the case of kidney problems, if waste material is not excreted through the urethra and instead enters the bloodstream, it can cause blood toxicity and life-threatening risks. In such cases, diaphoresis is necessary.
c. When the body swells, it produces toxic material that is eliminated through sweating.
d. Steam therapy with boiled chamomile water can be helpful in cases of severe pain and stiffness due to swelling of the body organs. This causes sweating and reduces both swelling and pain while also assisting in breaking down any morbid substances in the body that may be causing the pain.
e. In chronic skin conditions like vitiligo, skin spots, psoriasis, and others, it is helpful to increase blood circulation and sweating in the skin. An Inkabab/Bhapara (vapour bath) or hammam (bath) is usually used to initiate perspiration. Applying Zimad (external paste) or Tila (oil or liquid medication) immediately after diaphoresis maximises effectiveness. In many skin diseases, diaphoresis is utilised to dissolve the active matter of the skin.
f. In case of a severe cold, sweating is beneficial. However, in the initial stages, it is contra-indicated because it causes the retention of viscous substances (ghaleez Mavaad).
1. Imala[475] Mavaad (matter redirection): Diaphoretics can be used for treating kidney and intestinal diseases by redirecting matter. The blood vessels in the body are interconnected, so when the blood flow to one area increases, it decreases in another area. When the blood flow to the skin is increased through diaphoretics, the blood flow to the mucous membranes of the kidney and intestine decreases, which slows down their functions and provides relief. This technique also helps reduce swelling and congestion in these organs.

---

[472] To lessen the body heat. It is one of the methods of thermoregulation. There are several routes through which body heat is lost, e.g., perspiration/sweating/diuresis, etc.
[473] generalized accumulation of fluid in the interstitial space.
[474] a build-up of fluid in the abdomen.
[475] Diversion of morbid humours from the affected site to the other site or increase in the flow of humours towards a specific site.

g. Nourishment of Skin: Diaphoresis enhances the skin's ability to absorb nutrients and expel waste, thus promoting overall skin health. A diaphoretic bath can significantly aid in this process by stimulating the absorptive faculty (Quwwat Jadhiba)[476], making the skin more receptive to nourishment and detoxification.

Methods of diaphoresis:

There are various ways to cause sweating in the body. One method is by dilating the blood vessels of the skin. This can be achieved by stimulating the nerves with local heat, which can quickly dilate the blood vessels and easily cause sweating. This is why hot fomentation, Vapour baths (Inkabab/Bhapara), baths (hammam), and Sitz baths (Abzan) are all known to cause perspiration.

Another method is through an increase in blood pressure. This can be achieved by taking blood-diluting drinks and water, which can cause sweating.

Perspiration can also be induced by directly stimulating the nerve centres that produce sweat. Camphor (Cinnamomum camphora) is known to cause sweating in this way.

Lastly, reflexively stimulating the sweat-producing centres, as in using hot, spicy foods, can also cause sweating.

There are two ways to induce sweating: natural methods and diaphoretics. Natural methods involve increasing heat externally to relax blood vessels in the skin, increase blood circulation and induce sweat production and excretion. The perspiration rate is also affected by the atmospheric air temperature. For example, when the atmospheric air is dry, the perspiration rate will be low even if external warmth is provided, as in the case of summer. On the other hand, if the atmospheric air is humid, even a little external warmth will increase the perspiration rate, as during the rainy season.

The second method is the use of diaphoretics, which can be taken internally or used in the form of incense or vapour. Medical methods involving diaphoretics include hot foment, poultice, vapour, incense, hot baths (hammams), and Sitz baths (Abzan).

Fomentation:

There are two types of fomentation: dry and wet. Dry fomentation involves using hot water bottles or rubber bags filled with hot water. Wet fomentation requires two towels. The first towel is soaked in hot water and applied to the swelling. When its heat dissipates, the second towel is soaked in hot water and applied.

---

[476] One of the sub-serving powers of Quwwat Ghadhiya (nutritive faculty.) Its function is the absorption of food.

Poultice:

For treating tonsillitis, a poultice is usually made by kneading flaxseed (Linum usitatissimum seed – Alsi) flour with water and heating it. This poultice is then applied externally to the affected area, which leads to sweating and pain relief.

To prepare a vapour bath, a pot of boiling water is covered with a lid that has a hole in the middle. Next, a sheet or a thick cloth is wrapped around the affected organ and positioned over this hole to direct the steam to the affected part. If steam is to be applied to the whole body, the patient must sit on a stool. The opened pot of the vapour bath is placed inside the sheet, covering the body from the neck down. This affects the whole body and causes perspiration.

A prescription of a vapour bath that induces sweating and dissolves the active matter (Mavaad) is as follows:

Add 35 grams each of Baboona (Matricaria chamomilla flower), Ikleelulmalik (Trigonella foenum-graecum bud, Brinjasif (Achillea millefolium) and 18 grams each of Marzanjosh (Origanum majorana), to approximately 10 litres water. Bring to a boil until the volume is reduced by one-third, then use the decoction for the vapour bath.

Incense (Bakhoor):

Incense is made from burning dry herbs. It produces minimal smoke and can help induce sweating and bring smallpox spots to the surface. To use, boil equal amounts of Baboona (Matricaria chamomilla flower), Nakhoona (Carum copticum), Gul Banafsha (Viola odorata flower), Tukhme Khatmi (Althea officinalis), and wheat bran in water. Then, use the mixture for a steam treatment.

Hot bath (Har Hamam):

When excess sweating is required, then a longer bath should be taken, and more air should be used than water. Some patients experience headaches, nervousness and mild weakness from hot baths.

Sitz bath (Abzan):

Sitz bath involves immersing the patient in hot water or a decoction of resolvent and diaphoretic drugs up to the level of shoulders or below the navel.

Herbal formula for a Sitz bath to induce sweating. 18 grams each of the following: Tukhm Katan (Linum usitatissimum i.e., Flaxseed), Tukhme Teratezak[477] (Lepidium sativum seed), Tukhm Gazer (Daucus carota seed – carrot seeds), Tukhme shalgham (Turnip seed), Sudab (Ruta graveolens), Lablab (Hedera helix), Badiyan (Foeniculum

---

[477] Also known as Halim/Halyun in Unani.

vulgare – fennel seed), Barg Karafs (Apium graveolens leaf), Gandana (Allium ascalonicum herb). Plus, one karamkalla (Brassica oleracea - cabbage), 2 ½ onions and 400 grams of olive oil. Boil all of these in around 30 litres of water. Reduce it down to one-third and then strain it. Sit in lukewarm water for 1 hour. Then, wipe the body with a clean cloth and cover it with a warm sheet so the sweat does not evaporate easily. This should be repeated for a maximum of 3 days.

Internal drugs that can induce sweating:

Badiyan (Foeniculum vulgare – fennel seed), Kababchini (Piper cubeba fruit), Pudina Nehri (Mentha aquatica - dried water mint), Cardamom (Elletaria cardamomum seeds), Kalonji (Nigella sativa seed), Brinjasif (Achillea millefolium herb), Anisoon (Pimpinella anisum seed), Tukhm Sudab (Ruta graveolens – seeds), Berg Sudab (Ruta graveolens – leaves), Saffron (Crocus sativus), Black Tea (Camellia sinensis), Black Pepper (Piper nigrum), Blachher[478] (Nardostachys jatamansi root), Shokran (Conium maculatum herb), Kafoor (Cinnamomum camphora dried extract - camphor), Tobacco (Nicotiana tabacum), Affiun (Papaver somniferum), Shor qalmi (Potassium nitrate), Naushader (Ammonium chloride), Kaknaj (Physalis alkekengi - dried fruit), etc.

Increasing The Flow (Idrar[479])

Diuresis (Idrar-i-Bawl)

The primary purpose of diuresis (Idrar-i-Bawl[480]) is to purify urinary substances from the blood. The drugs used for diuresis are called Diuretics (Mudirat).

There are two types of diuretics:

1. **Urine stimulators (i.e., diuretics, Mudirrat-i-Bawl muharrika):**
    These drugs stimulate the structure of the kidneys, which produces more urine. For example, Kababchini (Piper cubeba fruit), Black Pepper (Piper nigrum), Zarareeh (Canthradin), Roghan pudina (Mentha arvensis - mint oil), Roghan Ajwain (Trachyspermum ammi oil), etc.
2. **Cooling medications that increase urine output (Mubarridaat bawl):**
    These drugs increase the fluid component of blood. Therefore, water, soda water, barley water, watermelon water, Shor qalmi (Potassium nitrate), etc., and Khari Namak (alkaline salt) increase urine volume.

Ancient physicians have divided diuretic drugs according to Kayfiyat (four natural properties) as barid (cold), har (hot), and motadil (balanced/normal); among them, cold

---

[478] Also known in Unani as Sumbul-ut-teeb.
[479] The process of increasing the flow of any liquid from body e.g., urine, menstrual blood, saliva, milk etc.
[480] Removal of waste products of the body through urination.

diuretics usually act similarly to refrigerants (mubarrada) and hot diuretics usually act similar to stimulatory (muharrika) diuretics.

Indications/uses of Diuresis:

Diuretics are used in the following conditions:

1. If a matter remains in the vessels after purgation and Fasd and it is necessary to expel it, then diuretics (Mudirrat) should be given.
2. Diuretics play a crucial role in treating kidney and bladder diseases because they help remove toxic materials from the body through urine. Normally, kidneys filter these toxins from the bloodstream and eliminate them. However, in severe cases of kidney disease, diuretics can be harmful to the kidneys. In such instances, waste materials must be expelled from the body using purgatives (Mushilat) and diaphoretics (Muarriqat).
3. If urine output is low in heart and lung disease cases, diuretics are recommended. This is because the relaxation of the heart can cause a decrease in arterial blood pressure, which reduces urine production and increases the risk of oedema. Diuretics are also useful in managing high blood pressure.
4. When heavy substances are produced in the blood due to weak digestion or morbid blood and can produce blood or stones, then diuretics are essential.
5. Diuretics are also used in oedema. Similarly, using diuretics is beneficial when bloody water accumulates in the cavity of the wound with six edges in pleurisy.
6. Diuretics can be used to treat hemiplegia, arthritis (Waja al-Mafasil), and swelling on the convex side of the liver (Waram-e-kabid Muhaddab[481]). Arthritis can be caused by toxic substances usually filtered by the kidneys and eliminated through urine. Therefore, diuretics can have a significant impact on arthritis. Additionally, diuretics can help reduce swelling on the convex side of the liver due to their interaction with the kidney.
7. If the urine is acidic, using cold or saline diuretics like cucumber seeds and Kharkhasak (Tribulus terrestris) is beneficial.

Drinking water while taking diuretics is beneficial, as pure water is also considered a diuretic. Furthermore, keeping the skin cool can enhance the effect of diuretics, while keeping the skin warm can improve the action of diaphoretics.

Examples of Diuretics:

Hot diuretics (Mudirrat Har): Hansraj / Persiyoshan (Adiantum capillus), fennel seeds, Khubbazi (Malva sylvestris seed), Zoofa khushk (Hyssopus officinalis flower - dried), Tukhme Sudab (Ruta graveolens - seeds), Anisoon (Pimpinella anisum seed), Brinjasif (Achillea millefolium herb), Qust e Shireen (Suassurea lappa root), Habbe balsan

---

[481] When liver inflammation is associated with kidney, diaphragm and spleen.

(Balsamodendron opobalsamum fruit), Kalonji (Nigella sativa seed), Ajmod (Apium graveolens), mint, Ajwain Desi (Carum copticum seed), etc.

Cold diuretics (Mudirrat barid): Cucumber seeds, Celery seeds, chicory seeds, Cucumber water, pumpkin water, watermelon water, barley water, Shor qalmi (Potassium nitrate), Sikanjbeen (vinegar and honey – oxymel), etc.

Moderate diuretics (Mudirrat motadil): A combination of hot and cold diuretics can produce a moderate diuretic effect. The combination of chicory seeds and fennel seeds can help regulate urine flow.

Emmenagogic (Idrar-e-haiz[482])

Menstruation is a natural and healthy monthly process in a woman's body. It involves the shedding of the uterus's inner layer, which helps maintain good health. However, if menstruation is reduced or stopped, it can be a sign of an underlying medical condition and can lead to other health problems. In such cases, an emmenagogue (a substance that promotes menstruation) may be necessary.

Emmenagogues help to excrete waste material from the blood, phlegmatic fluids from the uterus and related organs, and toxins in the menstrual blood. They are also useful for cleansing the uterus after childbirth or abortion.

During menstruation, women need to avoid heavy work and exposure to cold temperatures, which can cause retention of menstrual flow. If retention is caused by cold, warm measures like hot sitz baths and emmenagogues can be helpful.

Iron-rich foods and compound formulations such as Sharbat Faulad or Qurs Kushta Khabsul Hadeed should be consumed if menstruation has stopped due to anaemia.

Emmenagogue

Emmenagogues (Mudir haiz) are substances that can stimulate or increase menstrual flow. There are two types of emmenagogues. The first type consists of drugs such as Hing (Ferula asafoetida), Tukhme Karafs (Apium graveolens seed), Habbul Qurtum [483] (Carthamus tinctoria), and Mur (Commiphora myrrh gum), which mildly stimulate the uterus to increase menstrual flow.

The second type of emmenagogues affects the uterus indirectly by affecting the body in other ways. These may include compounds that improve blood flow, such as faulad or Khabsul Hadeed formulations. Some compounds stimulate the nervous system, such as those found in Kuchla (Strychnos nux-vomica seed). Additionally, drugs that cause discomfort in the organs adjacent to the uterus, such as purgatives containing Aloe vera,

---

[482] Increase in Urine flow. For drugs that simulate menses this is known as Mudir Haiz.
[483] also known as Kusum/Safflower.

can stimulate the intestines. This, in turn, may stimulate the uterus and increase menstruation.

Emmenogogic (Mudir-e-haiz) drugs:

Persiyoshan (Adiantum capillus), Post Amaltas (Cassia fistula fruit epicarp), Abhal (Juniperus communis fruit), Asaroon (Valerina wallichii), Tukhme Gajar (Daucus carota seed), Anisoon (Pimpinella anisum seed), Brinjasif (Achillea millefolium herb), Baboona (Matricaria Chamomilla flower), Tukhme Khayaren (Cucumis sativa seed – cucumber seeds), Tukhme Kharpaza (Cucumis melo seed), Habbul Qurtum (Carthamus tinctoria – seeds), Kharkhasak khurd [484] (Tribulus terrestris), Kharkhasak kalan (Pedalium murex[485]), Tukhm Sudab (Ruta graveolens – seeds), peppermint, Ajwain Desi (Carum copticum seed), Tukhme Karafs (Apium graveolens seed), Kababchini (Piper cubeba fruit), Mur (Commiphora myrrh gum), Kaknaj (Physalis alkekengi - dried fruit, marzanjosh (Origanum majorana), Castorium (Castor beaver secretion), saffron, Elva (Aloe vera dried juice of leaf), Afsanteen (Artemisia absynthium herb).

Galactagogic (Idrar-e-laban)

Galactagogic is an essential process for lactation, especially when the breast milk supply is deficient. Galactagogues are used in two ways: either by stimulating the breasts and increasing milk production, such as Anisoon (Pimpinella anisum seed), Shabbit (Anthium sowa), Sarson (Brassica nigra), etc. or by improving the quality of the blood and thus increasing milk production, such as nuts and seeds, Faulad (processed iron powder), etc.

Some foods that increase milk production include nuts, seeds, anise seeds, Anisoon (Pimpinella anisum seed), Musli siyah (Curculigo orchioides), Musli safed (Chlorophytum Borivilianum), Sataver (Asparagus racemosus root), Samagh Arabi[486] (Acacia arabica), Kunjud safed (Sesamum indicum – white sesame seeds), etc.

Expectoration

Expectoration (Naffeeth) is eliminating phlegm from the lungs in thoracic diseases. Expectorants, are drugs that aid in the expulsion of phlegm. They belong to different categories based on their varying qualities and are prescribed based on the individual case.

Stimulatory expectorants:

Stimulatory expectorants **(muharrika)** are used in lung diseases where respiration is impaired and the lungs cannot expel phlegm due to weakness. This is usually seen in chronic catarrh caused by irritation of vessels. In the case of acute diseases, such as Nazla

---

[484] also known as Gokhru khurd or 'small' Gokhru.
[485] also known as Gokhru kalan or 'big' Gokhuru.
[486] Also known as Babool, Kikar, Gomadar.

Haar[487] (a cold that is hot in nature), calming (masakkin) drugs like a decoction of 3 grams of Behi (Cydonia oblonga, quincy seed), 5 grains of Unnab (Zizyphus sativa fruit), and 9 grains of Sapistan (Cordia latifolia fruit) are given.

Use camphor compounds and Afiun (Papaver somniferum latex) with caution during peak illness when the patient is not weak.

If the phlegm is thick and scant, and little comes out, as in Nazla barid (A cold that is cold in nature), then for the tanqiya (elimination) of phlegm, a decoction of 7 grams of Gul Banafsha (Viola odorata flower), 5 grains of Unnab (Zizyphus sativa fruit), 9 grains of Sapistan (Cordia latifolia fruit), 7 grams of Tukhme Khatmi (Althea officinalis), and 5 grams of Gaozaban (Borago officinalis) is used.

If the phlegm is too thin, the severity and temperature are high, and there is a need to thicken the phlegm, a decoction of 3 grams of Behi (Cydonia oblonga, quince seed), 5 grains of Unnab (Zizyphus sativa fruit), and 9 grains of Sapistan (Cordia latifolia fruit) prepared with sheera maghaz kadu (sweet pumpkin seed syrup) can be used. This can also help reduce the weakness in the brain associated with catarrh.

Antispasmodic expectorant:

Antispasmodic (Tashanuj) expectorants are used to relieve airway spasms and narrowing, as seen in conditions like whooping cough or pertussis.

Emetic expectorant:

In some cases, emetic (Muqi) drugs can cause vomiting, which may exert pressure on the lungs and airways. This can also help to expel phlegm from the airways. This technique is often used with children who cannot expel phlegm through the mouth. When phlegm enters the mouth and throat during a cough, they tend to swallow it into their stomach.

Effect of heat on expectoration:

In catarrhal diseases, cold can usually cause harm, while heat is often found to be beneficial. As a result, medications for catarrh are recommended to be taken as a hot decoction. It is also important to keep the patient's bed warm, especially in winter, and a hot compress on the chest can be applied for the same purpose.

In case of weakness, it is necessary to use stimulants and tonics for catarrhal diseases. For this reason, the Khamira Gaozaban formula is often preferred in prescriptions.

---

[487] Nazla can be classified as hot (Nazla Haar - such as rhinitis in hot seasons), cold (Nazla Barid), or epidemic-like influenzas.

Reflex irritative cough

Reflex irritative cough is a type of cough that occurs due to nervous excitation and irritation. This cough is usually dry, so little or no phlegm is expelled. It can be so painful that the physician may need to give compounds of opium, such as the preparation Barshasha. Various factors, including liver, spleen, oesophagus, throat, larynx, trachea irritation, and nervous excitation of the lungs, can cause this type of cough. Therefore, in such cases, nervous excitation should be treated first through careful administration of opium compounds, as they can cause irregular breathing.

Shallow breathing:

When suffering from respiratory diseases, shallow breathing can cause pain and difficulty breathing. To help alleviate these symptoms, it is recommended to use powerful and stimulating expectorants that can reduce irritation in the respiratory tract and increase the expulsion of phlegm. Some examples of such expectorants include Aslussoos (Glycyrrhiza glabra root) and Kuchla (Strychnos nux-vomica seed), and opium-based medicines, etc.

Redirection of matter

Redirection (Imala) refers to diversion of morbid matter or humour from one part of the body to another or an increase in the flow of humours towards a specific site.

Aims and objectives of Redirection:

Sometimes, when we need to alleviate pain or inflammation, reduce nervous tension or irritation, strengthen the body's natural healing powers, dissolve inflammations, tumours, and glands, or absorb moisture or substances, we may need to redirect a matter from one organ to another. This process is called Redirection.

Adjacent and distant redirection

Blood and matter can be redirected to an adjacent or distant organ. For instance, when a patient is bleeding through the mouth, two treatment options are available. One is to divert and expel the matter towards the opposite direction. If the flow of matter is redirected towards the nose by causing epistaxis (nosebleed), it can stop the bleeding from the mouth. Similarly, the bleeding in piles will cease if the matter is diverted to the uterus through emmenagogic methods.

Regarding distant redirection, bloodletting from the male's lower body and the female's upper body can cease bleeding, which is a form of distant redirection.

In some medical cases, distant redirection is more appropriate than adjacent redirection. For example, in meningitis, elimination is more favourable. At other times, adjacent redirection is preferable, such as when a zimad laazi (a poultice with irritant herbs, i.e., 10g each of Triphala powder and Manjistha, and 5 grams each of Sandalwood, Bark of Babool and Henna powdered) is applied on the forehead for headaches or a zimad is applied over the location of the liver in liver inflammation. Sometimes, both adjacent and distant redirection can be used, as in the case of apoplexy, where errhines (drugs that cause sneezing) and enemas (Huqnayat) can be applied.

When madda (matter) has to be absorbed in the distant opposite direction, it is best that the two organs are not on the same side. For example, if the matter is in the right upper body, it is better to divert and absorb the matter in the right lower body than to absorb it in the left upper body.

Redirection rules:

1. Madda (matter) should not be in a place where it is easily excreted before it can be redirected for absorption.

2. If there is a risk of harm in diverting the madda towards a natural outlet, then it should be diverted to the other side.

3. If there is a risk of activating harmful mavaad (substances) that remain after expulsion of morbid matter through, for example, Fasd, etc., then redirection should be avoided.

4. The madda should not be diverted towards any supporting organ or organ that does not have the strength to bear this substance.

5. If there is a risk that the madda can cause crises in any organ while passing through it, then redirection should be avoided.

6. The organ towards which mavaad is being diverted must not have any pre-existing substance.

7. The primary absorptive organ should not contain more mavaad than its ability to absorb it to prevent crises after absorbing a large amount of substance.

8. The relationship between the primary and secondary absorptive organs should be considered during redirection to ensure easy absorption of the madda through nerves and vessels.

When redirecting or absorbing morbid matter, careful consideration should be given to its direction. It should be diverted to the opposite side from its original direction.

Types of redirection:

There are two types:

A. Redirection with elimination:

Redirection with elimination (Imala Istifragh) involves redirecting matter (mavaad) by eliminating it through various methods, such as:

1. Purgative (Mushil): Redirecting matter through the use of purgatives, directing the matter towards the intestines for elimination.
2. Diuresis (Idrar): Redirecting matter through diuretic methods, directing the matter towards the kidneys and bladder for elimination.
3. Diaphoresis (Ta'riq): Redirecting matter through inducing sweating, directing the matter towards the skin for elimination.
4. Emmenagogues (Idrar Haiz): Redirecting matter through the use of emmenagogues, directing the matter towards the uterus for elimination.
5. Ulceration (Taqarruh): Redirecting matter by creating or utilising an ulcer, directing the matter towards the site of the ulcer.

Sometimes, purgation is used to redirect matter within the body. For example, to stop uterine bleeding, fasd (venesection) of the basilic vein is performed. Similarly, excessive vomiting can be managed by inducing the elimination of stools, or excess stool elimination can be controlled by inducing vomiting.

B. Redirection without elimination:

Redirection without elimination (Imala bil Istifragh) involves redirecting matter without eliminating it. This can be done through various methods, such as:

1. By the use of astringent medicines, the mavaad (matter) is redirected towards the location of the site of inflammation.
2. With the use of Errhine (sneezing drugs), matter is directed towards the nose.
3. By causing swelling, the matter is directed towards the site of inflammation.
4. The process of redirecting matter can be accomplished by inducing pain (Ilam[488]) at a specific location. This induces an injury, which then attracts matter to that location.
5. By using cupping without scarification, matter can be directed towards the cupping site.

---

[488] To simulate the nerves, sometimes pain is induced by pressing or tying the organ or cupping the organ, etc.

Conditions in which redirection is helpful:

1. For calming and relief when there is inflammation. For example, using camphor (Cinnamomum camphora), mint, etc., produces internal and external inflammation, which causes redirection of matter and relief from internal pain.
2. In cases of swelling or inflammation, using escharotic[489] (Kawiya[490]) drugs can resolve swelling. Applying leech and superficial lancing is also favourable for the redirection of the substance.
3. Potent purgatives and enemas are used in inflammation of the brain's membranes, and Fasd is done to expel the blood, which causes redirection of the matter and provides relief.
4. Kawiya drugs and mumammir[491] (rubefacient) are applied to the skin to resolve the inflammation of glands and tumours - these drugs redirect and absorb any matter.
5. In order to stop elimination (Istifragh), for example, to stop idrar (the flow of any liquid from the body, e.g., urine), or to stop diaphoresis (Ta'riq) or emesis (Qay). In this case, one method of redirecting matter is purgation (Ishal).

Cauterization (Kaiyy)

Cauterization is a procedure that involves burning with heated metals, known as actual cautery (Kayy bi'l Nar). It can also be performed using escharotic drugs like boraqiya (compounds containing borax, such as sodium borate) until a vesicle filled with pus is formed. This method is called cauterization with drugs that are caustics (Kaiyy bi'l adviya). Cauterization is used to prevent the spread of diseases from affected organs to healthy ones, strengthen organs, dissolve waste products in organ structures, stop haemorrhage and the flow of fluids and catarrh, and expel putrid flesh. For example, if someone is experiencing hip pain, cauterization at the hip can help strengthen the affected organ.

The following are some principles to keep in mind when performing cauterisation:

1. When selecting a tool for cauterisation, a tool made of gold[492] is the best choice.
2. The person performing cauterisation should aim to limit the procedure to the muscle only and avoid affecting the nerves and vessels.
3. When cauterisation is used to stop haemorrhage, it should be potent enough to create a thick clot.
4. If a diseased muscle is being cauterised, the boundaries of the muscle should be taken into consideration.

---

[489] Drugs that usually remove skin or superficial growths like warts, leaving them to slough off.
[490] Singler - Kawi - An agent which destroys the surface of the tissue/ skin/organ.
[491] These drugs dilate the blood vessels and improve local circulation, due to which there is redness of the skin.
[492] cauterant, made up of gold for the purpose of cauterisation. It is used especially for curative or treatment purposes.

5. When cauterising bone and muscle, the process should continue until all the organs to the bone are cauterised, as done in corrosive and putrid ulcers. However, if cauterisation is only done in soft organs, it should not be done deeply.

Pain management

Pain induction

Pain induction (Ilam) is a treatment method that involves stimulating the nerves by inducing pain or irritation. This method uses stimulants (muharrik) and vasodilators (mufattihat) to increase blood circulation and dilate the vessels, which in turn stimulates the nerves.

Types of Pain induction:

Various types of pain induction techniques are used for different purposes. These techniques include massaging, squeezing, cauterizing, ulcerating an organ, attaching a leech, or superficial lancing. These techniques can be used for different reasons, such as dissolving inflammation, relieving pain, or arousing the medicatrix naturae (Tabi'at).

Philosophy for stimulating the Tabi'at (medicatrix naturae):

When a person experiences syncope or is under the influence of opium, their heart and lung movements may decrease. In such cases, pain induction is used to stimulate these movements. This is done by applying cold or hot water to the face, using mustard paste on the skin, or other vascular escharotics and irritants. These measures increase blood circulation and the nerves' motor faculties, improving function. The skin is irritated, excited, and injured by these measures, stimulating the brain and increasing reflexive movements, allowing the patient to regain consciousness.

Pain relief

To alleviate pain (Taskin e waja[493]), one must address the underlying causes (asbab) of the pain. This is why pain relievers (Musakkin-i-waja[494]) are categorized into three types: moderate (mutadil), matter resolvent (mavaad mulayyin), and anaesthetic (mukhaddir). The first two types relieve pain by addressing imbalances in temperament (Su-e-Mizaj[495]) and discontinuity (tafarruq-i-ittisal[496]), while the third type directly affects the sensory nerves and numbs them to relieve pain.

---

[493] Also known as Taskin Al-Waja (To relieve the Pain) Taskin-i-Dard. Pain is relieved in three ways: 1. By using narcotic drugs, e.g., opium; 2. Changing the temperament of the site of pain, e.g., cold fomentation 3. By acting directly on the cause of pain.
[494] Also known as Musakkin-i-Alam – Alam is pain, Musakkin is a relief.
[495] Also known as Mizaj Ghayr Mutadil. It is an imbalanced temperament and the main cause of disease in Unani medicine.
[496] The breach in the continuity of tissue.

Relaxation:

Relaxation (Irkha) can help relieve pain. To achieve this, relaxants (Murkhiyat) are used along with resolvents (Mulayyin). Together, they gradually dissolve any substance or matter (mavaad). Examples of these relaxants include Tukhme katan (linseed), Ikleelulmalik (Trigonella foenum-graecum bud), Baboona (Anthemis nobilis), Tukhme Karafs (Apium graveolens seed), Tukhme Khatmi (Althea officinalis), saffron, and various oils.

Emollients (Murakhkhiat) loosen muscle fibres, which helps reduce tension and dissolve any remaining matter (mavaad). This, in turn, helps alleviate pain. Zimad or external paste and foment are other measures that can help relieve pain. They create heat and increase moisture, which leads to relaxation.

Purgatives and relaxants may be potent or weak, and hot or cold. They are included in emollients and resolvents because they help expel the matter causing pain and facilitate the dissolution of any residual matter that remains after the initial expulsion. This, in turn, helps to relieve pain.

Pain management and conflict of drug action and treatment:

Pain management presents a complex challenge for physicians due to potential conflicts arising from drug action and treatment. Pain-relieving drugs may either have a slow onset of action, causing the patient undue suffering before relief is provided, or they may be fast-acting but have the potential to cause harm. For example, administering anaesthetic drugs during colic can lead to increased air retention and lung obstruction.

In this context, Ibn Sina suggests that physicians must carefully weigh the benefits of eliminating the source of pain against those of providing anaesthesia to relieve the patient's suffering. In such circumstances, physicians must evaluate the duration and severity of the pain and consider the risks associated with anaesthesia. Ultimately, the physician must prioritize the course of action that will most benefit the patient.

Given the complexity of the decision, physicians must exercise sound clinical judgment, carefully assessing the patient's medical history, current health status, and other relevant factors. The physician must also be mindful of the ethical considerations associated with administering pain relief and anaesthesia, ensuring that the benefit to the patient outweighs the potential risks.

Sedatives

Sedative (Tanwim) is a medication that can help with sleep. It is effective in relieving pain and numbness caused by pain (Takhdir).

Principles:

It is important first to identify and address the underlying causes of wakefulness. This could include pain, indigestion, fever, excessive anxiety, or other mental illnesses. If sleep issues are minor, then mild measures can be adopted to induce sleep, such as making the bedroom comfortable and dark, avoiding strong winds, washing the feet with warm water, massaging palms and soles, silently counting to a hundred, and listening to or reading uninteresting stories or books.

Use of sleep-inducing drugs:

If the above measures don't help, sleep-inducing drugs can be used. However, these drugs are often anaesthetic and toxic and should be used with caution in small doses. Initially, try using lettuce and poppy seeds, and if they don't work, then Afiun (Papaver somniferum latex) and its compounds can be used.

Treatment of Swellings

There are various types of Awram (swellings), such as Waram Harr (hot swelling) and Waram Barid (cold swelling). These swellings can be infective, soft, or hard.

Hot swelling (Waram Harr):

Waram Harr, commonly known as inflammation, can occur either as a simple inflammation without infection or as an inflammation accompanied by infection.

To effectively treat Waram Harr and swelling, it's important to address and fix their underlying causes. To relieve the swollen area, it's recommended to apply a splint. Swelling is a form of discontinuity, which essentially means it's a type of wound. Therefore, rest is crucial for the wound to heal. To alleviate pain and stress, it's important to reduce congestion and the accumulation of fluids.

For this purpose, the malfunctioning organ must be supported, blood must be expelled, or cold compresses can be used to reduce the swelling.

If the swelling occurs in an organ responsible for discharging vital matter, such as the lymph nodes near the ear that drain waste products from the brain or the inguinal lymph nodes near the thigh that drain waste from the liver and lower abdomen, then resolvents should not be used. According to Ibn Sina, using resolvents in such cases can result in the matter diverting towards the vital organ, which poses a risk. Therefore, we prioritise the importance of vital organs over the harm to the less vital organs and instead use drawing and absorptive pastes.

Heat can be very helpful in reducing swelling, and when combined with moisture, it can produce relaxation, which helps to reduce stress and pain. Relaxation can also be beneficial as it dilates the vessels, particularly the lymphatic vessels, which are responsible for absorbing and transporting fluids, and increases the function of the inflamed organ.

Different methods of using heat include wet fomentation (Takmeed ratab) and Harr zimad (hot paste). For example, Zimad Alsi (flaxseed paste) or a warm compress soaked in a hot herbal decoction[497] can be applied over the swollen part of the body.

Small cakes made from Urad bean flour can be placed on the area, or a dry fomentation (Takmeed ratab), such as a warm flatbread (roti), can be used on the swollen area.

Management of Infected Swelling

The principal objective in managing infected swelling is to eliminate the infection and destroy the infectious agent. The following methods are employed to accomplish these objectives:

External measures, appropriate medication, and diet should be utilised to enhance the natural constituents of the blood. This is because blood contains natural disinfectants and can neutralize toxins.

To promote healing, a method that coagulates blood at the site of swelling is applied to ensure fresh blood flow; such as applying a cold compress or using astringent herbal pastes (like those made from alum or witch hazel) can help coagulate blood. Therefore, it is essential to eliminate the cause of the infection as much as possible. For example, if an organism is the source of the infection, it should be treated accordingly. The swollen part should be kept in a comfortable and relaxed position to prevent the spread of toxins due to movement.

The swollen area should be elevated to empty the absorptive vessels; however, this should not be done for an extended period as it may impair its function. An incision is made to reduce the congestion of fluids, and a cloth bandage is applied to absorb excess fluid. Vasodilator (Mufattih-i-Uruq) drugs and measures are applied. When pus is observed, irrigation and injectable drugs should be used to eliminate infected matter that is decaying and destroying structures.

To enhance fresh blood flow, hot irrigation and paste should be applied, and the wound should be sterilized and bandaged to prevent external infections.

General treatment of hot swellings

General treatment of hot swelling includes measures to improve the patient's overall health and strength, which vary based on the severity of the condition and the patient's health status.

If the patient is strong, their blood pressure would be high. If the pulse is full (Nabd Mumtali) and large (Nabd Azim), then measures should be taken to reduce the blood

---

[497] such as: 10 grams of flaxseeds, fenugreek seeds, chamomile flowers, and marshmallow root, with 5 grams of liquorice root, fennel seeds, and ginger root in 1 litre of water.

pressure. These measures include diaphoresis (Ta'riq), which increases the function of the skin; purgation (Ishal), which increases the function of the intestines; diuresis (Idrar), which increases the function of kidneys; and venesection (Fasd), which reduces congestion and distention of the vessels.

In addition to these measures, plain and easily digestible food should be given. However, if the patient is weak, then a good diet and care should be given. Stimulants (Muharrikat) and tonics (Muqavviat) should be used, and weak diuretics (Mudiraat) and purgatives (Mushilaat) should be given.

Infectious diseases are often accompanied by a slight fever, which can be beneficial, contrary to popular belief. This is because the elevated temperature helps to eliminate toxic substances from the body, which can aid in the recovery process. However, it is important to note that this fever should not be too high, as excessively high temperatures may adversely affect the body.

Furthermore, it is recommended that refrigerants (Mubarridat), should not be used when the body temperature is very high. This is because refrigerants can have a negative impact on the body's ability to regulate its temperature. As such, it is recommended that alternative methods be employed to manage high body temperatures in cases where refrigerants are not suitable.

Where internal swelling is accompanied by congestion, two forms are distinguishable: one arising within an organ that serves as a discharge site for vital fluids and the other within an organ that does not. In the latter case, the initial use of resolvent (Muhallil) and diaphoretic agents is not recommended; instead, the priority is to treat the discharge organ responsible for the swelling. Should the discharge organ remain unknown, the entire body should be treated with purgation, diaphoresis, Fasd, and the like. If congestion throughout the body is the cause of the swelling, astringent and divertive (Radi) drugs should follow treatment.

As the swelling progresses, the amount of astringent and divertive medications should be reduced while the use of resolvent drugs should be increased. In the final stages, resolvent and deobstruent medications should be given. During the degeneration stage, resolvent and relaxant medications should be used.

If an external factor causes the swelling without any congestion of fluids, it is beneficial to use relaxants, resolvents, and diversion from the start. Patients with external swelling should only be given a soft and nutritious diet, especially if they have a fever and swelling.

Pus forms in purulent swellings and may be discharged spontaneously by applying flaxseed paste or an incision.

Outcome of swelling:

Swelling can have any one of the following outcomes:

1. Resolution (Tahlil): The swelling resolves by maturing and disintegration.

2. Pus formation (Taqayyuh): Pus forms in the swelling.

3. Hardening (Tahajjur): The swelling hardens.

Two ways to identify pus are:

1. If the affected area feels soft and easily compressible, it indicates pus formation. In some cases, even the layers of pus can be felt upon touching.

2. If the swelling has a white or whitish colour when inspected, it indicates pus formation. However, if the pus is deep, this condition will not be applicable.

Cold swelling (Waram Barid):

Cold swelling, also known as Chronic swelling, occurs due to the accumulation of thin morbid matter (Mavaad) at the site of inflammation. This type of swelling typically lacks the heat and redness characteristic of hot swelling and is often accompanied by coldness, pallor, and firmness. Chronic swelling persists for an extended period.

Unlike hot swelling, chronic swelling can appear dark or black, which is why scholars refer to it as black bile (Sawdawiyya) due to its blackish appearance. This type of swelling is caused by the accumulation of black matter at the site of inflammation, leading to slow changes and a prolonged course.

Principles of treatment of cold swelling

Cold swelling poses a more arduous and prolonged treatment process than hot swelling, resulting from a long-standing corruption in the Khilt (humour) and mizaj (temperament). The principles of treatment entail several key considerations:

Firstly, identifying and resolving the underlying causes of the swelling are paramount.

Secondly, relaxation of the affected organ is necessary. For joint swelling, restricting movement through the application of a splint is recommended. Slowing down the function of swollen glands and preventing irritation and excitation of sensory organs is also advised.

Thirdly, redirecting morbid matter through irritant drugs (Laaze[498]) is a viable option. Different types of redirection methods include massage, heating (Musakhkhin[499]) drugs, producing blood accumulation (Imtila Damawi) in an opposite organ, expectoration

---

[498] Laaze / Muhayyij (Irritant): These substances produce skin irritation and increase blood circulation. All Hakkak are Laaze. Hakkak (Irritant): These substances cause itching. They are hot and irritant, drawing irritant matter towards the skin and producing irritation. Examples include Konch ki phali (Mucuna pruriens fruit), Barg Bhindi (Abelmoschus esculentus leaf), and Utangan (Blepharis edulis seed). Nettle leaf has a similar effect.

[499] All those drugs, which increase body temperature.

(Tanaffus), ulceration through caustic (Akkal) drugs, suture tied onto the skin by a needle that prevents healing, or cauterization.

Fourthly, applying pressure on the affected organ can halt the exudation of fluid filtration. This can be achieved by applying a bandage or support to the diseased organ.

Fifthly, artificial congestion can be created through hot irrigation (Nutool[500]), massage, or exercise.

Sixthly, general body treatment through blood purifiers is a viable option.

Finally, in some instances, surgical intervention may be necessary.

Hard swellings (Waram Salabah)

If a solidified swelling has advanced beyond its initial stages, it necessitates treatment with resolvents and relaxants. These substances aid in the reduction of the heat and dryness of the swelling, thereby preventing the thick part from undergoing excessive decomposition and preparing the entirety of the swelling for decomposition. Subsequently, stronger decomposition follows. Once the components are receptive to dissolution, the potencies of the resolvents may be increased. If a possibility arises for the remaining portion to harden, it is imperative to soften it again and repeat the routine until total disappearance is achieved between softening and decomposition. This method will facilitate timely and effective resolution of the swelling, thereby averting further complications.

Transudative swellings (Waram Rikhw)

Chronic swelling can encompass transudative swellings[501], which may not manifest symptoms such as erythema, burning, warmth, and pain. These types of swellings result from sluggish blood flow and occlusion in the vessel. When blood flow is impeded in a specific area, the veins and capillaries become engorged, and the structures are abnormally infused with the serum of swelling, leading to an augmentation in the volume of the affected organ.

The principles of treatment for transudative swelling are as follows

Firstly, the real cause of the swelling, which is the obstruction in the vessel and flow of blood, should be eliminated. Additionally, the serum in the structure of the swollen organ must be dissolved and absorbed. The obstruction of vessels is usually caused by liver and kidney diseases such as liver swelling (Waram al-Kabid, i.e., hepatitis) or inflammation of the liver due to the predominance of yellow bile (Waram al-Kabid Safrawi - bilious hepatitis). Hence, these underlying diseases should be treated accordingly. If the cause of the pressure is a tumour or cyst, then treatment should be focused on it.

---

[500] Saline water or any liquid containing medicine is irrigated on any part of the body in a small quantity.
[501] Here, only fluid moves from the intravascular space into the extravascular space. There is no inflammation of the vessels.

Secondly, if the reduced blood flow is due to the weakness of the heart and lungs, then tonics and stimulants should be given.

Thirdly, local application of relaxant drugs and measures should be adopted for the absorption of serum. The absorption of serum can be facilitated through diaphoresis, diuresis and purgation.

Lastly, it is important to note that coldness is contraindicated in transudative swelling, as opposed to hot swelling, where it can be beneficial.

Points to note regarding swelling:

When addressing cold transudative swelling, it is advisable to employ resolvents more frequently than in cases of warm swelling. When using astringents to treat cold swelling, it is important to incorporate additional ingredients that provide some warmth, including Izkher (Cymbopogon jwarancus), Senna makki (Arabian Senna), Nakhoona (Carum copticum), to enhance the body's absorptive ability. This is because cold swelling requires less coldness than warm swelling.

Gaseous swelling (Waram Rihi):

Gaseous swelling is a form of inflammation characterised by the accumulation of air or gas in the interstitial spaces and crevices of organs, resulting in distension. To address this condition, warming or heating drugs may be employed to absorb and dissolve the gas. Purgation and sweating can also aid in the elimination of unhealthy matter. It is essential to utilize remedies that are gentle in nature and facilitate pore opening to relieve gaseous swelling and widen the pores, since that the root cause is concentrated air and closed pores. Furthermore, any unhealthy material causing the gas swelling must be treated.

Solidification

Obstructions in the body can be caused by various factors such as solid waste materials, thick humours, or an excess of humours. Structures or materials within a vessel or pressure leading to the closure of a vessel can also result in obstructions.

The treatment of obstructions varies based on their underlying cause. If the obstruction is due to an excess of humour, purgation can be used to expel it. However, obstructions caused by concentrated humour require lacerative drugs, and incisive drugs are necessary for obstructions caused by viscous humour. Resolving obstructions caused by a concentrated substance requires proper care, as a weak resolution can worsen the obstruction. In contrast, a potent resolution can lead to the evaporation of watery components, leaving behind concentrated and stiffened excess components.

Obstructions can have severe negative effects on the body, such as the interruption of nutrition and life within organs and the loss of sensation and movement in nerves. Vascular obstruction can lead to death, while obstructions of the spinal cord and brain can cause serious conditions like hemiplegia, epilepsy, and apoplexy.

Clearing obstructions requires the use of deobstruction drugs along with strengthening drugs to balance any potential harm from the resolving power of deobstruction drugs. For instance, Revand Chini (Rheum palmatum root) is an herb with vessel deobstruction and purgative properties that also increases intestinal contraction due to its astringent properties, making it a more suitable treatment option.

The action of deobstruent drugs

Deobstruent (Mufattih) drugs work by dilating vessels and tubes with the help of heat and moisture. This process liquefies thick and viscous substances, making them easy to expel. Conversely, cold temperatures can constrict vessels and create obstructions, while applying heat can alleviate them.

Discontinuity

Discontinuity (Tafarruq-i-ittisal) refers to various types of injuries that can occur inside the human body. One type of discontinuity affects bones and cartilage, such as bone fractures or joint dislocations. To address this type of discontinuity, it is necessary to correct the disunion and immobilize the joint. Rest is also recommended to promote healing.

Another type of discontinuity affects soft organs and is referred to as a wound. Soft organ discontinuity can be categorized into two types based on the cause. The first type arises from a prior cause, where morbid matter accumulates inside the diseased organ and is not transferred from any other organ. The second type is caused by a non-prior cause, where morbid matter flows into the organ from another organ.

When treating discontinuity of soft organs, three critical factors are considered:

1. Halting the flow of matter caused by discontinuity.
2. Closing the cut with a suture.
3. Safeguarding the discontinuity from infection.

To stop the flow of matter, the methods described in the topic of elimination should be utilized. Where feasible, the mouth of the wound should be approximated, desiccants should be given, and suturing should be done. If the wound is dry, a dry wrap is generally preferred.

To prevent the wound from becoming infected, it should be protected from dirt, germs, and other pathogenic organisms. Sterilized bandages should be applied, and the wound should be kept closed to prevent external matter that can cause infection from entering the wound.

Tonics and easily digestible foods that aid the natural healing process and facilitate recovery should be given. These foods can fill any gaps in recovery.

Ulcers

Ulcers (Quruh) are wounds prone to infection as they start to secrete pus. The main treatment principle for ulcers is to keep them dry. This is achieved by reducing the fluids and putrid matter flow from the ulcers and stopping their secretion. Fasd, softeners, and purgation are commonly used along with other treatments.

Concerning external treatment, getting rid of the pus and using sterilized, dry, and moisture-absorbing cotton or gauze is important.

The choice of desiccants (mujaffifat[502]) is based on the normal temperament of the organ and the ulcer involved. For example, if the organ's temperament is moist and the ulcer is not too moist, a low first-degree desiccant will suffice. Second and third degree desiccant drugs are required to restore the true normal temperament of dry-tempered organs and ulcers with significant moisture. Moderate measures should be used where both the organ and the ulcer possess a moderate temperament.

In addition to the organ and ulcer's temperament, the body's Mizaj (temperament) is also considered. If the body's temperament is moist and the ulcerated organ is dry, both should be treated according to their temperament. This involves producing desiccation in cases of excess moisture and less desiccation in cases of excess dryness.

The body's power is also considered when using desiccants. Desiccants help to grow flesh tissue by drying, which facilitates ulcer healing and the creation of new flesh tissue. If the ulcer is clean and free of pus or contamination, desiccants are sufficient. However, if the ulcers are infectious, corrosive drugs such as Zangar (Cupric sulfate), Borax, Lime, Tootia (Copper sulfate), Soap, concentrated acids, and concentrated alkalis should be used. If these drugs are not effective, cauterization is necessary.

Galen combined beeswax (Qairooti) and iron rust to balance their properties for ulcer treatment. Beeswax removes flesh but increases pus, while rust inhibits healing but increases burning. The combination aims to harness the benefits of both substances while mitigating their adverse effects. This approach reflects the Unani principle of achieving balance in treatment formulations.

Internal ulcers

Treating internal ulcers involves using honey in combination with desiccants and astringents. Honey is considered the most effective treatment for internal ulcers. Once the ulcers have been purified, they should be treated with sticky drugs and astringents such as Gile Makhtoom (Silicate of alumina, clay).

---

[502] These drugs produce dryness and decrease moisture, e.g., Habbul Aas (Myrtus communis fruit), Tabasheer (Bambusa arundinasia).

Simple and compound ulcers

Simple ulcers show no abnormalities such as abnormal pain, decay, infection, exudation of substance, or abnormal temperament. On the other hand, if any of these abnormalities are present, such ulcers are considered compound ulcers.

Sutures should be applied to seal small and simple ulcers that do not have decay or infection, and bandages should be used to protect them from dust and dirt. Over time, they will eventually heal. A dry bandage that does not involve toxic drugs, oils, and other substances is typically used in simple ulcers. If the ulcer is large and filled with pus, then the treatment method should be Takhaffif (desiccation). When desiccant drugs prove ineffective, an incision should be made to remove the infected and decayed fluid from the ulcer, after which desiccant drugs should be applied. A soft diet that promotes the production of normal blood and strengthens vital organs should be prescribed.

In cases where the morbid matter has reduced or dissolved due to ulcers, drugs promoting clotting, such as astringents, become necessary. Corrosive (Akkal) drugs also produce clots, but excessive use may worsen the wound. If the flesh or skin has already dissolved, then mild desiccant drugs (not exceeding the first degree) should be used to repair the flesh.

Several factors may prevent the healing of ulcers. Damage to ulcerated tissue must be corrected by addressing the temperament. In case of blood corruption, foods promoting blood production should be prescribed. If there is excessive blood flow towards the ulcer (which may lead to fluid buildup), elimination/purgation is recommended. If the bone beneath the ulcer is damaged and pus is present, rubbing and scraping the bone should be attempted if possible. Organisms present in ulcers should be removed. Congestion in the body, indigestion, anaemia, weakness, pain severity, and contamination of ulcers may also hinder the healing process.

Fistula

'After healing, if an ulcer repeatedly erupts, then this indicates that a fistula (Nasur) has formed. The physician needs monitor the colour of the pus and the edges of the wound.'
– Ibn Sina

If the pus/sore is white or of moderate consistency with no bad smell, and there is a reduction in quantity of the pus and the edges of pus are red, these are signs that the pus is settling well. Conversely, if the sore is of thick consistency, has a foul odour, and the edges of the wound are yellow, green, black, and scaly, these are signs indicating delayed healing of the ulcer.

Decayed organ

Cause:

An organ can decay or die due to the failure of a vital function. This can happen for various reasons, such as a lack of vital air/pneuma caused by severe swelling, constriction, or arterial obstruction. It can also occur due to extreme heat or cold, toxic conditions, obstruction or strangulation.

When decay occurs in bones, it is known as Spina ventosa[503] (Rih al-Shukah). When it occurs in other soft organs, it is called Shafaqalus[504] (moist gangrene). If the decay process is incomplete, it is termed dry gangrene (Ghangharana[505]).

Treatment:

In the initial stages, an incision can help treat a corrupted organ due to its temperament (mizaj), with or without matter (madda). Subsequently, therapies like hijama (cupping) and leeching can be beneficial. Additionally, Gile Makhtoom (silicate of alumina, clay), Gile armani (Arminium bole), and a liniment (tila) made of vinegar and rose can be used.

However, if the organ is not treated with an incision and liniments, then the only option left is to cure it by dissecting and cleaning the decayed flesh. If the decay has spread further, the only option is to remove the organ.

Advice on which treatment to start first

Ibn Sina, the prince of physicians, says that in cases where multiple diseases occur simultaneously, it is essential to prioritize treatment based on certain criteria. Firstly, priority should be given to the ailment that is hindering the treatment of other diseases. For instance, if there is an ulcer and swelling, the swelling should be treated first to eliminate abnormal temperament (Su-e-Mizaj), which could impede the healing of the ulcer. Subsequently, the ulcer must be treated. Secondly, if one disease is causing another, such as obstruction causing fever, the obstruction should be treated first as it is the root cause of the fever. Warmers or desiccants may be used to remove the obstruction without worrying about the fever, which is impossible to treat while its cause persists. Thirdly, priority should be given to the more severe disease. For instance, if a person is experiencing continuous fever (synochus) and hemiplegia, synochus should be treated first using coolants, even though coolants are harmful in hemiplegia.

---

[503] Tuberculous infection of metacarpals, metatarsals and phalanges is known as tuberculous dactylitis. There is a spindle-shaped expansion of the short tubular bones due to tuberculous granuloma. Hence it is also known as spina ventosa.
[504] A Greek word meaning decomposition of organs. It is a decomposed inflammation caused by putrefied or without blood.
[505] An initial stage of moist gangrene (Shafaqalus), in which the colour of the affected part slightly changes due to decayed and putrefied blood. There is no loss of sensitivity of the part. The innate energy of the part remains preserved, i.e., there is no destruction of tissues of the affected part.

Diseases are generally treated rather than their symptoms, except when they become more dangerous. In such cases, fasd of the symptoms should be performed without worrying about the disease itself. For example, in severe colic, where the colic becomes difficult, anaesthetics may be given, even though it may affect the colon adversely. Fasd may, however, be delayed due to stomach weakness, existing diarrhoea, or nausea. Alternatively, partial Fasd may be performed in spasmodic episodes, leaving some of the humour to allow the spasmodic movement to break it down without affecting the innate heat.

FURTHER RESOURCES

College of Unani and Alternative Medicine (CUTAM) Courses

Manchester, UK

Phone: (+44) 0161 945 0418
WhatsApp/Text: (+44) 07415810582
Email: admin@cutam.org.uk
Website: www.cutam.org.uk

Comprehensive Diploma-Level Courses in Unani and Eastern Nutrition Available Online and In-Person for Beginners and Professionals

Foundation in Unani Medicine

Designed for Beginning Unani Medicine Students

This part-time course (one day a month) runs from September to June, providing a solid foundation in Unani Medicine. Students will explore:
- The history and development of Unani Medicine.
- The relationship between mankind, nature, and social environments.
- Key concepts of Unani lifestyle factors.
- Theories of disease, including signs, symptoms, and diagnostic methods.

Assignments and an examination will be conducted at the end of the academic year.

Diploma in Unani Medicine
For In-Depth Knowledge and Naturopathic Practice

This two-year course covers eleven modules through formal lectures, group discussions, and presentations.

First Year:

- In-depth Unani theory and practical applications.
- Preparation to become a skilled practitioner.

Second Half of the First Year:

- Enhanced knowledge and skills with a client-centred approach.
- Topics include herb identification, preparation, energetics, and Unani formulations.
- Therapies covering Eastern nutrition, food energetics, diet treatments, cupping, fasd (pricking), and bodywork benefits.
- Case studies focusing on maintaining health and treating diseases

Nutritional Courses

Naturopathic Nutrition Advisor Diploma

- **Format:** Online with filmed lectures and an exam.
- **Outcome:** Qualification to practice as a nutritional advisor (Level 4).

Diploma in Naturopathic Nutritional Therapy and Eastern Nutrition

- **Format:** Online with some live teaching.
- **Registration:** Level 5, registered with the FNTP.
- **Outcome:** Eligibility to register as a nutritional therapist.

SELECTED BIBLIOGRAPHY

The Book of Sufi Healing, Hakim Chishti, Healing Arts Press, 1988.

Canon of Medicine Book II Materia Medica by Hakim Ibn-Sina, Department of Islamic Studies, Hamdard University, New Delhi, India, 1998

Canon of Medicine Book I General Principles of Medicine Assessment Regimen in Health and Disease by Hakim Ibn-Sina, Department of Islamic Studies, Hamdard University, New Delhi, India, 1993

The Canon of Medicine of Avicenna, O. C, Gruner, 1930.

Canon of Medicine, 5 volumes. Ibn Sina, trans, Laleh Bakhtiar, Kazi Publications, Inc., 1999.

The Traditional Healer's Handbook: Hakim Chishti, Healing Arts Press, 1991.

The General Principles of Avicenna's Canon of Medicine, Mazhar H Shah, Naveed Clinic, 1966.

Avicenna's medicine: a new translation of the 11th-century canon with practical applications for integrative health care, Mones Abu-Asab, Hakima Amri, Marc S. Micozzi. Healing Arts Press, 2013.

Firdaws al-hikma, Ali ibn Sahl Rabban al-Tabari, Urdu translation, Fazlur Rahman Chishti, Pakistan, 1952.

Avicenna's Single Drugs: The Second Book of the Canon of Medicine, Mones Abu-Asab, 2020.

Usool-e-Tibb Syed Kamaluddin Hussain Hamdani, 1998.

Pulse - Let's Understand and Practice, Mudasir Khazir, Educreation Publishing, India, 2017.

Makhzan-ul-mufradat, Hakeem Mohammad Kabiruddin, Pakistan, 2014.

"Pain alleviation in Unani medicine – A conceptual analysis" Mirza Ghufran Baig, International Journal of Pharma Sciences and Research (IJPSR), Vol 5 No 12 Dec 2014

"Venesection (Fasd)", Naheed Begum and A.A. Ansari, Department of Kulliyat, Govt. Nizamia Tibbi College, Hyderabad, India. Hamdard Medicus, Vol. 55, No. 1, 2012.

UnaVerse 1.0, Dr Waish, Ahmed. 2022.

Meezan Ul Tibb, Hakim Muhammad Akbar Arzani, (Trans, Hakeem Kaber ad Deen) 2010.

Amur E Tabiya 2 Vols Hakim Md. Aslam Khan, Idara Kitabushshafa, 2008.

Hamdard Pharmacopoeia of Eastern Medicine, Sri Satgurun publications, India, Hakim Mohammed Said, 1997.

The Medical Formulary or Aqrabadhin of al-Kindi, Trans, Martin Levey, University of Wisconsin, Madison, 1966

The Medical Formulary of Al-Samarqandi, Trans, Martin Levey, Noury Al-Khaledy, University of Pennsylvania press, 1967.

INDEX

A
Abscess 107, 169, 208, 223, 240, 391
Acute diseases 113
Af'al Haywaniyya .... See, Vital functions
Af'al Nafsaniyya .... See, Mental or psychic functions
Af'al Tabi'iyya .... See, Vital functions
Air
    Abnormal changes in Ambient air 124
    Celestial factors 124
    Earthly factors 124
    Effects of different types of air 128
    Seasons 122–24
    The effects of living in different locations and habitats 126
    Wind Direction and its effects 127
Akhlat .... See, humours
Amenorrhoea 214, 231, 391
Amrad Hadda .... See, Acute Diseases
Amrad Khassa .... See, Specific diseases
Amrad Murakkab .... See, Compound Diseases
Amrad Muzmina .... See, Chronic Diseases
Amrad Shirka .... See, Secondary diseases
Amrad Su-e-Tarkib .... See, Structural Diseases
Amrad Zahira Wa Amrad Batina ... See, External and Internal diseases
Anaemia 52, 163, 167, 228, 366, 398, 415
Anasir
    their states and their existence 39
Angina 155, 158, 388
Antagonistic drugs 323
Anxiety 141, 167, 199, 279, 385, 407
Apara .... See, Swollen/Bloating
Appetite 168, 251, 286, 339, 345, 383
Arkan .... See Elements
Arrhythmia 190
Arthritis 231, 238, 296, 365, 367, 369, 397
Asbab badan .... See, Bodily causes
Asbab Fa'iliyya .... See, Efficient Causes
Asbab Ghair Daruriyya .... See, Non-essential Causes
Asbab Ghayr Daruriyya .... See, Non-essential Factors
Asbab Hafiza .... See, Maintaining causes, See, Modifying causes
Asbab Maddiyya .... See, Material Causes
Asbab nabd .... See, Causes of pulse
Asbab Sitta Daruriyya .... See, The six essential factors
Asbab Sitta Dharruriyya ... See, The Six Essential Factors
Asbab Suriyya .... See, Formal Causes
Asbab Tamamiyya .... See, Final Causes
Asbab-i-Sihhat-o-Marad ... See, Causes/means of health and disease
Asthma 93, 101, 140, 213, 229, 299, 391
Awram .... See, Swellings
Awram Balghamiya .... See, Phlegmatic swellings
Awram Saratan .... See, Carcinoma swellings
Awram Sawdawiyya ...... See, black bile swellings
Awram Sulb .... See, Hard Black bile swellings
Awram Ma'iya .... See, Watery swellings
Awram Reeh .... See, Gaseous swellings

B
Back Pain 123, 389
Boils 168, 367, 391
Bone Fractures 413
Bronchial Asthma 213
Burns 119
Buthur .... See, Eruptions

C
Causes of pulse types
    Cause of Weak pulse 200
    Causes of a Cold pulse 201
    Causes of a Empty pulse 201
    Causes of a Full pulse 201
    Causes of a large pulse 199
    Causes of a long (Taweel) pulse 202
    Causes of a narrow pulse 199
    Causes of a Spasmodic Pulse 203
    Causes of a Warm pulse 201
    Causes of an Irregularly irregular pulse 201
    Causes of an Irregularly regular pulse 201
    Causes of Ant-like pulse 202
    Causes of broad pulse 199
    Causes of Deer-leap Pulse/Jerking Pulse 202
    Causes of Dicrotic Pulse 202
    Causes of elevated pulse 199
    Causes of Frequent pulse 200
    Causes of hard pulse 200
    Causes of Infrequent pulse 200
    Causes of Intermittent Pulse 202
    Causes of Irregular pulse 200
    Causes of long pulse 198
    Causes of low pulse 199
    Causes of Millipede/Vermicular pulse 202

Causes of Mouse-tail Pulse 202
Causes of Normal/Natural pulse 201
Causes of pulse with abnormal rhythm/dysrhythmic pulse 201
Causes of Rapid pulse....................... 200
Causes of Saw-teeth like Pulse 203
Causes of short pulse 199
Causes of small pulse......................... 199
Causes of soft pulse 200
Causes of Strong pulse 200
Causes of Trembling Pulse 203
Causes of Wavy Pulse/Bounding Pulse 202
Differences in the pulse of men and women 204
Effects of a Country's Climate on the Pulse 206
Effects of age on the pulse 203
Effects of Bathing on the Pulse......... 207
Effects of emotions on the pulse....... 209
Effects of exercise on the pulse 207
Effects of food and drink on the pulse 206
Effects of pain on the pulse 207
Effects of pregnancy on the pulse 207
Effects of seasons on the pulse 205
Effects of swelling on the pulse......... 207
Effects of temperament on the pulse. 204
Causes of pulse types....................202–3
Cauterization 404
Chronic diseases.............................. 113
Colic. 55, 57, 94, 153, 155, 158, 214, 223, 224, 228, 236, 239, 357, 359, 372, 374, 380, 381, 382, 386, 391, 406, 417
Complex and Simple Disease Classifications 113
Compound pulses
　Ant-like pulse/Pulsus formicans........ 195
　continuous mouse-tail pulse 194
　Cord-like pulse/Pulsus Chordosus.... 196
　Deer-leap/Jerking pulse 194
　Dicrotic /Pulse with two beats 194
　elapsed mouse-tail pulse 194
　Intermittent pulse/Pulsus intercidens 193
　Millipede/vermicular pulse/Pulsus vermicularis..................................... 195
　Mouse-tail pulse- Pulsus myurus 194
　Pulsus serratus 195
　Pulsus tremulus 195
　recurrent mouse-tail pulse 194
　Spasmodic pulse................................ 195
　Spindle-shaped / Tubercular pulse ... 193
　Supernumerary.................................. 193
　Twisting pulse/Wiry pulse/Pulsus retortus.. 195
　Wavy/ bounding pulse/Pulsus fructuous 195
Compound pulses................................192–96
Concoction..368–71
　Benefits of concoction 368
　Black bile humour concoctive 370
　Duration for concoction.................... 368
　Phlegm humour concoctive............... 370
　Principles of Concoctives 369
　Signs of concoction 369
　The need for the concoction.............. 368
　Yellow bile humour concoctive......... 370
Condition and diseases of body and their pulses types.. 210
Congestion ... 11, 117, 138, 150, 154, 156, 159, 167, 201, 213, 228, 333, 341, 389, 391, 393, 407, 408, 409, 411
Constipation....... 127, 130, 131, 135, 255, 260, 323, 338, 340, 348, 359, 372, 373, 380, 381, 386
Cosmetology..110–11
Cough .. 97, 127, 159, 234, 299, 359, 361, 377, 383, 400, 401
Cupping therapy
　Cupping Location points and benefits 391
　Rules and Conditions for Cupping... 390
Cupping therapy.....................................389–91

D

dalk ....See, Therapeutic massage
Dawa Ghayr Mu'tadil.... *See*, Abnormal/Change causing drug
Dawa Mu'tadil........................*See*, Normal drug
Debility (General Weakness) 228, 346
Decayed organ.. 416
Definition of medicine................................. 31
Dementia.. 92
Depression... 195
Diabetes... 231
Diaphoresis
　Fomentation 394
　Incense... 395
　Methods of diaphoresis 394
　Poultice.. 395
Diaphoresis..392–96

Diarrhoea 54, 97, 102, 122, 123, 126, 130, 131, 135, 158, 165, 236, 238, 255, 258, 261, 266, 267, 323, 325, 354, 363, 364, 365, 366, 379, 386, 417
Diet Therapy
  food in terms of tenuity and concentration.............................. 346
  Types of dietary treatment 344
  Types of reduced diet 345
Diet Therapy 344–47
Digestive faculty
  Alimentary digestion 80
  Expulsive faculty 82
  Hepatic digestion 81
  Vascular digestion 82
  Waste material routes 83
Digestive faculty
  Four stages of digestion 80
Discontinuity 413
Disease 91–92
Disease conditions as seen through the pulse 212
disease transfer 113
Diseases 95–96
Diuresis
  Examples of Diuretics 397
  Indications/uses of Diuresis 397
Drug adminstration
  administration of external drugs 307
  administration of internal drugs 305
  Internal drugs 305
Drug adminstration 305–8
Drug function and characteristics 325
Drug substitutes
  Abdal Advia 313
Drugs
  Absolute Poisons 252
  Action of drugs on parasites 289
  Adverse Effects of Gas-Creating Substances on the heart) 273
  Adverse effects of resolvents on the heart) 273
  Antiseptic 288
  Blood purifiers 287
  Calorifacients/Heat-Producing Agents 291
  Classification of Drug Potency 251
  Collection of drugs 308
  Composition of drugs 248
  Drug Potency Levels 250
  Drugs affecting female breasts 269

Drugs affecting female reproductive organs 268
Drugs affecting hair 283
Drugs affecting the intestines 265
Drugs affecting the liver 267
Drugs affecting the reproductive organs 268
Drugs affecting the stomach 264
Drugs affecting the urinary organs ... 267
Drugs that Decelerate Metabolism ... 287
Effect of Drugs on Blood Vessels 275
Effect of Drugs on Disease Substances 290
Effect of drugs on metabasis and metabolism of the body 283
Effect of drugs on sensory nerves 278
Effect of drugs on the blood 277
Effect of drugs on the brain 279
Effect of Drugs on the nose 281
Effect of drugs on the sensory organs 280
Effect of drugs on the spinal cord 278
Effect of Drugs on the Tongue 282
Effect of the drug on the skin 282
Effect of the drugs on the respiratory centre 279
Effect on the Mucous Membrane 282
Effect on the Olfactory Nerve 281
Effects of drugs 253
Effects of drugs on innate heat 291
Effects of drugs on respiratory organs 275
Effects of Drugs on the Ear 281
Expiry period of drugs 310
Expiry period of drugs in terms of their sources 311
Explanation of forms of drugs 296
Guidelines for Determining Drug Potency Levels 250
heart 269, 272, 273
Hypothesis 260
Hypothesis – through Colour 262
Hypothesis – through Consistency and weight 262
Hypothesis – through physical and chemical properties 263
Hypothesis – through Smell 262
Hypothesis – through Taste 261
Hypothesis and experiments 257
Issues in hypothesis 264
Mechanism of Tonics 286

Metabolism Stimulants 285
Metal drugs 311
Mineral drugs 311
Non-Metal drugs 311
Nuanced Understanding of Dosage .. 252
Physical properties of drugs 255
Plant drugs 311
pneuma 269
Principles for Experiments on Drugs 259
Properties of drugs 249
Refrigerants 291
Shapes of drugs 292
Stone and Clay drugs 311
Storage of drugs 309
The action of deobstruent drugs 413
Tonics Based on their Function) 286
Toxic Drugs 252
Use of drugs with Heart exhilarants and tonics) 272
Utilization period of drugs 310
Drugs
　Active parts of drug 247
　Definition of a Drug 243
　Difference between Drug and diet 244
　Drug Classifications 243
Drugs
　Drug substitutes 313–19
Drugs
　Beneficial and adverse effects of drugs 319
Drugs
　Correctives 319
Drugs
　Treatment with single and compound drugs 320
Drugs
　The mixing and synthesis of drugs ... 324
Dysentery 228, 361, 375, 381, 391
Dysmenorrhoea 391
Dysuria (Painful Urination) 123

E

Eczema 214
Efficient Causes 33
Elements 35–37
　Conflict among scholars 37
　Physical qualities 37
Emesis
　Appropriate measures after emesis 385
　Benefits of emesis 383

Emesis contraindication 383
Emesis guidelines 384
Emesis issues and their treatment 385
Emesis requirement 384
Emesis timings 384
Emetic drinks 386
Emetic prescriptions 386
Emesis 383–86
Emmenagogic 398
Enema 379–82
　Enema guidelines 381
　Enema Procedure 380
　Enemas for dysentery 382
　Laxative enema 382
　Steps during an enema 381
Epilepsy . 93, 113, 131, 160, 166, 279, 386, 412
Evacuation 365
　Aims and objectives 366
　Conditions of Evacuation/Elimination 366
　Instructions 367
Excessive Sweating 328
Expectoration 399–401
External and Internal diseases 112

F

Factors of Existence 34
Fasd .... See Venesection
fatigue
　Distension fatigue 145
　Inflammatory fatigue 146
　Ulcerative fatigue 145
Fatigue 145
Fever(s) 31, 57, 94, 97, 113, 117, 123, 146, 152, 159, 160, 167, 168, 169, 187, 199, 208, 215, 216, 221, 222, 223, 224, 228, 229, 230, 231, 238, 239, 289, 290, 291, 292, 322, 326, 328, 347, 348, 349, 359, 360, 361, 362, 363, 364, 372, 374, 376, 379, 386, 388, 391, 407, 409, 416
Fistula . 102, 228, 266, 269, 308, 317, 321, 332, 373, 374, 377, 378, 382, 399, 415
Flatulence 155, 240
Food and drinks
　Effects food and drinks 131
　Types of Types of diet 134
　Types of water 129
　Water 129
Food and Drinks 129–35
Functions
　Compound functions 87

Mental or psychic functions 85
Physical/Natural functions 86
Single functions 86
Vital functions 86

G

Galactagogic 399
Gastritis 165
Gout 113, 229, 296, 369, 389, 391
Gudad Sal'at .... *See*, Glandular tumours

H

Hadima Kabidi .... *See*, Hepatic digestion
Hadima Mi'di .... *See*, Alimentary digestion
Hadm Udwi .... *See*, *See*, Organic digestion
Hadm Uruqi .... *See*, Vascular digestion
Haemorrhoids 126, 167, 359, 361
Haraka wa Sukun Badani *See*, Bodily Movement and Repose
Headache .. 31, 57, 94, 141, 160, 169, 212, 213, 221, 230, 233, 277, 357, 362, 375, 383, 388, 391, 395, 402
Health 91
Hepatitis 290, 411
Hernia 383
High Blood Pressure 184, 185, 397
Hijama .... *See*, cc
humours
   abnormal phlegm humour in terms of taste 53
Humours 48
   abnormal phlegm in terms of consistency 53
   Black Bile Ailments 58
   Black Bile Humour 57
   Blood Humour 51–52
   Phlegm Humour 52
   Phlegmatic Ailments 54
   The absorption of the humours into the organs 50
   The creation of humour 49
   The definition of humour 48
   Yellow bile Ailments 56
   Yellow Bile Humour 55
Huqna .... *See*, enema
Hypertension 185
Hysteria 231

I

Ibn Sina 31, 139, 159, 358, 363, 364
Idrar 399

Idrar-e-haiz .... *See*, Emmenagogic
Idrar-e-laban .... *See*, Galactagogic
Idrar-i-Bawl .... *See*, Diuresis
Ihtibas Wa Istifragh .... *See*, Retention And Evacuation
Ilaj bil Didd .... *See*, Heteropathy
Ilaj bil-Misl .... *See*, Like for like treatment
Ilaj-bil Ghiza .... *See* Diet Therapy
Ilaj-bil Tadbeer .... *See* Regimental therapy
Ilm al-asbab .... *See*, Study of Causations
Imala .... *See*, Redirection of matter
Increasing The 'flow'
   Diuresis 396
Indigestion .. 135, 165, 229, 230, 239, 374, 407, 415
Infected ulcers 289
Infection 11, 35, 52, 53, 55, 106, 117, 126, 129, 130, 138, 156, 215, 224, 268, 275, 280, 281, 288, 289, 326, 407, 408, 413, 414, 415, 416
Insanity 302
Insomnia 165, 215, 221, 251
Intermediate state 93
Intiqal Amrad .... *See*, disease transfer
Irsaal-e-alaq .... *See*, Leech therapy
Ishal .... *See*, Purgation
Istifragh .... *See*, Evacuation

J

Jaundice 56, 214, 220, 228, 235, 290
Joint Pain 362, 365, 389

K

Kaiyy .... *See*, Cauterization
Khilt Balgham .... *See*, Phlegm humour
Khilt Dam .... *See*, Blood humour
Khilt Safra .... *See*, Yellow Bile humour
Khilt Sawda .... *See*, Black Bile Humour
Kidney Stones 130, 221

L

Leech therapy 392
Leprosy 113, 148, 150, 216
Leucorrhoea (Vaginal Discharge) 263
Liver Diseases 365, 383, 389

M

Malaria 228
Malarial Double Fever 238
Malarial Fever 229
marad .... *See*, Disease
Material Causes 32
Medicatrix Naturae 34

Menorrhagia (Heavy Menstrual Bleeding) ..126, 131, 387
Menstrual Blood............................365, 396, 398
Menstrual Flow............................269, 391, 398
Mental faculty..71–76
    Five external senses..............................73
    Five internal senses........................73–76
    motivating faculty 71
    Motor faculty..71
    Receptive faculty 71
    stimulating power/efficient faculty 72
Metabolism
    Causes that increase or decrease metabolism......................................284
    Classification of Drugs Based on Metabolic Impact............................285
    Understanding Factors That Affect Metabolism......................................284
Migraine...154
Miscarriage 227, 384
Missed Periods...221
Mizaj Awali................ See, Primary temperament
Mizaj Thanawi........See, Secondary temperament
Mulayyin .... See, Softeners
munzij sufra See, Yellow bile humour concoctive , See, Phlegm humour concoctive , See, Black bile humour concoctive
Mushil-i- Balgham............. See Phlegm purgative
Mushil-i- Sawda............See Black bile purgative
Mushil-i-Safra ....See Yellow bile purgative
Muslehat......................................See, Correctives

N

Nabd 'Arid..................See, Causes of broad pulse
Nabd 'Azim ....See, Causes of a large pulse
Nabd Da'if ....See, Cause of Weak pulse
Nabd Dayyiq .... See, Causes of narrow pulse
Nabd Dhanab al- Far 'A'idSee, recurrent mouse-tail pulse
Nabd Dhanab al- Far Thabit ...... See, continuous mouse-tail pulse
Nabd Dhanab al-Far.. See, Mouse-tail pulse, See, Causes of Mouse-tail Pulse
Nabd Dhanab al-Far Munqadi .... See, elapsed mouse-tail pulse
Nabd Dhu'l Fatra .... See, Intermittent pulse
Nabd Dhu'l Qar'atayn....See, Causes of Dicrotic Pulse
Nabd Dhu'l Qar'atayn.......... See, Dicrotic pulse
Nabd Dudi .. See, Millipede pulse, See, Causes of Millipede/Vermicular pulse
Nabd Ghazali....................... See, Dicrotic pulse
Nabd Ikhtilaf......... See, Causes of Irregular pulse
Nabd Layyin ....See, Causes of soft pulse
Nabd Mawji .... See, Wavy pulse, See, Causes of Wavy Pulse/Bounding Pulse
Nabd Minshari See, Pulsus serratus , See, Causes of Saw-teeth like Pulse
Nabd misalli .... See, Spindle-shaped pulse
Nabd Mukhtalif Ghayr MuntazimSee, Causes of an Irregularly irregular pulse
Nabd Mukhtalif Muntazim ..... See, Causes of an Irregularly regular pulse
Nabd Multawi ....See, Twisting pulse
Nabd Munkhafid.......... See, Causes of low pulse
Nabd Murta'ish .. See, Causes of Trembling Pulse
Nabd Murta'ish ....See, Pulsus tremulus
Nabd Mushrif........ See, Causes of elevated pulse
Nabd mustawi .... See, Equal pulse
Nabd Mustawi... See, Causes of Normal/Natural pulse
Nabd Mutafawit See, Causes of Infrequent pulse
Nabd Mutashannij......See, Spasmodic pulse, See, Causes of a Spasmodic Pulse
Nabd Mutawatir ...See, Causes of Frequent pulse
Nabd Mutawattir................ See, Cord-like pulse
Nabd Nabd Dhu'l Fatra .... See, Causes of Intermittent Pulse
Nabd Namli .. See, Ant-like pulse, See, Causes of Ant-like pulse
Nabd Qasir ....See, Causes of short pulse
Nabd Qawi .... See, Causes of Strong pulse
Nabd Radi al-Wazn ......See, Causes of pulse with abnormal rhythm/dysrhythmic pulse , See, Causes of Deer-leap Pulse/Jerking Pulse
Nabd Saghir .... See, Causes of small pulse
Nabd Sari' .... See, Causes of Rapid pulse
Nabd Sulb .... See, Causes of hard pulse
Nabd Taweel ....See, Causes of long pulse
Nabd tibbi .... See, Normal pulse
Naffeeth................................ See, Expectoration
Natural/Physical faculty
    Digestion of food 79
    Nutritive faculty..................................77
    Personal faculty 77
    Reproductive faculty 76
    Transformative faculty 78
Natural/Physical faculty................................77
Natural/Physical faculty
    Absorptive faculty 79
Natural/Physical faculty
    Digestive faculty.................................80
Nausea......... 122, 131, 214, 266, 366, 387, 417
Non-essential Factors
    Exercise 143

Hammam 139
Oiling... 141
Splashing water................................ 141
Sunbathing....................................... 140
Therapeutic massage........................ 141
Non-essential Factors.............................143–45
Nudj...*See*, Concoction

O

Obesity 102, 111, 362, 365
Oedema..77, 97, 105, 109, 113, 123, 128, 140, 147, 158, 200, 220, 224, 228, 235, 258, 364, 365, 383, 397
Organs
Classification of Compound organs... 61
Compound organs............................. 61
Serving and Receiving Organs 65
Simple organs 61

P

Pain 152–56
Causes of pain 153
Effects of Pain.................................. 155
Factors Leading to Cessation of Pain 154
Fundamental approach to pain management................................. 155
Using of hypnotics for pain 154
Why abnormal humours cause pain. 155
Why air causes pain 155
Why movement can cause pain........ 155
Pain management
Pain induction................................. 405
Pain management and conflict of drug action and treatment..................... 406
Pain relief 405
Sedatives.. 406
Palpitations..........................213, 271, 331, 337
Paralysis 160, 369, 383
Parameters of the pulse 190–92
Parameters of the pulse
Amount of Expansion of Pulse 180
Parameters of the pulse
Strength of Pulse 184
Parameters of the pulse
Duration of the movement of Pulse. 185
Parameters of the pulse
Period of Pause................................ 185
Parameters of the pulse
Texture of the Arterial Wall............. 186
Parameters of the pulse

Emptiness and Fullness.................... 187
Parameters of the pulse
The Feel of Touch 187
Parameters of the pulse
Uniformity and Variability 188
Parameters of the pulse
Regularity and Irregularity............... 190
Parameters of the pulse
Measurement................................... 190
Pharmacotherapy
Apparent conflicts in treatment 359
Drug resistance 357
Examples of general acting drugs 360
Factors to consider when prescribing 351
Heteropathy 348
Law on drug timings........................ 355
Law on quality of drugs 348
Like for like treatment 349
Managing hyperaesthesia 358
Pain relief is a priority in treatment.. 357
Principles Of Treatment and other Considerations............................. 357
Restrictions on the use of potent anaesthetics................................. 358
The faculty and function of an organ 351
The intensity of a disease 351
The law of quantity of drug............. 349
The location of the organ 350
The nature of the organ 349
The structure of the organ 350
The temperament of the organ 349
Treatment in cases where the diagnoses is difficult 360
Use of potent therapies 357
Pharmacotherapy..347
Phlegm Disease..54
Piles..... 101, 114, 131, 137, 164, 388, 391, 401
Practical aspect of medicine 32
Psoriasis 153, 392, 393
Psychological and emotional illness.................92
Psychotherapy...358
Purgation
Additional instructions related to purgatives 374
Afteemoon pills as a purgative........... 379
Ailments related to purgatives.. 375, 376
Ayarij purgative 379
Black bile purgative 378
Contraindications of purgatives 373
Cooling after purgation 376

Majun Senna as a purgative 379
Managing issues with purgatives 375
Measures to be taken during purgation
.... 374
Phlegm purgative 377
Purgative powder 378
Purgative prescriptions 377
Salateen pills as a purgative.............. 379
Softeners 373
What to do after purgation............... 376
When to take purgatives................... 373
Yellow bile purgative 377
Purgation................................... 377–79

Q

Qay.................................... See, Emesis
Quruh .... See, Ulcers
Quwwat Dafi'a .... See, Expulsive faculty
Quwwat Hadima .... See, Digestive faculty
Quwwat Haywanniya .... See, Vital faculty
Quwwat Jhadiba .... See, Absorptive faculty
Quwwat Mughayyira .... See, Transformative
   faculty
Quwwat Nafsaniyah .... See, Mental faculty
Quwwat Tabi'iyya . See, Natural/Physical faculty

R

Redirection of matter
   Conditions in which redirection is
      helpful...404
   Redirection rules 402
Redirection of matter............................... 401–4
Regimental therapy........................ 344
Ruh
   Locations and routes of Ruh (pneuma)
   69
   Types of pneuma............................. 70
Ruh (pneuma) 68–69

S

Sciatica 123, 229, 367, 389, 391
Secondary diseases........................ 112
shiyaf .... See, Suppository
Signs and Symptoms.............................. 169–71
signs and symthoms
   Signs and symptoms of plethora/fullness
   166
   Signs indicating a temporarily acquired
      temperament................................ 165
   Signs indicating temperament 163

Signs of a balanced temperament 165
Signs of disease................................ 159
Signs of external diseases 160
Signs of health................................. 159
Signs of internal diseases.................. 161
Signs of loss of continuity................. 169
Signs of obstruction 167
Signs of reeh................................... 169
Signs of swelling/inflammation 168
Signs that indicate a dominant humour
.... 167
Sihhat .... See, Health
Sinusitis.. 392
Skin Diseases 106, 300, 392, 393
Spasms 113, 128, 139, 195, 220, 221, 275, 278,
   326, 400
Specific diseases 112
Sprains.. 149
Stages of Disease 111
Stool 239–40
   Colour of the stool 240
   Consistency of stool 239
   Properties of an Ideal Stool 240
   Quantity of stool........................... 239
Study of Causations
   Bodily causes 116
   Causes of abnormal movements 149
   Causes of congestion 156
   Causes of discontinuity/separation ... 150
   Causes of increased size and number of
      organ... 150
   Causes of infection 156
   Causes Of Obstruction And
      Constriction Of Ducts 148
   causes of retention and evacuation.... 156
   Causes of swelling 151
   Causes of ulcers............................. 151
   causes of weakness of organs............ 157
   Causes Related To The Four Qualities
   146
   Disfiguring causes 147
   External causes 151
   Internal causes............................. 150
   Maintaining causes........................ 118
   Other causes of weakness................ 158
Study of Causations................................ 116–19
Subject matter of medicine 32
subsitutedrugs
   Substitute drug list 314

su-e-mizaj .... *See* treatment for abnormal temperaments
Su-e-Mizaj .... *See*, Impaired temperament
Su-e-Mizaj Maddi .... *See* abnormal temperament with a substance
Sufuf Mushil .... *See* Purgative powder
Suppository 382
Swellings 105

T

Ta'riq .... *See*, Diaphoresis
Tafarruq-i-ittisal .... *See* Discontinuity
Tahabbuj .... *See*, soft gaseous swellings
Temperament
    Abnormal Temperament 43
    Temperament according to age 46
    Temperament of Organs 45
    Temperament types 41
Temperament of Drugs
    Abnormal/Change causing drug 245
    First type of temperament of drugs .. 245
    Normal drug 245
    Primary temperament 246
    Second type of temperament of drugs
    246
    Secondary temperament 246
    Types of Secondary Temperaments . 248
Temperament of Drugs 244–48
The benefits of using only single drugs 320
The Four Pillars of Nutritive Faculty 285
The Pulse
    A pulse cycle 174
    Causes of pulse 197
    Conditions for examination of pulse 176
    Definition of Pulse 174
    Equal pulse 196
    Methods of examining the pulse 178
    Movement of pulse 175
    Normal pulse 196
    Reason for examining the pulse at the wrist 178
The Six Essential Factors
    Bodily Movement and Repose 135
    Food and Drinks 129
    Mental Activity and Repose 136
    Retention And Evacuation 137
The Six Essential Factors 122–39
    Air 119–20
The use of compound drugs 321
Theoretical aspect of medicine 31
Tonsillitis 123, 395

Treatment of abnormal temperaments 362–64
Treatment of Swellings
    cold swelling 410
    Cold swelling 410
    Gaseous swelling 412
    General treatment of hot swellings ... 408
    Hard swelling 411
    Hot swelling 407
    Management of Infected Swelling 408
    Outcome of swelling 409
    Points to note regarding swelling 412
    Solidification 412
    Transudative swelling 411
Treatment of Swellings 407–13
Tremors 103, 141, 147, 149, 150, 160, 167, 168, 383, 385
Tuberculosis 66, 193, 223
Types of diseases 97–103
Types of Diseases
    Compound Diseases 105
Types of Simple Diseases
    Structural Diseases 101
    Su-e-Mizaj (Impaired temperament) .. 98
Types of Simple Diseases 97–103
Types of swellings
    Black bile swellings 107
    cold swelling/ chronic swelling 107
    Eruptions 110
    Gaseous swellings 109
    Glandular tumours 108
    Hard Black bile swellings 108
    hot swelling/acute swelling 106
    Phlegmatic swellings 108
    soft gaseous swellings 109
    Swollen/Bloating 109
    Watery swellings 109
Types of swellings 110–11

U

Ulcers 11, 95, 103, 123, 130, 149, 151, 167, 214, 226, 229, 234, 277, 283, 289, 297, 307, 308, 351, 391, 392, 405, 414–15, 414, 415
    Internal ulcers 414
Urine 227
    Colours of urine and related condition and diseases 228
    Complex Urine colours 222
    Haematuria 226
    Indications from colours of urine 219

Urine and Fevers 231
　　Urine density 223
　　Urine froth 224
　　Urine of pregnant women 227
　　Urine sediments 225
　　Urine sediments and Diseases 229
　　Urine smell and Mizaj 229
　　Urine types and Diseases 230
Urine Infections 268
Urine Retention 101, 169

V

Venesection
　　Important veins for fasd 388
　　Principles of Fasd 388
　　Rules of Fasd 387
Venesection 389
Vertigo 212, 232, 233, 391
Vital faculty 76
Vitiligo 77, 111, 303, 393
Vomiting 22, 54, 56, 57, 122, 137, 160, 167, 214, 217, 236, 258, 265, 266, 306, 319, 336, 349, 357, 362, 363, 365, 374, 375, 383, 384, 385, 386, 387, 400, 403

W

Waram Barid .... *See* Cold swelling
Waram Barid*See*, cold swelling/ chronic swelling
Waram Harr ... *See*, hot swelling/ acute swelling , *See* Hot swelling
Waram Rihi .... *See* Gaseous swelling
Waram Rikhw .... *See* Transudative swelling
Waram Salabah .... *See* Hard swelling
Warts 110, 404
Worms .. 55, 123, 267, 289, 314, 332, 340, 379, 381

Z

Zulkhassa 244

www.ingramcontent.com/pod-product-compliance
Lightning Source LLC
Chambersburg PA
CBHW080213040426
42333CB00044B/2640